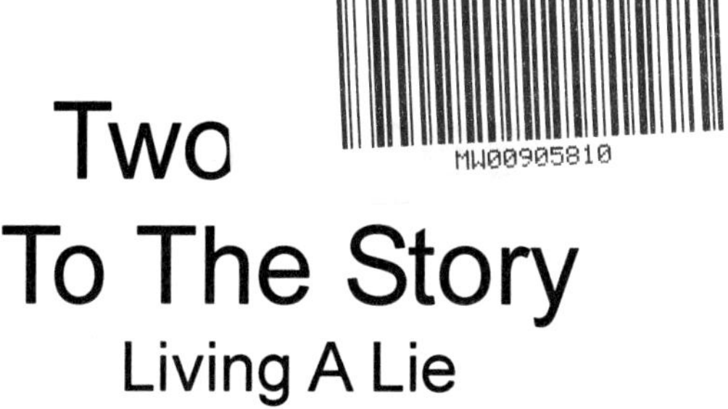


# Two

# To The Story

## Living A Lie

## A Battle With Mental Illness

Chris Nihmey

**chipmunkapublishing**
the mental health publisher

Published by
Chipmunkapublishing
United Kingdom

**http://www.chipmunkapublishing.com**



ISBN 978-1-84991-942-5

Special thanks to Jenn McMillan, Graphic Designer for cover: my vision, your design ... spectacular.

Chipmunkapublishing gratefully acknowledge the support of Arts Council England.

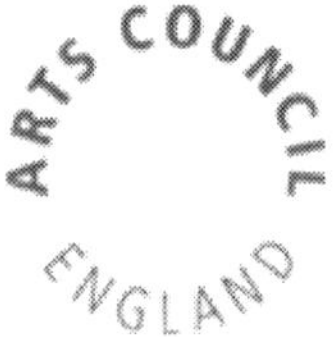

She represents the millions of deprived victims worldwide, both on and off the street, who have been abandoned by family, friends and society because of their illnesses, living with an emptiness which we cannot fully appreciate.

Sally, this book is dedicated to you.

# ACKNOWLEDGEMENTS

A special thanks to those who have helped make this book possible, because of the wonderful support and hope they provided throughout the most difficult times of my life. Thank you, God, for your love, inspiration, continued guidance and wisdom. Thank you, Mom, Dad and Julie, for your unconditional love. You never gave up on me no matter how much I put you through. I couldn't have done it without you. Dad, for your countless hours of editing over coffee and cookies; these are moments I will never forget. Finally, thank you, Dr. Boyles. You were a blessing in every way. I put my complete trust in you, not only for my healing, but also as a friend. Your knowledge and discernment were invaluable, and your approval of this book has helped make me confident in its accuracy and authenticity. You never stopped believing in me and my desire to step beyond my ailments.

Without all of you, this dream would never have been possible. I love you all and, again, I thank you for your strength and support through this difficult journey.

# TABLE OF CONTENTS

# INTRODUCTION

There are two sides to everyone's story, and my life is no different. To many of you who know me, or thought you knew me, reading this story will come as a surprise. I was living as a teacher, an author, a friend, but I was living a lie, a big part of me that you just didn't know. It's time you knew my story. I can no longer keep it a secret. This is my story and, like all others' stories, it has two sides.

## THIS BOOK'S PURPOSE

When I started writing this book, I had a vision. I knew that I wanted to educate people on the effects of mental illness on a person's life and on those around them. I wanted to inspire and give hope to all, by teaching about my challenges and my accomplishments: my "ups and downs", you might say. However, as I proceeded, I realized that something important was missing. I knew that there was a greater purpose in writing this book. I finally realized why I needed to finish it. With that, I completed *Two Sides To The Story.* It is not a doctor's manual or a "cure-all" recipe. It is simply my story, but it is a story that will bring you hope and inspire you to take the first step into making changes for the better, so that you can feel the amazing freedom that I feel today.

I wrote with three visions in mind. The first was to educate the reader on the effects of mental illness on a person and their loved ones. That was a vision I knew I could achieve, because I had been through the whole experience and I knew the cold hard facts.

The second vision, I knew, would be a difficult one to achieve. It began with a hope I had for all. I hoped to be one, among many, who dares attempt to dispel the terrible stigma surrounding mental illness, to break the bonds that have held those who suffer for so long. Living with a mental illness does not, and should not, make a person different from those who suffer from other various illnesses. Mental illness is a sickness like any other, be it diabetes or Parkinson's, heart disease, asthma, or even cancer. Most often it is genetic, inherited from family. The sufferer need not be feared. The difference is that you can't easily categorize a mental illness and predict its repercussions. Mental illness isn't "worn on a sleeve" like other illnesses. That is why it is such a difficult thing to live with and to heal. People just don't understand what they may not ever have to deal with. The tendency is for one to fear the ramifications of the illness and to shun the sufferer.

Finally, I hope to drop a pebble into the social pool in order to start a ripple, thereby creating more ripples. This would result in a decided change in people's thinking with regard to how to perceive mental illness and ensure that people who suffer receive proper treatment and loving support.

In summary, I hope to open your eyes to understanding and appreciating mental illness for what it really is, and the devastating effects it has on a person's life and their loved ones. At the same time, I want to offer hope to the sufferer and their significant others that one can heal and thrive. Come and witness my story.

# PROLOGUE

*I watched a little girl today while having a coffee at a Tim Hortons donut shop. She really was an image of peace and serenity, no more than five, as she sat with her mom in front of me, eating a sparkled donut, the kind that most kids like to eat. Her mother mixed a hot chocolate with chocolate milk, so that her drink would be just as sweet, but not so hot. I watched her sitting there so attentive to her donut. I remembered a time when I needed to be told to wipe my mouth and not slurp my drink, when I had to be reminded to take my shoes off when entering the house. When going out at night felt like going on a week's vacation. You were completely absorbed in every moment and nothing else mattered, not yesterday's failed test, not tomorrow's trip to the dentist, not the biggest of snowfalls. All that mattered was the moment you were in, and what you were sharing with the people you were sharing it with. Growing older, I've realized that life is not that simple, and I found out the hard way.*

*Life is weird that way. You know, I never felt at any time in my life that I had it all, that I had everything. But I can say this. Whatever I did have, it was taken away from me quickly, quietly and abruptly without notice or even the slightest bit of warning. God, we never saw it coming; but when it came, it came hard and it felt like it would never leave. It never did leave and will linger for a lifetime.*

*You never really know what you have until you lose it. And I did. I lost my life, as it was, never to be the same again.*

***"I never had any friends ... like the ones I had when I was twelve. Jesus, does anyone?"***

***Stand By Me, 1986, Stephen King,***
***Bruce A. Evans, Raynold Gideon***

# PART I

# LIVING THE 'HIGH'LIFE

## CHAPTER 1
## LIFE IS A HIGHWAY

This book begins with a moment to moment account of someone who is experiencing the peak of full-blown mania in 2001. My doctor called me the "perfect patient", and I was, in every way.

At four in the morning I stirred in bed, staring up at the ceiling searching for answers, answers that I knew would be difficult to find. My head was racing, so I put on some light music and reflected on everything that had just happened to me. Wow, it was almost too much to take in. I couldn't believe what I had just experienced. I was so full of energy and excitement, I literally felt like blowing up! How could anyone sleep after having realized what I did tonight? You just couldn't. It was beyond anything I could have ever imagined.

I lay awake the rest of the night, trying to figure out what it all meant. My thoughts were racing uncontrollably and I wanted to tell everyone what had happened. I wanted to wake my roommates up and shake their heads with my hands and look them in the eyes and say, "HEY! Guess what?" But I decided to wait. I didn't think it would sit well with them and the last thing I needed was to confront two tired and cranky roommates.

I turned on my side and switched on my light. I was now being hit with the definite possibility that maybe I was being chosen for something. Could you imagine that? I'd thought of this possibility a few times before but, after tonight's events, I was really starting to believe that I was special in some way and that God was using me for something big. I didn't know what, but He definitely was ... wow! What did it all mean?

I was so excited. I felt like a secret agent embarking on a covert mission, what with the endless coincidences I was experiencing day after day and the dozens of connections that I had experienced tonight. I was being guided most definitely, but why? Why was I the one being chosen? I knew the answer would come soon, but when? I needed to know! God! God!

I listened to some spiritual music for the next couple of hours, which calmed me down a bit, but when I stared at my clock at 7 am, I sighed and grinned, realizing that another sleepless night had occurred: another one, no different from the others that week or weeks previous. Who needed sleep anyway? There was so much to do!

I jumped out of bed and looked out the window. The sun was beginning to rise in the distance. A new day had finally arrived and I just couldn't sit still. I yawned, stretched and then started to walk around my room. I began to praise and pray to God, thanking Him for last night's revelations. I knelt at my bedside and gave Him my full attention and my thanks. "God, show me," was all I needed to say. We had a special bond, Him and me. Then I took my big clunky discman (no such thing as Ipods or MP3s at the time), and I put on a spiritual CD, one that I had listened to over and over the last while. I was surprised it wasn't worn out already; I'd used it that much!

I started to hum to the music as I walked around my room, pointing up to the clouds and singing prayers out loud. My pacing had now taken the form of circles around my room and, at that moment, as I looked up into the sky, I knew God was listening. I just knew it. And it was then that I realized that God wasn't the only one listening. My roommates were also, and it was seven in the freakin' morning ... on a Saturday! They would not be forgiving, so I gave my head a shake, grabbed my discman and slowly opened the door. Thankfully, my roommates' doors were both closed. Phew, I thought, as I carefully crept down the creaky stairs. I knew that the basement would be the best place to sing and pray. I'd never thought about it before. I knew that God would be downstairs too, and I needed Him badly! I had to figure out what had happened to me last night. I went downstairs and headed to the far corner of the basement. I closed my eyes, pressed play and began to pray again in song.

"I need You now ... You're all I ever needed. Dear Almighty, God ..." Now, it wasn't that song exactly, because I really just made that one up for this part, but it was something like that. It had the word "You" in it and "Almighty". I know that for sure!

So as I sang, I started to lose complete awareness of where I was and what I was doing. This was often the case. You might say I was "caught up in the spirit"!

As I prayed and sang away, I didn't realize it (because I had the headphones on), but I was singing very loudly. I mean

REALLY loud! So loud, in fact, that in what seemed like only seconds, my roommate came stomping down the stairs to see what was wrong and what all the ruckus was about.

"Chris!" he said to me.

Since my eyes were closed and the headphones were on, I didn't see or hear him. I just continued singing, raising my arms in the air and closing my hands in prayer. He yelled again, very loudly, and this time I heard him. I opened my eyes, stopped the music and looked at him. I could see right away that he was NOT a "happy camper". Off came the headphones.

"What the ... what the hell are you doing?" he belted out angrily. If steam actually came from our ears, now would have been the time! He had seen this strange behaviour for almost two months now, and he had no clue why I was doing what I was doing or where it was coming from. No one understood me at the time, even my family. I just had a whole new way about me and it felt great.

"Nothing," I said looking down. "I'm, uhh, just singing."

"It's not nothing, Chris! It's something! You woke the whole damn house up, and probably our neighbours too!"

"Sorry man. I didn't realize I was singing that loud. I had these on."

"Well, Chris, I ... I don't know what to say!" He then trailed off, telling me why he was mad and how stupid I was acting lately, and other stuff like that—you know, all that "feel good" kind of stuff. He had seen a lot over the last while, but this time he was really letting me have it! So, within a minute or so of him telling me all of this stuff, I sort of zoned out and wasn't listening to a word he was saying. Blah, blah, blah, blah, blah ... he went on. I put my mind on better things, like God, and all that had happened only hours before.

I thought of telling him what had happened, but I knew he'd just think I was crazy and wouldn't understand. Most people would feel the same, but I knew better. So instead, I let him drill me out for singing so loudly. And it was then that the weirdest thing happened. To this day, I cannot explain it, but I remember it happening, and when it happened, I was blown away by it. Now that's a whole lot of happening!

As he continued to berate me for my rude behaviour, I suddenly felt a small surge of energy building up in my right arm. It began in my elbow and slowly it made its way towards my hand. I felt it rise and build in my whole arm. It felt truly amazing, so freaky, but so cool. It was nothing like the feeling you have when your hand falls asleep. I'd had that happen hundreds of times in my life, but this was a completely new feeling. It was very different from that, and much more intense.

Slowly, as he continued to chastise me, I felt this surge build up in my arm. I couldn't believe it! Oh my God, I thought. What's going on? This energy made me feel more and more electrified inside, to the point where I truly believed that if I touched him at that moment, I would shock him and knock him right over. It felt that extreme and intense! I'll never forget it; I never told him about it when it happened. I kept it to myself. It felt so real and so pure.

To this day, I still can't come to grips with what happened in that basement. It was really incredible and it only lasted minutes. By the time he was done his rant, it was gone. I sort of wish I had tested it out on him when it happened, like a taser gun on a guinea pig, but I didn't. He told me he was going to take a shower and then that he wanted to have a "talk" with me. He was red in the face and not happy, but I could see that he looked worried, which worried me. Maybe he was going to give me the boot. It wouldn't have surprised me after the last couple of months. As soon as he left, I started to feel anxious about everything. What would he say? What would happen? I started to panic, and became very agitated. I knew I had to get out of there, and right NOW!

I hopped up to my room. My other roommate was still dead asleep, door closed, as always. I heard the shower running in the other room. I grabbed my purple University of Western Ontario bag and threw some clothes inside. I grabbed my Bible, wallet and discman and put them in the front pocket of my bag. I left my cell phone behind! I grabbed my hat and my keys and quickly rushed downstairs, two steps at a time. In my mind, everything was aroused, but this was crazy.

Everyone would be out to get me after hearing about this morning, everyone: my parents, my friends, maybe even the police if my roommate had had intentions to call them. I was becoming paranoid, and worried that this was likely. They were all part of the problem; they were so hard-headed and stubborn. They just didn't know. They didn't get it! I had to head off to find people who would understand what was happening to me. The last few weeks comprised some of the most exciting days I had ever experienced, but everyone was telling me I was wrong. Screw them all! I thought to myself. Things seemed really strange to them, but I knew it was right. So with that, I hopped into my car, revved up the engine and looked up at my window. Bon Voyage, everyone! I was gone, with no intention of ever returning.

I drove through town and knew deep down that I needed to leave this area, but where would I go? This mission was developing. Maybe I needed to leave this city, and leave it right now! They really would be after me; they would try to stop me. So with that, I made my final decision. I was leaving Ottawa to find safety and security elsewhere.

And so began my long journey to the biggest city in Canada: Toronto. Toronto was big time and I was ready for it. And it was ready for me! I didn't have to worry about food, since only five days ago, I had begun a fast for God! I couldn't afford to stop anyway, when so many were out to get me. I looked at the rear view mirror to make sure I was alone. At 8 am, running on an empty belly, I headed out of Ottawa towards the wild blue yonder. I left my family, my friends and others, who would only be a hindrance to my mission, a mission that was now taking shape. This was my life! Not theirs! How could they be so obtuse? They really were!

Toronto was next on this adventure to who knew where? I turned on the Christian music station and pumped up the volume. I tapped my hand on the dash and realized I was now finally free. I looked one more time in my mirror. No one was there. I breathed a huge sigh of relief. The sky was the limit, and I spread my wings and flew. As Leo had said on his *Titanic* voyage, "I'm the king of the world!" Corny, but you get the idea. I was free, and I was taking things one moment at a time. It was all so spontaneous and, although I was making one rash decision after another, it all felt completely right, never truer than this moment. I was finally free and I loved it. Dear world, I was ready to make a splash.

## CHAPTER 2
## MIRACLE ON ICE

As I left Ottawa, early Saturday, my hands started to shake at the wheel. I don't know why, but they were shaking uncontrollably. Maybe it was the excitement of it all or maybe the craziness of what was happening, but either way, I was trembling. I may have been a bit nervous about what I was doing. My hands barely gripped the steering wheel. I laughed to myself because it felt really weird. I pulled into a convenience store just before entering the highway. I quickly filled the car. I grabbed a bottle of water and my hands were shaking so much that water was spilling out! I drank some and wiped my brow. I was sweating too, and as I left the store, I took another quick look in my mirror to make sure I wasn't being followed. So far I was safe. My biggest fear was whether the police were tracking my whereabouts. Was I being hunted? I couldn't be more relieved as I approached highway 416 and branched off. I was finally leaving Ottawa!

Minutes into my drive, my shaking slowed, as I started thinking about different things. I felt sure now that I was safe. As my mind relaxed, I started to reminisce about the truly incredible night I had experienced only hours before. What a special night it had been.

[*Friday, February 23$^{rd}$, 2001 marked the fifth day of my fast. It had begun on the previous Sunday when I spent a whole night praying with my hands over a newspaper. I remember being in tears, balling uncontrollably, as I prayed, looking with dismay at countless stories of despair in our world. I was very emotional and my tears were dripping onto the newspaper causing it to run.*

*In between prayers, I grabbed my journal and lay my ink-filled hands down on the open pages. My handprints were clearly visible. I then started to draw a picture. I closed my eyes and let God guide my hand. What formed on the page was an image of a large cross planted atop a hill, with dozens of little round stones below. Slowly, my hand drew more and more of these small circles one by one. I then shaded certain stones, firmly believing the Holy Spirit was guiding me to do so. Finished, the image lay before me. What did it mean? I wondered. I would soon find out.*

*Over the next hour, 4:30 am on, I prayed to God and asked for discernment and guidance to help me to understand what all of this meant and why I was being chosen for something. I felt the Holy Spirit speaking to me. "Chris, you have been chosen to travel the world in My name. Each stone represents a different country. The shaded stones indicate where you will go. Trust in the Holy Spirit, Chris. It will guide you. Bless you."*

*It was at that particular moment that I truly believed that God was calling and had some sort of mission for me. In turn, He was asking me for an immediate favour, and it was: "Chris, please starve yourself for Me and for your world. No more food." And with that, the decision was made. I would begin my fast that moment, however long it might be. I was thinking 40 days or possibly longer.*

*That whole week, my stomach had been aching so much, and by Friday night I was a bit woozy. Yet I was getting used to the hunger pangs. I'd never done something like this before. I had adopted a pattern of drinking water and juice all week, and had started to drink more coffee. At the time, I never thought much about coffee being a diuretic. You can imagine!*

*Friday night arrived and it was a night I'll never forget ... ever. It affected me in so many ways. I had been waiting for a call from Denis, a close friend of our family, and former student of my dad's. We were planning to go to an OHL hockey game together.*

*I had a half hour or so before leaving, so I lay on my bed and put my hands behind my head. I threw on the same spiritual CD I'd been listening to for weeks and closed my eyes. Everything I did now was connected to God and my faith. For months, I'd been barely sleeping because I was so busy praying. I would head to work most times without any sleep at all, but I always seemed to have enough energy to get through my days. I truly believed my gift of energy to be God-given, since I felt He was overseeing my every moment. Again, I can't emphasize enough how everything in my life was about God. My motto at the time: "Let Go, Let God."*

*I was just so excited about my intense faith fever and was too high-strung to sleep. At the time, I never thought it unusual. If anyone had told me that I was sick or there was something wrong, I'd have laughed in their face. As far as I was concerned, things were as normal as they could be. God had a purpose and a plan. In time, I would know what it was.*

*Denis and I were planning to see the Ottawa 67's play. I loved going to see them, and I especially felt excited in the state of mind I was in. I wanted to see and meet anyone … actually, everyone! And I knew I could meet thousands of people at a hockey game!*

*I didn't know what it was at the time, but I especially liked to meet new people. My friends were okay, but they seemed to avoid me because they couldn't understand the "new me". Screw them, was my attitude, and I avoided hanging around with them mostly because it only stressed me out. They had too many questions.*

*I was just so high on life that I wanted to connect with whomever I could. Maybe it was because new people had no expectations or judgments about me. I could be whoever I wanted to be with them. With friends and family, I felt restricted and pressured. I couldn't live like that. I needed freedom, like a butterfly coming out of a cocoon. My wings were fluttering and I needed to move forward. I didn't need a net around me!*

*At 7:10 pm, my phone rang.*

*"Hello?" I jumped up and said, clearing my throat. I had drifted off. "Hello?"*

*"Hey man, it's Denis!"*

*"Denis! How come you're calling so late? It's after seven! The game starts in less than thirty minutes!"*

*"It's takin' me a fucking long time to do things. Man!" I heard something bang. I could tell he was extremely frustrated and flustered.*

*"I know, Denis. I know. No worries, okay?"*

*Yes, Denis did use the f-word. Get used to it. You needed to understand Denis, and I did. Denis was very sick. He was suffering from diabetes and, at the time, I didn't know he was dying. Denis had not taken the disease seriously for years, even after losing his left eye from it, along with over 200 pounds! He'd been a rebellious child, wild and free, not thinking about the consequences of his actions. Even at thirty, he acted child-like, like a kid who knew no boundaries. Lately though, his body was keeping him from acting in any way. He was now subject to two walking canes, with bruised, battered and bleeding legs. He showed me them several times against my will, gross to see. It was so hard to see him this way.*

*Having been through so much, he had a tendency to complain ... about everything. We all need that but, when Denis complained, he used very colourful words. One started with "f", another with "s", two words you can probably guess, and sometimes you'd hear a combination of the two. As I look at his life, and all he had been through, I couldn't blame him for his choice of words.*

*Denis was an integral part of my mania and I'll never forget this special night. Who would have thought that this night would change my life forever, and that Denis would be a big part of it. He was a special person, even though he was not with us long. He passed away only a year later.*

*"Alright, guy! We gotta get going! Are you ready?"*

*"Yah!"*

*"Alright, I'm on my way!"*

*I threw on a hat. Who didn't wear a hat to a hockey game? I grabbed my coat, my keys, and left my watch in my drawer. Lately, I wasn't even using a watch or setting my alarm—hell, I was up most nights! I was trusting God to take full reign of my life and to guide me in everything I did, and that included wake-up calls! Funny thing was, I was never late for anything at that time, including work!*

*I headed into the freezing cold and raced down street after street. It was not uncommon for me to speed at the time, as I tore through town heading towards the east side of Ottawa. I was always anxious to get to where I was going. I needed to talk to someone, anyone, and would often talk on my cell phone to ease my mind. Hands-free laws were not in play as of yet, thankfully! At 7:20 pm, I knocked on Denis' door.*

*"Hey man, let's get going! We're late!" I told him. Denis didn't like my pushy attitude one bit.*

*"Fuck man, gimme a break! I'm goin' as fast as I fucking can!"*

*"I know, I know. Settle down, we'll be okay. Where's your coat?"*

*I reached for his black leather coat, the one he always wore, winter and summer. It was draped over an old stained couch. As I grabbed it, I took a quick look around the room. Denis' first floor apartment was a sorry sight, a pig sty. The room was littered with papers, girly magazines and garbage. He had a broken TV in one corner and a dirty couch and coffee table in the other that I would never, in a million years, lay anything on. His room had an awful smell too. These were all reasons that my family had a soft spot for the poor kid.*

*Denis needed help with his walking canes, and I had to hold him tightly under an arm to help him into the car. At the time, I thought to myself, how the hell is he going to survive a hockey game? He can't even walk down the driveway of his house! I actually hadn't realized that Denis was suffering this much, but he was. I slammed the door shut and hopped in.*

*"Throw the heat on, man! It's fucking cold!"*

*I pulled out of the laneway. "And how are you doing, Denis?" I said and smiled.*

*"I'll be better when we're out of this goddamn cold!" Denis said, folding his arms in disdain. He tucked his hands into his armpits. I opened the glove compartment. "Here, I got these. They'll help." I handed him a pair of thin winter gloves.*

*"They'll do fuck all!" Denis said, as he threw them on the floor. You had to love Denis. Never a dull moment, or a dull word.*

*We drove into downtown and headed towards the arena. It was 7:50 when we pulled into the parking lot. The game had already started. We parked and began to make our way. Denis was right, though. It was "fucking cold", excuse my language. There was a strong wind, but it was a crisp and clear night. We arrived at some stairs that we'd have to climb to enter. I hopped onto the first step and turned to face Denis.*

*"Where you goin', man? I ain't climbing those fuckin' stairs," he said, pointing with his cane.*

*"But Denis, we've got to, or we'll have to go all the way around this parking lot. That would take us a hell of a lot longer, and there are stairs there, too! If we go up here, we'll get in much faster. I think there's even a chance we can get in through one of those glass doors right up there." I hoped we could, because I didn't want to keep Denis out in the cold much longer. It was damn cold, and he was complaining constantly. He was very bitter, and staring at him helplessly resting on his canes at the base of the stairs, I tolerated his rude and obnoxious behaviour.*

*I grabbed his arm and we slowly made it up the first step.*

He moaned and groaned. After that, with Denis r help, it took us over five minutes to climb the nex Denis was whining and bitching the whole tir everything off, when I reached the top, I realized tha glass doors along the top level were locked. Ugh! This time, I was the one swearing. And yes, Denis, halfway up, continued in his usual fashion.

"What are we gonna do, man? I'm fuckin' dyin' here! I might as well fold up and die. This is fucking shit, man!" he complained, as he hung onto the metal railing halfway up the staircase. "I ain't goin' up no more of those goddamn stairs, and there's no way I can make it way over there to the front." He was right. At the rate he was moving, we'd take over an hour to get to the front, and by then, we'd have to be thawed out!

Looking back, I honestly didn't know what to do. I had to think quickly. Denis was freezing and he was in a lot of pain. Even those few steps were taking a toll on his body. Think, Chris, THINK! What could I do? I had that burning feeling in my stomach, and it was not hunger this time! I stood there with my hands on my hips, trying to think. I looked up into the sky ... God, give me a break!

"Aw, man, this is fucking ridiculous. I should just lie down right here, because I ain't goin' anywhere else. I wanna to go home! You'll have to fuckin' carry me back to the car. I'll never make it on my own!"

I didn't know what to do. Here I was, going out of my way for this guy, and I had to sit here listening to him complain. Could it be worse? I was convinced that there was nothing worse. I needed a miracle here, even if it was just a small one.

I took a look inside. It was intermission. People spilled into the open hallway, going this way and that. There was buying, and there was selling. Kids ran through the hallways, while other kids chased them, while parents chased them! The hallway was packed, as we stood on the outside looking in. I stared inside looking for something, anything. I didn't care what it was. I waved to people, I rapped on the glass windows and doors, but no one would answer. And why should they? Who the hell were we?

And then it happened ... my mini-miracle. I couldn't believe it! It came in the form of my cousin. Let me explain. It is part *of a much larger plan that I will share with you.*

*Amidst the people in the arena's hallway, I noticed a particularly tall gentleman walking through the crowd. He was a distance from the window and passed by me and continued on. For some reason, he seemed to stand out from everyone else, even though surrounded by so many. I took a closer look at him, and screamed his name. It was my COUSIN! Unfortunately, he wasn't looking my way at all, so with a desperate attempt at getting his attention, I started banging the glass. That didn't work either, so I started doing jumping jacks, hoping for something. I don't know why I thought of jumping, because my cousin had already walked passed me, and all hope seemed to be lost. But, miraculously, for some reason, he turned back and saw me outside. I was floored! I just couldn't believe it!*

*He made his way over to the glass exit door. I was standing there with a very agitated Denis a few steps down. We were both freezing our asses off and we needed to get inside. I had my mini-miracle, wow! My cousin yelled out, "Hey guys, come in here. What are you doing out there?" I quickly helped Denis to the top of the staircase. He didn't argue.*

*"We were stuck, cuz. You're a blessing! I thought we'd be stuck out here all night!"*

*"Fuck man, just let me inside," Denis said, as he pushed me aside and slowly waddled through the door.*

*"Excuse the bitterness. Former student of dad's," I laughed, and he let us both inside. I introduced Denis and we stood in the hallway talking.*

*I gave him a big hug. "Thanks so much. Thank God you saw us. We were like ice cubes out there. I thought you were going to miss us! Something must have caused you to look our way, because you were practically gone. Did you hear me banging on the glass?"*

*My cousin had a look of bewilderment on his face. "No, and I really don't know why I looked. I just happened to turn and look back and you were there!" He smiled, and then a look of distress appeared on his face.*

*"Sorry, Chris, I gotta leave you guys. I was actually leaving the arena when I walked passed you. I just got a call from home. My little guy is sick. I gotta leave now. Where you sitting?"*

*I took out my tickets. "Section 310, S-23, 24."*

*"Oh, you guys are way around the other side, and up at the very top. Here, why don't you take these tickets? I gotta leave anyway." It was our second miracle of the night. Surprisingly, and thankfully, he told me that his seats were in the section right to our left. We were already there!*

*"The seats are right in the top row of the lower deck. We have some season tickets there. We share these with friends from the company. Enjoy the game and give my best to your family."*

*I smiled and stared at the tickets. I gave him an even bigger hug and he headed out.*

*"Well, are we gonna sit, or what? My legs are killin' me."*

*"We're going to sit, Denis. We're finally going to sit," I said, rolling my eyes.*

*We took our seats in the top aisle of the lower deck. We were conveniently on the end of the row, too, which was perfect for Denis. He needed to spread his legs out and lay down his canes. I looked at my old tickets and ripped them up.*

*"These tickets ARE way up there!" I said, pointing across the arena. "God, thankfully we bumped into my cousin. I still can't believe how that all happened so perfectly." I knew deep down, for sure, that it had to be God's choosing and His path. I quietly gave praise to God. Denis wasn't much of a spiritual person, but I know he believed. He actually wore a cross around his neck. It meshed nicely with the Harley-Davidson pin on his lapel!*

*"My legs, Chris," Denis said, relieved. "I'd be best to leave them right fucking here!"*

*He laughed. I laughed. It was the first time he had felt at ease since I picked him up: me too! Oh, and you know what else? He was no longer complaining. Well, okay, maybe he was, but it was about other things, like what he wanted to eat, or the players being too small, or what souvenir I should buy him. Denis loved to complain about everything, but I miss him now. It's amazing how you get used to someone and learn to love them despite their shortcomings. Denis had a lot of them, but deep down, he meant well. And you know what? I know he loved me. He just had a weird way of showing it.*

*I'd like to say that the night ended and we won the game*

*and everyone went home happy, but I'd be lying. Little did I know, at the time, that my night was only just beginning.*

## CHAPTER 3
## IT'S A SMALL WORLD AFTER ALL

*The puck dropped for the second period. Denis was enjoying himself and so was I. He finally had a smile on his face for more than a few seconds. I wished I'd had a camera. Smiles didn't come often for Denis, and looking at him sitting there, I could see exactly why. I couldn't believe how thin he'd become. He was losing weight every time I saw him, probably weighing in around 110 lbs. He had weighed close to 300 pounds only a year prior! Diabetes can do that to a person, especially when one didn't take care of themselves. He was dressed as a punk-ass kid. But that's all he really was, a kid who never got to grow up.*

*We scored a goal and took a 2-1 lead. The fans were happy, and you could feel a buzz in the arena. As we watched, another strange thing happened. Call it chance, call it coincidence, call it whatever you want. Either way, you'll agree that it was "strange". It was a case of being in the right place at the right time. Again, I knew it to be God's path, but many hearing that would think that that was just crazy talk.*

*There was a couple sitting in the seats next to us. We'd already exchanged "hi's" and smiles but that was all. After the second goal, the man for some reason looked over and just started to talk to me.*

*"Nice game, eh guys?"*

*"Sure is. I love this place. Do you come to games often?" I asked him.*

*"These are our seats. We have season tickets here."*

*We exchanged names and I introduced Denis, who cared less. I struck up a conversation with them. Suddenly, the strange thing I mentioned began, and it started with a group of little girls who came running up behind us.*

*"Mr. Nihmey!!!" they yelled. I turned around to find four of my former students from my first teaching job several years before. They were so excited and so was I! I hadn't seen them in a while! I had taught them in grade four and they were now in … hmm, grade seven!*

*"How are you, girls?"*

*"Good," a few of them responded. I stood up and stepped into the aisle to talk with them. We chatted for several*

*minutes. We exchanged hugs and they ran off, and that's when the strange thing actually occurred. The gentleman beside me said, "I heard the girls say Mr. Nihmey. Listen, you'll have to excuse me, but I have a funny thing to ask you. Does 509 Bronson Avenue ring a bell for you?"*

*I thought for a moment. "509 Bronson ... no, not really. Why?"*

*"Well, I may be way out in left field on this one, as there are, I'm sure, many people with your last name, but we live at 509 Bronson. I'm positive that a Nihmey lived in our place at one time. Lily Nihmey?"*

*"Oh my God! That's my grandmother! Yah! That used to be her place! You live there now?"*

*"We moved in recently and the only way I knew it was your grandmother's place, was that we found some old papers with her name on them stashed in the fireplace. I guessed she had moved out many years ago. Wow, this is really weird," he said, scratching his brow.*

*Then it dawned on me why this was BEYOND weird and I said to him, "What might be even crazier ... do you know the guy who has tickets right here beside you?"*

*"Yes we do!" the wife chimed in excitedly. "He's been here with his two little kids many times!"*

*"Well, you won't believe it. He's my first cousin!" I said, as the man looked at me with a startled look on his face. He was taken aback, just as I was. I couldn't believe it! We couldn't believe it! And when I told him what events had transpired and the reason we were sitting there, we all scratched our heads.*

*Talk about strange coincidences. What were the odds of all these events happening the way they did tonight? Here we were, sitting next to a couple who lived in my grandmother's old house, and my cousin, a Nihmey, who has season tickets beside them, had never realized it! And to top that off, the only reason we're sitting beside them now is the smallest of chances that we'd meet him outside the glass doors, stranded in the cold. And the only reason we see him is the fact that we are LATE for the game! Good God, the strangest of coincidences were happening over and over again tonight, as they had been for months. Things were just falling into place like a puzzle. It was really fantastic! What are the chances that in a whole building of thousands of people, let alone a city of almost a million, that we would bump into my cousin the way we did, when we did? Add to that, sitting next to a couple who lived in our grandmother's old house!*

*The energy I'd been feeling over the last month was brewing inside. I was seeing this kind of stuff all the time! I concluded that these events were definitely miracles in themselves. The man beside me told me that I was welcome to come by to see the papers sometime. I later took him up on that. It was my grandmother's old place. Wild!*

*At intermission, I walked out into the busy hallway and headed towards the concession stand to get Denis something to eat. Oh, and a souvenir, which he insisted I buy him. And then, as I walked around, talk about a small world or "coincidence" or whatever you want to call it. In that hallway alone, I actually ended up meeting person after person after person that I knew! It was crazy and hugs galore! I was feeling so high on life lately.*

*One after the other, person after person, everywhere I turned, I bumped into someone I knew! I must have said, "What a coincidence!" or "What a small world!" dozens of times! These incidents were happening way too often for me to believe that these meetings were just mere chance. Later that evening, and weeks following, I realized that these were part of a much larger plan that was developing rapidly. God had great plans for me and I was the perfect vessel for him, willing to do anything. Anything.*

*I returned to our seats and cooled down a bit. So much to take in, so many familiar faces.*

*"Here you go, Denis," I said, as I handed him the food. He started munching on the popcorn even before it left my hand! Don't ask me how, but he found a way!*

*"Crunch, crunch." Then, with his mouth full of popcorn spilling out, he asked, "Did you get the souvenir?"*

*"Yes, here you go." I handed him a little hockey figurine to put on his key chain.*

*"Hey, thanks, man." At least he was appreciative. It was nice to hear thanks instead of fuck for once!*

## CHAPTER 4
## STRANGE HAPPENINGS CONTINUE

*The hockey game ended. The crowd left happy with a home team victory. I was especially proud of our boys, because one of the 67's defensemen was my second cousin. Yah, another cousin! I hadn't seen him play in awhile, so I was hoping to meet him before I left the arena. I wasn't sure I'd be able to because of security. However, feeling as good as I was, I felt that nothing could get in my way. I was so fired up and I had to make it happen. This was indicative of my life at this time. If my mind was on something, it was going to happen and, more often than not, it did!*

*We slowly began to make our way to the far side of the rink. This was where the players exited their dressing room. Denis was complaining incessantly about how tired he was and how he just wanted to go home. I hate to say this, but I was getting a little tired of hearing it all. However, looking back at things now, I'd have to admit that I deserved a good kick in the ass that night. I wasn't being fair to him at all. He hadn't been out in months and this was a lot for him to handle.*

*"Fuck, man, I'm way too tired to keep goin'! Do you have to see another cousin?"*

*"I'd like to, Denis. It's been a long time since I've seen him."*

*"Well, I'm going to sit right fucking here until you're done. I ain't goin' nowhere. My legs are killin' me! Can't we just go home?" Denis was starting to whine, but after all I'd seen and experienced so far tonight, I didn't want to stop now. I really felt I was being guided, and I couldn't put an end to things just like that. I was finding that there was something special behind every corner, and I wasn't about to give up any of it. Big things were happening, and I couldn't explain them. I had to go on. So, I made a quick or, you might say, selfish decision, and looked Denis in the eyes. It may not have been fair, but it didn't matter. I was as high as a kite, and I needed to see where all of this was taking me.*

*"I'll be right back, Denis." I had to be stern and to the point with him. He wanted things his way and only his way. So did I, I guess, but he could wait for me and, besides, he had his*

*souvenir to look at. It cost me ten freakin' bucks!*

*I left Denis and headed towards the front of the arena where the locker rooms were. In order to get downstairs to the lockers, you had to pass security, so things were not going to be easy for me. However, the players did come up that way, and there was a table they usually signed autographs on. As I walked up to the waiting area, I was shocked by the number of people that had gathered to see the players. I estimated close to 200!*

*"Did any come up yet?" I asked the security guard standing by the table.*

*"Not yet, can you please step back, sir?"*

*I stood back and grinned, "Actually, I'm not "sir", I'm Chris."*

*The security guard chuckled. We chatted for a minute and that's when things got bizarre again. I will tell you, but first, I'm going to sidetrack for a moment.*

[*Being on a manic high, although at the time I didn't know I was, is like being on a drug, but without coming down into withdrawal. You don't come down until your chemicals shift and you hit the other* ***"side of the story"*** *... depression. I hate that word! On your high, you always feel great and it feels really good. If anyone could sell that feeling in a bottle, they'd make a fortune!*

*Because I was so high, I wanted to meet everyone! And I mean EVERYONE! I truly felt that everyone who crossed my path was important, and that they were someone I must meet. I believed, and still do, that every person in your life is there for a reason, not just by mere chance. At the hockey game that night, I was slowly realizing that this was most certainly the case and, during the next months of my mania, that was true hundreds of times over.*]

*Now, where was I? Oh yes, the security guard.*

*"Have you worked here a long time?"*

*"Just started, actually."*

*"Well, nice chatting with you. By the way, I'm Chris." I stuck out my hand.*

*We shook hands. "Clark," the man said, as I looked at his name tag. I noticed that his last name was Kelly, which definitely struck a chord.*

*"Kelly. Hey, my mom's a Kelly!"*

*"Really?" he answered, intrigued. I had his attention.*

*"I know it's a big family, but my mom's family comes from Manotick."*

*"So does mine! We actually have a picnic there each year!"*

*"I know! I wouldn't miss it! You know what? We're cousins!"*

*What were the chances? There was a reason for this and I knew it.*

*After a little more chat, we laughed and went our separate ways, and promised to catch up at next year's picnic. Clark told me that the boys would be up soon. I was getting more excited about how this night was unfolding. It was a lot to take in, and I was loving every minute of it! God was enjoying this, too, I could tell. If the theory I was developing was right, I was surrounded in this part of the arena by people that were meant to be in my path and who I'd connect with in some way.*

*It was time to test my theory further. Since the players weren't up yet, I started to strike up a conversation with a woman beside me, decked out in 67's gear.*

*"I'm Chris Nihmey. It's nice to meet you."*

*"Nihmey?" The woman looked up and closed her eyes. "Hmm … a Mr. Nihmey taught me at Commerce, years ago."*

*"That's my dad!" I said excitedly. "I can't believe it! What a small world!" Although I still didn't believe in the small world thing, I just said it anyway.*

*"I can't believe you're Mr. Nihmey's son. Wow!"*

*"Mr. Nihmey?" a man jumped in when he heard the name. "I worked with Mike over at Highland Park." Well, that floored me! What were the chances? And of all places, that was where my dad had taught Denis!*

*"So you both know my dad! It's weird, eh, that we'd meet this way," I said.*

*"I know, what are the chances you'd meet both of us at the same time?" she said.*

*"Better than you think," I snickered. And then, feeling like my ball of energy was about to explode, guess what I did? I decided to make my way through the busy crowd to meet as many people as I possibly could. I started to talk to everyone, to test my theory that, somehow, everyone had a connection with me. I started to jump from person to person kind of like a jack rabbit. It would have been funny to see from above. I*

*moved around and threw questions at people all over the entrance way. My conversations were short, because I was talking a mile a minute. I got my fix and my theory was proved. Honestly, I know it's hard to picture, but I went from one person to the next, as high as ever, to look for some type of connection between me and them. I found connections everywhere! Imagine! Cousins, friends of my parents or sister, people with whom I'd worked, even former students. The list of connections went on and on. As I said, it was truly unbelievable to be surrounded by so many. I must have met close to a hundred people in that entrance way alone! In my overly friendly way, yes, I hugged them all! I even ended up standing behind the autograph table!*

*Suddenly, a kid called out my name, "Mr. Nihmey!"*

*I recognized him from a school I had taught at. He introduced me to his father. Then the funniest thing happened. The boy actually asked ME for an autograph. Here goes, I thought, and I signed his ticket stub. After signing his stub, I looked up, and several kids had made their way to the table. They, too, began to ask me for my autograph! So, I started signing a bunch of autographs! The security guard couldn't believe it. I raised my shoulders and eyebrows and we both laughed. "I'm just a teacher, kids!"*

*After signing eight or nine stubs, I remembered something. DENIS! Oh my God! I'd forgotten about Denis! I'd been down here for at least a half hour! I signed one last autograph and ran back into the arena. I guess I wouldn't be seeing my cousin tonight!*

*Denis was right where I left him and he was not happy at all, sitting with his arms crossed. I was too charged up to care that much.*

*We headed away and I drove Denis home. He was not happy, but I didn't care. All I really wanted to do was to get him home and be on my way. One, because he was complaining constantly and, two, I wanted to continue to test my theory of connections and find out what God was trying to tell me. Who would I meet next? I had to find out and I knew Denis couldn't keep up. I helped Denis inside and left him sitting on his couch. It was a little rude but he was home.*

*"I gotta go, Denis." I had tried to explain things to him on the way home, but he just thought I was a lunatic. I knew he wouldn't understand the "theory", so I just left. It was 11 pm,*

*and I was more revved up now than I had ever been. I was ready to go at any time of the day, because that's what a high is all about. I, however, believed it was because I was chosen for greatness in some way. Who knew where this was going to take me?*

## CHAPTER 5
## REALLY, I'M NOT CRAZY … TRUST ME!

*As I left Denis' place, I started to think deeply about what I had experienced so far tonight. Was I right? Were there connections and coincidences all over that others were missing? Were they too caught up in their own lives? It looked like this was the case and, in time, I had convinced myself of this. I could not let this thought go. God was complex but I was starting to think I had Him figured out.*

*I drove down a busy St. Laurent Boulevard and came to a Tim Hortons. It was booming inside: well, as booming as a donut shop could be! I contemplated a coffee and a donut when I entered. Actually, I really just wanted to test my theory. Besides, I couldn't eat anyway! Five days and counting, no food whatsoever!*

*"A medium double-double, please," I told the cashier. I looked closely at her. Was there a connection or coincidence here? She was wearing her regular Tim Hortons apron, but I could see a shamrock through the white material. BINGO!*

*"Do you go to St. Pat's?" I asked. She smiled and said yes.*

*"Do you know Mr. Nihmey?"*

*"Yah!" she said excitedly. "He taught me History last term! I loved having him, he was an amazing teacher!"*

*"That's my father!"*

*"Really? That's your dad? What a great teacher he is!" I always heard that about my dad. I took my coffee and sat in one of the few empty seats (pews?).*

*As I enjoyed the coffee, I looked around the store. There were dozens of people sitting in groups of their own. I started to wonder what connections they had with each other or with me. If I tested that out, I'd probably be kicked out, but I didn't care! I continued my quest of finding coincidences and connections with people. God would protect me!*

*Of the fifteen or so people I interviewed, each had a connection with me in some way! Wow! Amazing! I left the shop even more charged than when I came in.*

*I ran across the street and entered a McDonald's. I abruptly walked up to a group of five guys sporting leather jackets, sitting at the back. I was getting really good at this, and I knew exactly what to say, without getting my head kicked in!*

*I pointed at each of them and asked, "Where did you guys go to high school?" They looked at me rolling their eyes and said, "St. Pat's. Why?" By the way, St. Pat's was nowhere near.*

*"Do you know Mr. Nihmey?"*

*There was a stir at the table. All five knew him. Just as I thought. This was getting very interesting. It seemed like God was placing the right people in my path, but why?*

*I left the group and walked up to the cash.*

*"I'm not ordering, I just want to ask you a question." Like I said, I was starting to get real good at asking astute questions. It felt like God was directing me to say what He wanted me to say, to prove His point.*

*I asked a "way out there" question, "Do you live in the Hunt Club area?"*

*"Yah, I do, why?" she responded, puzzled.*

*"What street do you live on?"*

*"Blohm," she replied. "Can I take your order?"*

*"One minute. One minute. Do you know the school in that area?"*

*"It's an elementary school. Actually, my cousins go there!"*

*We chatted for one more minute, and I found out that one of her cousins had graduated from there last year.*

*"That's amazing. She probably knows me! I taught there last year! It's Mr. Nihmey … here, write it down and say hi! Sorry for not ordering."*

*"That's okay. I will say hi! Small world!"*

*I had to keep this going. This was fantastic! Connections were everywhere!*

*I left McDonald's and headed over to a pool hall in the strip mall behind McDonald's, Dooly's. I walked in and, right away, as high as I was, zoned in on a pool table and walked up to two guys playing. In a mere minute, I found a connection between us. I zoomed to another table and did the same thing. It was then that a bit of trouble happened. I noticed that the owner, a tall burly man, was on to me. He didn't like what he saw. For some reason, what I was doing was "wrong". Yah, I know, I don't get it either.*

*"You'll have to leave, sir."*

*"What? Why? What's the problem?" I was beginning to raise my voice a bit. I was becoming agitated. During my*

*high, this was sometimes the case when people came at me the wrong way.*

*"You're bugging the patrons!"*

*"Bugging! No I'm not!"*

*"Yes … you are."*

*"I'd like to see the manager!"*

*"I'm the owner, so piss off! Get out of my bar!"*

*I got very angry, and I slammed my hand on the pool table. Ouch! Have you done this before? Don't!*

*"These guys aren't bothered. Guys, are you?"*

*They eyed the owner and said nothing. I put my head down and slowly walked out. I looked back and the owner just stared me right in the eye. I gave him a friendly wave but I was fuming. I got into the car and sped away, never to go back. At the time, I thought that I was as right as right can be. I could do no harm, and this was something that my high had taught me. I was ALWAYS right. And when things didn't go my way, I let people know it!*

*It was nearing 1:30 am by the time I left the pool hall. I raced down St. Laurent and drove up Walkley. I pulled into another McDonald's. A popular place! The same things happened, connections everywhere. I was getting really good at this. I was finding a connection with people after only two questions. Two! It was really incredible! God must be guiding my thoughts and my words and my path! At McDonald's, I struck up a long conversation with one of the custodians. We talked about all kinds of things and he thought I was a bit loopy with my theory. I don't know why I told him. In this state of mind, I often said and did things without thinking them through. That's what happens when you're manic. But at the time, I felt I was completely normal. Wasn't I?*

*I arrived at a Denny's restaurant on Bank Street. They were always open late. It was nearing 2:30. I walked past the hostess, ignoring her greeting, and went right into the dining area. I zoned in on a table of five and pointed to one of the guys. I found a connection in three simple questions. I walked to the other side and did the same. Connections! I walked to the back, and again, connections! The people were so fascinated with my energy and my discoveries. I was as high as I'd ever been, and I looked like a magician with a clever deck of cards. I was very entertaining and, again, I was talking a mile a minute.*

*As I walked around the restaurant finding connections everywhere, I noticed that a man, maybe the manager, was talking with the hostess. She came up to me and told me that I'd have to leave.*

*Ignoring her request, I asked her two questions. I found out that she was a Christian, and I told her I was, also. We knew the same church.*

*"I'd love to chat, but … you gotta leave, like right now! See my manager over there!"*

*I looked over. He didn't look happy. He was pointing to the door. I made my way out but, before I did, I asked the girl if she wanted to chat sometime about faith.*

*"I'm married, eh."*

*"That's okay. We have something more important in common."*

*She shrugged her shoulders. "What the heck. Here's my number." And over the next couple of months, I would spend time with her, her husband and their beautiful baby daughter.*

*I looked over her shoulder. The manager was fuming. He was holding up a phone. I gave her a hug, and left her quickly with a smile.*

*"I'm calling the cops, sir!"*

*"Okay, okay, I'm leaving!" He started to dial. I laughed and raced out as fast as I could.*

*My trip to Denny's and the next few coffee shops had taken me to 2:45 am. It was late, and I was getting tired. I decided to head home. I had to take all of this in. It had been an amazing night, one that I would never forget and pivotal to my quest towards understanding my mission from God.*

*Oh, and get this! This was the grand finale, the cherry on top of the scrumptious dessert. I pulled into a gas station, a block from my house. There was a teen standing beside the pumps with his car hood up.*

*"Can I help you?"*

*"Actually, my dad is on his way."*

*"What happened?" I asked, holding the nozzle.*

*"My car just stalled on me. I got here from the arena and it died."*

*"The arena?" I said.*

*"Yah, I play for the 67's."*

*Well that just about floored me! I left the station flying, the highest I'd ever felt! I arrived at my place at exactly 3:30. I headed upstairs as quietly as possible and I lay back on my bed. I wanted to wake up my roomies and tell them everything, but I couldn't. I held it in. Then, with my arms behind my head, everything began to hit me. It was odd, but it felt great. I wouldn't sleep at all that night.*

*What was that all about? I thought to myself. I couldn't believe what had happened tonight. This was greater than any "small world" theory, or coincidence. This went far beyond that. For some reason, I was in the exact right place at the exact right time. I was on some sort of path of God. I was being guided by something far greater than me. It was clear to me that these connections were happening for a reason. I just had to figure out what that reason was. I spent the rest of my night deliberating. It would take a long time to get a clearer picture.*

*As I lay there, I started to think about the probability of all these things happening tonight. Was it just mere chance or was there something greater? What was the probability of having all of these "coincidences" happening over and over again? Astronomical, far beyond any number we could ever calculate. There are connections everywhere in our lives, whether you call it God's path, a higher power, a "small world" or coincidence. For me, I found out that there is a definite reason for where we are, and who we're with. There are connections everywhere, each helping us to better relate with each other and to form friendships and relationships. These connections do happen, and this night proved that to me. Had I just been subject to the true meaning of life itself in one evening of hockey? It was fantastic and totally crazy at the same time! I lay there, a burning ball of energy staring at the ceiling. Until 7 am.*]

## CHAPTER 6
## MY WAY AND THE 'HIGH' WAY

Okay, I'm back. 8 am. The drive to Toronto ... remember?

I flew down Highway 416 heading towards Kingston. The highway was not busy at this hour, but none of that mattered to me right now. What mattered most was that I was finally free, and no one was going to get me. If I felt unsafe, I had to leave. Those who loved me most were those who wanted to stop me. They were now in my past, and I had the future before me. I had left them all behind. I finally started to relax a bit. I turned up the heat and the Christian music and I sailed forward while tapping my hand on the steering wheel. I felt like a huge weight had been lifted from my shoulders. My roommates, my friends, my parents ... they were all a hindrance, so I had to go. Problem ... solved.

After an hour or so of driving, I turned the heat down and turned the radio to a low mutter. It was prayer time and I needed peace and tranquility to talk to the "Big Guy", whom I would later call, ominously, Dad.

*"God, it's me ... again. I lay my life down before Thee, oh gracious and wonderful maker. I don't know where I'm going or what is happening with me, but I do all of this for You. Protect me with Your love and help me to trust You in everything I do from this day forward. Continue to show me the signs that tell me I am on Your path. I believe in all my heart that You will deliver me to safety and that I will fulfil Your plan for me. In Jesus Christ, I ask this. Amen."*

Driving along, I approached Highway 401, one of Canada's major highways. I looked ahead and noticed something in the distance. As I got closer, I realized that it was a man standing on the side of the road, thumb up, in the cold. A hitchhiker! I didn't know how I felt about hitchhikers and had never picked up one before, but, at the time, I knew that God was guiding my way, and if a hitchhiker was in that path, I would stop. He was there for a reason, obviously. So I pulled over. I gulped, thinking to myself, "What if he's an axe murderer?" I shrugged my shoulders and said, "Oh well, then it must be God's choosing!" In other words, I was going to stop no matter what, so I did. I rolled down my passenger side window.

"Hi!"

"Hi! Can I get a lift?"

"Where you heading?" I asked, not that it mattered. I knew deep down that he'd be part of my journey, regardless. He was there for a reason and I knew it. Man, was God ever great! He was giving me another opportunity to connect with someone. Another sign.

"I'm heading up to Kingston, to my brother's place."

"You been here long?"

"Yah, a few hours at least. I'm frozen. Can you help me out?"

"You know what? I can. I'm heading to Toronto. I can probably make a quick stop in Kingston. Hop in!"

I turned the heat up as he sat inside. I reached for the extra pair of gloves I had earlier given Denis and introduced myself. He accepted them more graciously than Denis had.

"I'm Chris."

"Andy," he said to me, as we shook hands. "You know, I really appreciate you picking me up. People just don't trust hitchhikers anymore, but when you're stuck, you're stuck. I've travelled this road many times in many different cars. Trucks, too! When you're working with very little means, you gotta do what you gotta do."

I then laughed in his face and told him that I didn't trust them either, and I threw him out into the moving highway. Kidding!

Here's what really happened.

We exchanged pleasantries and rode on towards Kingston. I learned that Andy was a struggling carpenter in Ottawa and had been for years. He lived downtown and expressed how hard it had been to make ends meet. He was trying to run his own business and money was not flowing his way. Working long hours with little pay was definitely difficult, so visiting his family in Kingston had to be achieved by hitchhiking. I felt for him and wished I could help him out. I reached into my pocket for some money, but $40 was all I could give him. I had nothing else on me. He was very thankful for my generosity.

When we arrived in Kingston, he was so grateful for the ride that he decided to take me on a small tour through the town. We visited many of its oldest parts and travelled along some of its canal locks. I spent several hours with him; we had some good chats. I briefly touched on my story. I didn't want to go into things too deeply.

Although Andy was not in my life much following that day, he did play a vital role. He became a lifeline to my parents. I found out later that he had been suspicious about my state of mind.

"Please, give my folks a call and tell them I'm okay, that everything is fine. Here's their number. Tell them that I'm going to see Mark in Toronto. They may be worried, but tell them you were with me and I am totally fine."

"Thanks, Chris. You've been a real lifesaver. I couldn't take that cold much longer. Thank you and God bless you on your journey."

"Yes, He has," I said solemnly. I waved goodbye and headed back on to the 401 and didn't stop again. I had my water, my music, my heat and my God carrying me. I headed right into Toronto and after a few misdirections, I thankfully found Mark's apartment. I had an idea where he lived because I had visited before, but never on this short notice—actually, no notice at all! I pulled in around 7 pm. I stood at his apartment with a bag on my shoulders. I rang up.

"Hello?"

"It's Nihmey!"

"Nihmey! What are you doing here?" he said, surprised, but excited.

"I'll tell you all about it. Let me up! It's darn cold out here!"

He laughed and buzzed me in. I walked up the stairs and into his apartment.

"What up, G?" he said, giving me a big hug. That was what he always said. "G". I never really understood it but it sounded natural.

"Good to see you, Marky," I gave him a hug back.

"What in God's name are you doing here?" he asked.

"It's a long story, Marky, but you know that I'll tell you everything."

I looked over at the couch. There was a man sitting there. He stood up and walked over to meet me. His name, Tom, a pastor from Whitby. Ah, just what I needed at the time. Man, God was so neat. If ever I had a sign that I was in the right place, it was this. What were the chances that Mark would have a pastor visiting him on the day I left Ottawa? Wow, it was freaky, just like all of the things that were happening! It made me extremely excited for what might come next. Mark's cousin popped into the room to say hi. In spite of his living there, we saw him very little.

"Marky, wait 'til you hear what happened to me last night! You will NOT believe it! I'll tell you everything! Man, I'm so glad I'm here." I hugged him again, and we sat down and had a cup of tea. They listened to my story, and all that I had been through. I told them about the strange coincidences and connections I had been experiencing over and over. I asked them to help me tie it all together. They listened intently and said nothing. I couldn't believe all that I was telling them—it just sounded so crazy. I'd even drawn a map of the Civic Centre arena on the back of my ticket stub to show them how it had all developed.

"So, I don't know what to think. Doesn't it all sound so weird?"

Mark and Tom looked at me, and Tom said, "It is, Chris, but I believe it. With God, anything can happen. You are definitely chosen for something. You just need to find out what. I have seen a lot of things and people in my life that have been touched by God. You are another. For now, relax and take your mind off things. Put your feet up and rest. You've travelled a great distance. Are you hungry?"

"Actually, I'm on a fast! I have been for six days now. I've only been drinking liquids. God called me to do this last week. Wait until I tell you about last Sunday. God was calling me in a big way!"

You've probably guessed it by now, but Mark and Tom were devout Christians. They trusted God in everything they did. We all did. I felt that Mark was one of the only people who would truly understand what had transpired over the last month or so. He was my Christian brother, and I trusted him. We hadn't spoken to each other in a while, but I knew that I was in the right place. You know when you feel like everything is right? Well, that was how I felt, as I sipped a green tea.

Mark and I headed off to a Swiss Chalet restaurant. I talked and he listened to more of my story. He ate; I drank water. It was tough watching him eat, but the burning that I was feeling was God working within me, not hunger, and I knew that the rewards would be plentiful.

I did not hear from my parents that night, but it didn't really matter to me that much. I knew that God had delivered me to a safe place. I would sleep well tonight, reassured by the fact that I was exactly where I was supposed to be. Tired, yes, but excited nonetheless. My mission was developing so quickly, it was amazing. As the lights in the apartment went out, I prayed in thanks and asked for discernment. I felt God's reply, smiled, and nodded off.

## CHAPTER 7
## AMAZING GRACE

That night, again, after only a couple hours of sleep, I woke to the howling wind of a cold February morning. I looked at the clock beside me. 3 am. I remember lying in Mark's living room listening to the wind. It was loud. It seemed to repeatedly punch the wall by my head and then swirl away. I also remember my state of mind at that moment. With as strong a connection I felt I was having with God, I believed in all my heart that I could rebuke the wind with my hand, by telling it to settle. I honestly thought I could stop the wind from blowing! And even though I really wasn't, when it momentarily ceased, I felt deep down that I had. That's how great I felt and how high I was. I believed I was connected directly to nature through God. This was common for me at the time. It made me believe I could do the impossible and that I could do no wrong. Rebuking the wind was a symbol of the invincibility I was feeling. It reminded me of how Moses felt when he had been given great powers by God. I knew that I could do great things with God's hand upon me. It was only a matter of time and it would come ... soon.

I looked at the clock again. 3:23. I sat up and looked down at Tom who was in a sleeping bag by the couch. He had given up his couch for me. I lay there looking at him sleeping so comfortably, and I was about to wake him up; I decided not to. He was snoring so damned loud! I stood up, made my way past him and tiptoed to the washroom. I wasn't tired at all. It would be another sleepless night. I closed the bathroom door and turned the light on. When my eyes adjusted, I looked in the mirror and smiled. It felt so good. I felt a surge of joy in my belly as I stared at myself. I truly felt that God was with me and I could do no wrong and that I would do great things with His help. Why was I chosen? I thought to myself. I just felt that I was perfect for Him. At the time, I would do anything for Him. And I mean anything!

I turned the light off and stepped into the hallway. I tiptoed back through the kitchen and dressed. It was then that I decided that something had to happen. At that moment, as I eyed the door, I felt the need to go somewhere. I didn't know where, but I just had to go. I had to take my mission further. I

NEEDED to take my mission further. I felt good about what I'd discovered so far. Who knew what else God had planned for me? As the Bible says, *"... with God, everything is possible."* I was excited to see what "everything" might be, even in a city I knew very little about.

As I put my second shoe on, Tom rolled over with his eyes wide open. I looked down at him and all I said was, "I gotta go."

He smiled, coughed and replied, "I know." Then he rolled over and was asleep again in seconds. Tom knew that something was up. He had heard my story. He had heard the facts and like Mark and me, he was fascinated and convinced that God was using me for great things.

I opened the front door and headed down the stairs to the world that I believed needed me. Someone was calling, someone was in need, and I was getting an idea of what my mission was intended to be. This would develop more over the next few days.

I walked to Spadina and zipped my coat up. It was very cold and the wind blew fiercely. After walking for a few minutes, I felt that I was being spiritually pulled down a dark alleyway. I remember feeling a bit nervous as I stared to my left and right at the austere townhomes. Although I was a bit tense, I remember also feeling that I was safe and secure because God was with me. It was dark and lonely but I felt God's hand on me. To ease some of the tension, I started to do something that I knew would bring relief. It was simple: a call to God for protection and guidance. I began to sing.

***"Amazing Grace,***
***How sweet the sound,***
***That saved a wretch like me.***
***I once was lost, but now am found ..."***

First it was low and under my breath but, as I walked on further, for some reason, I started to sing a little bit louder, and then, even louder. Within a short time, I got to a point where I was singing at the top of my lungs! I was praying, knowing that God would never leave my side. On both sides of me, several house lights switched on. I didn't care.

And it was at that moment, I had one of the most outrageous thoughts I'd ever had. It was one of the most frightening, but it didn't scare me. I was feeling, for the first time in my mania, and believing it in all my heart, that if someone came up to me with a gun and pulled the trigger, the bullet would veer around my head, kind of like in *The Matrix*. Isn't that crazy?

Continuing down the alleyway, I was starting to feel more and more invincible in everything I did. I felt that nothing could hurt or stop me. Nothing. I even felt that I could avoid death. I felt completely invulnerable. It was a first at the time, but it would stay with me for a long while.

I continued to the end of the alleyway and came out onto a main street once again. Finally some light, but the road was near empty. There wasn't a car in sight. I walked for about five minutes and came up to a Coffee Time donut shop. Outside of the shop, there was a man who was panhandling. I asked him if he wanted a sandwich and a drink. I invited him inside the shop and he took a seat. I went up to the counter and ordered a sandwich and a coke and brought them to him. I could smell alcohol on his breath when he thanked me for the food. He was very grateful and we started to chat. I found out that his name was Ralph. It was nice to put a name to his face. He told me about his life and how he ended up, not only losing his job, but also his family. He hadn't seen his kids in over ten years and missed them dearly. He told me he had resorted to alcohol to numb the mental anguish he was going through. It was a means to cope. I also found out that Ralph had lived in Ottawa years before! I had found a connection between the two of us! I knew now that we were meant to meet. Wasn't God fantastic?

Before parting, I told him briefly about my story and my mission which was becoming much clearer. Yah, he probably thought I was crazy too, but more importantly was the fact that I didn't feel this. I knew there was a reason I was in Toronto, and a reason for where I'd go next and, in time, I would understand everything. I waved goodbye and wished him well. And being touched by his story, and wishing I could do more, I left him with the last bit of money I unexpectedly found in my pocket. That twenty would get him some more food. He promised he'd use it wisely.

It was 4:30 am. As I walked along, I felt I knew my mission. Meet as many people as I possibly could and find connections between their lives and the lives of others, in hopes of helping them to find faith in God. I really felt that was it. These strange coincidences and connections were just God's way of using me to reach out to people and show them that He was there for them.

I passed two more homeless people and threw them a couple bucks, which I miraculously found, and continued down the street. It was quiet around me, but the homeless were always there. With that feeling of invulnerability getting stronger and stronger, I walked into a corner store and grabbed a juice. My stomach continued to grumble. I hadn't eaten in seven days, the longest seven days I'd ever spent. I was so hungry at the time, that I would have licked the floor for crumbs. I went up to the cashier and started to have a conversation. I told him to remember my face because, one day soon, he would see it all over the news. He would be able to say, "Wow! That's the guy I met in my store!"

At the time, I really believed this would happen, that all the world would soon know me. I knew I had been chosen for something extraordinary and that God was using me for His greatness. I would make His glory shine.

My mission was becoming much clearer. Eventually, at some time in the near future, God would use me to connect all people through my story and my mission. I ultimately would bring the world to Christ, through salvation. I was excited to see what God would do. Everything was incredibly real to me. Nothing was impossible.

I zipped my coat all the way up. I walked a fair distance for almost a half hour and checked my watch. 5 am. God, it was cold. I was fortunate to have on what I did, because I had met many people that morning who were inadequately dressed for winter. It was difficult to accept, but I did my best to comfort them as I made my way through the city.

I came upon a van that was parked with its back doors open. There was a small line-up of people dressed in tatters. Each of them was receiving food and water from a woman in the van. I ran up to the line and started to introduce myself. As was always the case, I started asking questions. Many of them started to talk. I had opened them up! When the line finally cleared, I walked up to the van and inquired about what she was doing. She told me that their truck tours around Toronto and offers food to the homeless. I was surprised to find that out. Toronto did, however, have many times the number of homeless people than other cities. It was so nice to see the goodness that was out there, because all we ever really hear about are the bad things.

The lady then asked, "Sir, would you like a sandwich?" As always, I started to share my story with her, about my seven day fast, and my mission to save the world. She smiled and said, "WHOA, man, all I asked you was if you wanted a sandwich!"

I laughed and shook my head and told her that I was heading towards downtown TO. She went to the front of the van and spoke to the driver. She returned and invited me to take a ride. They were heading my way. I hopped in the van and she closed the doors. I proceeded to the front of the van and struck up a conversation with the driver. We talked about their work, as we headed downtown. As I watched the street names change, I wondered where this adventure was taking me. What did God have planned next? It was approaching 5:30 and I was nowhere near Mark's. From the looks of things, I had no clue where I was or where I was going. But I didn't care. God was taking me on this adventure!

When we reached downtown, I said goodbye and headed off. As I walked down the street, I remember taking note of the people I passed and I tried to see connections. Were all the people we meet part of a larger plan? As I came to a homeless shelter, I stood in front and tried to gain my bearings. I felt lost. I didn't know which way to go. I walked around a few streets, trying hard to find the direction towards Mark's, but everywhere I turned made me feel like I was lost even more. Finally, I remember stopping and looking up to the sky that was starting to brighten. It was 6 am, and my feet were killing me and my legs were growing weary. Like Jesus? I stared into the sky and yelled, "Father, take me home!"

It was then that I noticed a sign that had an arrow pointing straight ahead. It was the first sign I had noticed, so I walked by it. Five minutes later, I noticed another sign with an arrow on it pointing left, so I cut down that street and kept on walking. I turned right after seeing another arrow and I kept going. That morning, and I can't explain it, I walked down dozens upon dozens of streets without knowing where in the world I was going. But I trusted God to get me back by following the signs that I knew He was providing for me. And these signs actually led me back to Mark's house and back to his couch by 8:00 that morning, well before the guys woke up. I lay back on the couch, relieved to be in the warmth. God had protected me all night. Consider the danger I had put myself in, in one of the worst parts of Toronto, Canada's largest city, six million people. I can think of countless things that could have hurt me that night, countless. *Amazing Grace*? It was crazy, but I was safe. God had obviously been by my side.

***"I was the perfect vessel for God. I'd do anything for him, even if I had to die. I was ready to lose my life."***

## CHAPTER 8
## HOLY ROLLER

That morning, after two hours of pain-staking lounging, rolling and ceiling staring, I finally gave in and woke Tom up. It was nine. Late for me. I had to tell him everything! Even when I got in earlier, I wanted to jump on him and then jump on Mark's bed. I wanted to grab both their heads, give them a quick shake and tell them what had happened. That's how excited I was! Funny thing was, I felt this way in almost everything I experienced at the time. I just had to talk to someone ... anyone.

Mark came into the living room shortly after, and sat on the couch to listen. He and Tom were once again amazed at my passion for God but, for the first time since I'd been there, they expressed some concern after hearing what I had done only hours before.

"Three in the morning?" Mark couldn't believe it!

"Yah, three in the morning! Tom saw me leave!"

"I did?" Tom questioned. He was half-asleep at the time, so I couldn't blame him for not remembering.

"Yah man, you spoke to me! Anyway, I just headed out and that's what happened out there! My mission continued!" I exclaimed with much excitement.

"Chris, you got to be really careful! This is a very dangerous part of Toronto," Tom warned, belatedly. "I know of many incidents ... in this one area alone! One guy got mugged just down this street!" Mark agreed that I had taken a big chance heading out there at that time.

I heard their advice, but I ignored it. I would hear nothing of it. I started to go on a philosophical rant, to show how safe I was with God. I stood up like a coach and lectured them, waving my arms all over the place. I pointed to each respectively.

"Marky, Tom, God is with me. God is with you. He protects his disciples. He always stands up to bat for us, and gives us the helmet we need for protection. You know it, I know it! I know this is not the safest place around, but God will not let His disciple be harmed. He puts a hedge of protection around those He loves, those who follow His heart. Look ... no cuts, no bruises. Praise God!"

Mark and Tom heard my case. Although they knew that God was doing great things in my life, I could tell they were starting to worry about my over-excitement for God: my expressive zeal and spiritual zest. Even these men of strong faith were now questioning my actions. What did I think of this? I realized that maybe I was getting a sign which was telling me that I wouldn't be with them for long. Like the others, they would soon slow me down. The traps would be set again and I'd have to flee Toronto, as I did from Ottawa.

I really didn't care what either thought. I knew I was chosen and I would soon know why and for what. Something great was coming my way; I was convinced of this. I just didn't know what, but time would soon tell. So many signs were pointing in the right direction.

Following their breakfast and my glass of water, Tom went home. Mark and I were going to attend a church in a suburb of Toronto. It was a charismatic church, similar to the many I had been attending back home. Charismatic churches were now my ONLY churches. You might say I had a strong "craze for charismatic"!

We drove the highway for a while and, as I had done since I arrived in Toronto, my lips started smacking the minute we rolled out, and I talked Mark's ears off! He couldn't get a word in edgewise. I was very expressive as usual; I was delirious! I was like a Chatty Kathy doll with a pullout talking string! Talking a mile a minute, I was imparting my deep thoughts on "coincidences" once again, and sharing more spiritual revelations that I had been having. My thoughts were scattered as I spilled them out to him. As he was the night before, Mark was very supportive and listened carefully, as we bobbed and weaved through the busy traffic. Much of the conversation was way out in left field, typical for me of late, but Mark was kind and understanding. As he nodded, I felt more and more reassured that things were normal. When I look back now, he would have been better off pulling the car over and yelling, "Chris, shut the fuck up, you're freakin' loony!" Of course, that didn't happen, but it probably would have been the best thing to say to me at the time ... or ... maybe not. Being a Christian brother, he'd never use quite those words! Had he ever? Yes, of course. I met him in university!

We arrived at the church and I got out of the car and looked up at the building. I never told Mark at the time, but I remember thinking to myself how bland the dark brown building looked, morbid-like. It was not a pretty sight, but all that really mattered was the cross above the entranceway door. I knew then that it was a safe place.

We were greeted immediately by two overly friendly teenagers who handed me a brochure. This was often the case at these churches. It felt like home.

"Chris, I'll be right back," Mark said, as he took a brochure and went over to meet some of his friends. He left me standing in the middle of the open hallway talking to two complete strangers.

"Welcome to Holy Faith Church (yah, just made that one up, forget what it was called. Good name though, eh?). Is this your first time attending?"

Unfortunately, I nodded yes, and this time they gave ME the earful! I should have said no, but that would be lying. So, because I said yes, the two of them started to tell me everything about their church and everything that was happening there! Blah, blah, blah, blah, blah! Like all the churches I attended during my high, one was always bombarded with these "happy" individuals. And as they spoke to me, I knew it was coming. I knew it! Out of the mouth of the young girl came "THE QUESTION" that all charismatic parishioners asked you. And I mean ALL! I had heard it numerous times in numerous churches!

"Are you born again?" she asked.

"Yes," I said confidently, but honestly, to tell you the truth, I was never too sure when asked this question. However, I was getting really darned good at sounding like I was the "biggest and baddest" Christian around! And so, now that they were done, I began MY rant.

"Well, Christ came into my life a few months ago. Praise the Lord. Alleluia!" I yelled out. Many people looked over, but they all smiled and gave me their approval. "Christ answered my call and saved me from the evils of the world. Christ is amazing! Christ is life! God bless you both."

They both smiled and I grabbed them and hugged them. You know how much I liked to hug!

"Enjoy church and may Christ be with you!" one of them said.

"And you too!" I smiled back.

"Born again" or "saved" ... what do they really mean? The boy and girl used these terms interchangeably. The charismatic and several other branches of Christianity believe that you need to be "saved" to go to Heaven. They believe that anyone who is not "saved" or "born again" as they sometimes call it, will end up in the other place, never to see the face of God, and kept away from Him eternally. During these months, I believed this with all my heart. That was why I tried with all my might to preach to friends, my family, my students and everyone I met. I honestly never felt secure in my own salvation, so I ended up praying these prayers many times, over and over to God. It became a huge obsession for me, which was true of many things. Although I was told that you just had to believe it in your heart, watching others talk about their faith always made me ask myself the question, "Am I "really" saved?"

After a bit more chit-chat with other members of the church, Mark and I took our seats. We sat at the end of a row. There was a large wooden cross at the front centre of the room. There was a band and a carpeted stage where the pastor would speak. It was exactly as I had seen at other charismatic churches. They all seemed to look the same. It reminded me of a particular church I had attended several times over the last while.

The last few people filed into their seats and proceedings began. The pastor called out, "Alleluia!" The congregation repeated after him and several patrons stood up and raised their hands in praise to God. You could hear people praying and mumbling, with their eyes closed. I looked around the room; people of all ages were there.

"Christ is King! Alleluia!" the pastor continued.

I had to have heard the words "Alleluia" and "Amen" twenty times in the first few minutes, and you know what? I also said them out loud, every time. I still had the fear of God in me, and I wasn't sure whether I was actually saved, so I said every darned word they called out! Who could guarantee salvation? Not me. Who knew what line you needed to cross to ensure you were saved? YIKES!

I could also hear people around me praying in tongues, using many different languages in their prayers. I had never heard the words before, but I got used to hearing these mumblings. "Huminamumina Moolimucoka," or something like that.

Then I noticed a lady across from me moaning out loud, making sounds like she was giving birth or something. I had never seen that and it kind of freaked me out. Mark said she was "birthing" the Holy Spirit. Whatever, I said to myself. I didn't know who was birthing what, but it all sounded weird, even in the state of mind I was in.

"Alleluia, praise God!" The pastor continued to talk about how great everything was and how thankful they all were, and then, in only minutes, baskets went around the church to collect tithes. Saw this coming, I thought—I had seen this back home. They read a verse that said that you must give your tithes to the church. I was pulled right in, and I took 60 bucks (another trip to the bank machine!) from my wallet and threw it in the basket. Never thought twice about it. Besides, I'd go to hell if I didn't. I knew that for sure!

Music followed and people stood and waved their arms; some danced on the spot, raising their hands to the sky. And then ... I saw him. Who is him? Let me explain.

Him was a man named John, in a wheelchair, who was sitting a few benches behind us. He was probably in his late forties, and he sat patiently while others danced about him. The music came to an end, and I told Mark I'd be right back. As the pastor started to speak again, I stood up and walked over to John. I introduced myself and went down on a knee. Surprisingly, to him, I placed my right hand over both his legs, closed my eyes and then ...

"You are great and wonderful, Almighty God, giver of all. I raise John to You now in prayer and ask You to lay Your healing hands upon him. Send Your Holy Spirit to his body to heal him whole."

I continued to pray over him and hadn't realized that the pastor was now giving his sermon. Even though he was speaking, I continued to close my eyes and pray over John's legs. And, for minutes, I prayed and prayed and, yes, for the second time in a couple of days, I felt some kind of electric surge in my right arm. Wow! So I damn well laid my right hand on both his legs, and I spoke with authority. The words came flowing out of me! And little did I know, I was being heard all over the church! Even the pastor could hear me and he had to speak louder to be heard by the people, but I didn't care. I was going to heal this man today! I knew it! I was the "chosen one"! Hallucinatory? Delusional? Psychotic? I didn't think so.

I started to hear people behind me commiserating, and saying how rude I was being. I heard them and when I opened my eyes, I saw their displeasure, but it didn't matter. I kept on praying with my eyes closed. I was convinced that their views represented the devil's. And I was convinced that I was going to heal this man right here ... in this church ... TODAY!

I started saying again, with authority, to spite their disapproval, "Keep the devil away, Dear Lord! Don't let him near! I cast out the devil in the name of Jesus Christ!" People continued to show their scorn and Mark actually told me later that many stood and walked out of the church. Again, I didn't care what was happening around me. I was going to heal this man, right here, right now! As I finished my prayers, I opened my eyes and noticed that most of our section was empty ... oops! I felt a bit foolish, but I knew my intentions had been good. God would be pleased.

I'd like to tell you that a healing had happened that day, but it didn't. I left John by telling him that one day he would be healed. I actually told him that he'd walk to the front of this church one day, with his wheelchair raised above his head! I truly believed it would eventually happen thanks to my prayers of healing, since it had not happened this day. I felt that special, a "chosen one" for sure.

I thought I'd hear a thanks for my prayers of healing that morning, but you know what John said to me? He said, "You know, in the future, maybe you shouldn't do that during the pastor's talk."

"Yah, I guess," I said, a bit embarrassed. He did thank me, though, and I got my hug!

No, there was no miraculous healing that day at Holy Faith Church. But I still believed it would happen. Only a matter of time. You're probably wondering, but I never saw John again. I hoped that one day my prayers would be answered, and that maybe I'd hear or see, on the news, some guy walking through a church with a wheelchair above his head and smashing it down on the floor, like a wrestler. Something like that. I could only hope.

At the end of the service, members and visitors of the church were invited to come up to the front to pray with the pastor and elders of the church. They implored people who were not "saved" to come forward. I didn't want Mark to think that I wasn't saved, because I felt I probably was, so I told him I was going to the washroom. Then, when he wasn't looking, I darted to the front of the church to participate in the prayers of salvation ... once again. I had to be sure. Any opportunity I had, I took. I was sure God would be pleased with his special child.

I believed that these "born again" prayers were the only way to God and eternal life. I felt in all my heart that anyone who did not pray these prayers and believe this would be damned eternally. This led me to believe, in my state of mind, that I had to go out and save every single person I met! Let's think about that for a minute. Good loving people were going to burn if I didn't reach them right NOW! Riddled with sickness, I became "beyond extreme", lacking all reason, control and sensibility.

## CHAPTER 9
## ALL IN THE FAMILY

That afternoon, Mark took me around Toronto and we had a good chance to catch up on our lives. Before this weekend, we hadn't been in touch for a year or so, so it was great to finally see each other again. I'd known Mark from the University of Western Ontario, where we formed a strong friendship. I never knew of his faith in those days, as we both lived pretty separate lives and mainly hung out in bars or restaurants, never at church. But years had passed and, as everyone knows, distance can really stall a relationship.

We drove along the Don Valley Parkway and Lakeshore Boulevard and visited several sites, the most impressive being, of course, the CN Tower. Every time I saw it, it looked more impressive. Maybe we could build one in Ottawa? I wondered. Maybe I could? I had grandiose financial visions that winter. I was convinced that I'd put them into play sometime very soon.

We got back to Mark's neighbourhood close to 6 pm and Mark didn't take us straight home. He wanted to talk about something, so we headed to a local café he knew well. He ordered a burger, and I had the usual ... coffee and water!

"You know you shouldn't be drinking all that coffee ... don't you think? It can't be good for you."

"Bhaa! I'll be fine buddy. I love coffee! I couldn't go without it."

"Chris, at church, did you find you were acting a bit strange?"

"Like how?" I asked, taking a swig of water.

"Well, I'm a little worried about some of the things that have been happening since you arrived. I mean, don't get me wrong, I really believe you are meant for great things, but don't you think maybe you're moving a little, I don't know, too fast? I mean, what happened with that guy at the church? What was that all about? I could hear and see everything that was going on in there. I couldn't believe it, honestly!"

"Hand of God, Marky! Hand of God! You know it, I know it. I felt it, man, I felt that feeling in my hand again. Maybe you've never experienced it, but I felt the energy. I really knew that God wanted me to do that. God was calling and I answered."

"But you never healed him!" Mark argued.

"Well, no, it wasn't in God's plan today, but who knows what the future holds for that man. I told John that one day he would walk down that aisle with his wheelchair over his head!"

"WHAT? You said that to him!? God, Chris, that's what I'm talking about! Seriously, don't get me wrong. Tom and I think you are chosen for something, but I don't know if walking the streets and healing parishioners are what you're supposed to do right now! I guess what I'm getting at, is that I think you should come to my church tomorrow so we can talk to my pastor. He's a wonderful man and I know he can give you insight, guidance and direction. What do you think, man?"

I could feel tension and agitation building in my body. It started in my head and made its way down. I felt anger towards Mark. How could he think this? How could he be so dense? First, it was my family who questioned my new spiritual path, and then, my friends, and now it was happening with a person who I thought I could put my trust in!

I sat there feeling like my back was against the wall. Accusations were being expressed, making me very uncomfortable and I knew in my heart that maybe this was a sign I needed to go on. I suddenly got very defensive and even a bit disrespectful with Mark, who was only trying to help. Yet, I saw it as no help at all!

"Marky, you've got it all wrong … my friend. I know for a fact that God is sculpting my path as we speak. You know it too! He is paving the way and I trust He'll show me where to go and what to do. The signs are there! They're all there and you know it; you've heard it all. I don't know why, but God has chosen me for something bigger than both of us! I must and I WILL stay the course. You can't stop me, you nor Tom, or my parents, or my friends! No one will, because God's put me in a big bulldozer and nothing will get in OUR way!"

By now, I was standing and slamming a fist and Mark told me that we had better leave.

"You aren't jealous, are you Marky?" I said, just to piss him off. I got up and I was trembling and was very frustrated. I felt deceived by him, by everyone. We got in the car and it was a silent ride back to his place.

When we arrived, there was a huge surprise waiting for me. It was a surprise I never, in a million years, expected, and it came to me on the sidewalk before we entered Mark's pad.

"Chris? Chris?"

I looked over and there he was. I couldn't believe it. It was my dad! He had travelled five long hours to find me.

"Dad! What are you doing here?" I asked, completely baffled.

He had shown up and was so relieved to see that I was alive and okay. He noted how thin I looked. Remember, I hadn't eaten anything since the previous Sunday and he had not seen me all week. To him, I looked sick, and you know what? I did look sick when I think about it. I would soon find out how sick I really was. Mark had already gone inside and my dad and I stayed at the curb by his car talking.

"Chris, please come home. We're all worried sick. Mom and Julie too."

"But I'm fine, Dad! Really, I'm completely fine!"

"Please ... son? Will you?"

I shook my head and pointed to Mark's apartment. "I'm not leaving, Dad. I need to be here right now. Great things have happened and I got to continue." My dad was sceptical, but he accepted that nothing would bring me home at that moment, except God himself reaching down and picking me right up! They trusted God in everything, but could this be something other than faith? At the time, none of us knew what ***bipolar disorder*** was.

We chatted a bit more in front. I did everything in my power to convince my father that things would be just fine. Although he didn't feel completely reassured, he knew that he had to accept it. I wasn't coming home, and I told him I would be gone for awhile. At the time, I was convinced of this. This was his son and he had to trust that God would watch my back. With his last bit of desperation, he asked one more time, "Chris, won't you join me? We can talk all about things on the way home."

"No."

My dad gave me a big hug and a kiss on the cheek, and as he got into his car, I could have sworn I saw tears in his eyes. At 8 pm, he waved goodbye and turned the corner at Spadina. He was gone and I was free again.

Wow. Talk about real love. Does love come any deeper than that ... a man travelling five hours just to hug his son? It doesn't. It really doesn't come any stronger. God bless my parents. I only wish that I had appreciated it when it happened. I do now as I look back at that night.

That evening, in the apartment, since more people back home were finding out about my escape to Toronto, I received a few calls. One was from my mom, who was also inquiring about my dad. I told her he was on his way home. She sounded so worried and I did my best to comfort her. It was difficult, but I knew I was doing the right thing. She told me that she'd had a visit from two of my closest high school friends, who had come to express concern about my unusual behaviour over the last while. As well, I got a couple of calls from my sister and friends who also cared but, to me at the time, were just a nuisance. I reassured them also that I'd see them sometime in the near future; I just didn't know when.

We cashed in that night around 10 pm. Mark and I were on speaking terms again, but I could feel the tension. It was something I had to think strongly about that night, and I prayed on it. I knew in my heart that I was definitely leaving soon, very soon. Mark being angry, phone calls from home, my dad showing up ... these were all signs telling me that I needed to go safely to a place where I could not be tracked. Those thoughts rested in my head that night and I remember once again that I couldn't sleep. Thank God for TV.

## CHAPTER 10
## BAPTISM BY FIRE

On Monday, the eighth day of my spiritual fast (yes, the eighth!), even McDonald's was looking like a gourmet meal. My stomach was on fire, yearning for nourishment, but I teased it by giving it only some water, some coffee and the odd fruit juice. These would only satisfy me for so long, however, I was constantly brought back to recurring thoughts of mounds of french fries, loaded pizzas and bowls of ice cream. Chocolate, of course! God, I was even dreaming of food now, and that only made things worse. Food was on my mind WAY too much!

That afternoon, Mark and I decided to go to another church to search out guidance for my mission. He was definitely convinced that I was on a mission from God, and he knew that I needed direction for it. He could only help so much and knew that I needed advice from someone more versed in faith than he. We had talked for a few hours that morning and he told me that he finally figured out what I needed to do.

"Chris, I got it! I know exactly what you've got to do! You NEED to do this. You're looking for direction, right? Well listen to this! There's no better place to get direction than what I'm about to share with you. You've told me numerous times since you got here that to be sure you are truly saved, you also feel the need to be baptized again. Well, I think it's time!" Mark stood up and put a hand on my shoulder. He looked me straight in the eyes and said, "My buddy, I think it's time for you to be baptized, but this time you need to do it right. You need to be baptized by the Holy Spirit as Christ Himself was!"

When he told me this, he said it with great enthusiasm and emphasis, and hearing it made me feel better about everything. It really pumped me up! Like I really needed that! Mark was right! This was exactly what I had to do and I had known this for a while now. I had been thinking about it over the last few months, but I just wasn't sure. Deep down, I strongly felt the need to be baptized again. You might say I needed to be "re-baptized". It was all making sense now and

I was finally seeing that it had to be done. This time, the "right" way.

Spiritual books I had read had told me so; spiritual friends I had met had told me so; spiritual shows, movies and prayer lines had all told me so. They had all pointed me in this direction, showing me how to do things the "right" way. I slammed my fist into my hand and said with authority.

"Let's do it, dammit! I mean, darn-it! Sorry God!"

As we drove off to the church, I laughed to myself, because I was finally seeing the light. My baptism at birth had been most definitely ineffective; I felt it really meant nothing to me or to God. I had thought that for awhile, but now, as we drove along, I really knew it. I needed to do this for me, and for all I'd meet on my spiritual mission. I needed to be baptized once again to make everything right with God and to, more importantly, save myself eternally! I believed I HAD to do it! Besides, I thought, what if the world was to end tomorrow? Then I'd be locked out forever! This thought drove me to tell Mark several times to step on the gas!

When we got to the church, I noticed how busy it was for a Monday night. I looked at Mark nervously, and he read my mind instantly.

"Chris, I know, you're nervous, but you got to trust me. What you're doing is essential to your life and your journey. I'm proud of you for agreeing to do this. Let's go! You'll thank me after."

We got inside and noticed quite a buzz in the hallway. There were people all over the place. I noticed several wearing long white robes, holding Bibles under their arms.

"Chris, those people are being baptized. I'm going to talk to the pastor over there and see if we can make this happen. Gheesh, I forgot that you will need to get wet to do this."

"Wet?" I questioned, thinking of the Catholic baptism, which involved wetting the infant's forehead solely.

"Take your pants off, Chris!"

"What, are you serious?"

"No, just kidding," he laughed.

Wow, Mr. Christian boy can joke! Who would have thought? I laughed to myself.

"We'll find you a robe and a bathing suit." Mark asked an elder in the church if he could lend us a suit and a robe. He gladly handed us the robe and headed in back to get a suit for me and to talk with the pastor who would conduct the ceremony. He actually went home to get one! After a few minutes, Mark joined me at the entrance to the auditorium.

"Chris, are you ready for this?" Mark asked, seeing that I was still a bit nervous.

"I am. God is with me. This is right. I know it."

The man came back with the suit and I went to change. When I returned, people were gathering inside the church. Mark and I took a seat near the front and then he directed me to a group of robe-wearing, Bible-holding people. Mark grabbed a Bible from a bench and threw it in my hands.

"God bless you all!" the pastor said to the crowd. I turned around and noticed that the room was packed! Wow! I thought to myself. I was going to do this, and do it BIG!!! The pastor addressed the crowd.

"Today is a very special and blessed day. Eleven fine people will be receiving their baptism today, where they will turn their trust to God and choose to follow in the footsteps of our blessed Jesus Christ."

The audience applauded and cheered. It was very loud for a church, I thought. As the pastor continued, people were raising their arms to the sky. Some moved and some danced, and all called out words of praise.

I stood beside my fellow supplicants who were going to be baptized with me by the Holy Spirit today. I counted eleven others. In fact, the pastor had to correct himself when he noticed that I had joined the group.

"We actually have twelve, twelve blessed individuals being baptized today! One more has just joined. Twelve! What a blessed number to have twelve! Alleluia!"

The congregation and its pastor were thrilled I had joined the group. Standing there, I thought about the number twelve. It really was special. I realized that it was the same number as the number of disciples that Jesus had! Wow, and I was the twelfth! Was Judas the twelfth? I wondered. I hoped not.

The pastor called us to the front of the church. As I rose to the top of the steps, I couldn't help but notice a whirlpool at the front. A whirlpool! What the heck was that doing there? What I was seeing was the water in which we were all going to be baptized. This was not going to be a "water over the forehead" baptism, as I had had at birth. This was going to be a "full body" baptism, like the one that Jesus had received in the Jordan! No wonder I needed a bathing suit. I was going swimming for godsakes!

One by one, each of us entered the pool of water.

"You are blessed in the name of Christ Jesus, our Saviour and our Lord."

People cheered and praised God as we were all baptized. Before each was, we were given the opportunity to say a few words to the congregation. I was feeling filled with the Holy Spirit (but also as high as ever!), and when it came to my turn, he held out the microphone. I actually yanked it from him and this was what I said. I'll never forget it. I was so animated and charismatic. I felt like the preacher himself!

"I'm a swimmer, everyone!" They cheered. "I do swimming laps for exercise!" They cheered again. "But I realize something today, as I stand here in this water, warm if you're wondering, quite comfortable. It doesn't matter how many laps you do going up and down the pool every day, it will NEVER, EVER put Jesus into your heart!"

The crowd erupted in praise and glory to Christ for those fine words, I must say. People were yelling and singing praise. Some were even lying on the floor, flailing. It was like a freakin' circus in there, and I was the ringmaster! I was so excited, as they lay me back to dunk my head and body into the water. I could barely contain myself!

The pastor said a few words and then he brought me up out of the water. They put a towel on my head and congratulated me on my life-saving decision. The crowd continued to cheer us on as we rejoined the congregation. It really was a fantastic night! I was NOW safely and happily a true member of God's family! At the time, it felt so right. Days later, I would doubt my salvation once again. In my unstable mind, it was never enough.

## CHAPTER 11
## THE BIG APPLE, HERE I COME

I woke up on the ninth day of my fast. It was a Tuesday, and what a great Tuesday it was! I had been baptized for "real" and I felt amazing! My old self was now gone and the new Chris Nihmey was finally here. I felt great about myself and my mission. For the first time, I felt the next step of my journey had arrived. I came to Toronto lost and now I was found, most definitely. I knew where I had to go, and just the thought of it made me crazy, but crazy in a good way! I was having a coffee when Mark woke. I pulled him aside to talk.

"Marky, I gotta talk to you."

"What's up, G?"

"Come sit here."

We sat on the couch. I felt a flame deep within my soul and I couldn't let it fizzle out. I was nervous and excited at the same time.

"Listen, buddy, I gotta go."

"Go where? Oh, you mean you got to go home?"

"No, no, I'm actually not going home at all, for who knows how long. I was praying last night and God told me that it was time to leave and that my journey here is over. He is calling me to leave today and I got to get going, now."

Mark looked at me and smiled, "Are you sure, Chris? I kind of feel like I've known this for a while, but are you sure it's time now?"

"It is," was all I said, touching his shoulder. "You've been so good for me, brother. Thank you for everything. You've shown me a door I would never have found on my own. Without yesterday's baptism, I would be lost. You've been a light to me and a great friend."

He stood up and asked, "Do you know where you'll be going?"

"Yes," I said, and that's all I said. I remember standing up and grabbing my car keys. I was chalk full of energy and excitement and was trying to contain myself, but it was tough. We chatted a bit more as I packed my things and helped fold up the futon.

I knew exactly where I was going and what I needed to do, but I kept that between God and me. Mark didn't need to know, and besides, I didn't want to leave any trails behind me that might leak back to home. I had already sent my father packing, and I didn't want him going to the next place I was heading. It would be much further! I would tell no one else about my journey. I knew myself that I was heading for New York City! Toronto was great, but New York was greater. New Yorkers needed to be saved and they needed to know me and, now that I was baptized, I could change many more lives. I would be back later to do more in Toronto, I was sure, but God was calling me out to the big time. I had met so many people here, and they had touched me in so many ways. I also saw connections and coincidences all over again, signs that God was with me and that I was in the right place at the right time, all the time. In the short time I was in Toronto, I had met dozens of people, some of whom I knew from my past. A few in a city of millions! What are the chances of that happening? I took these as deliberate signs from God that I was where I was supposed to be. Not to mention, the baptism that went off flawlessly, in spite of my spontaneous appearance. Who does this happen to? No one. I was the "chosen one"!

I said bye to Mark, got into my car and threw my bag into the trunk. I backed out and headed down the street. I was now starting the next leg of my mission. I was hopping with energy! New York was a dream which was now finally becoming a reality. For months I had been thinking of the Big Apple, and now I was actually going to do it and it felt great! I was going to leave the comfy confines of our "home and native land", and embark on a journey south, a journey that would not only affect me in a large way but, more importantly, affect so many others who I'd meet. They needed to hear my stories, they needed to witness my new powers to transform every person in my path through God's message.

How interesting. First it was Toronto, and now this. No one knew my plans, not my family, my friends, nor Mark, not anyone. This journey was not on paper, it was scribbled in my head, and only God and I knew the direction it was going. With God, anything was possible and the Bible told me so!

***"... with God everything is possible." Matthew 19:26***

***New Living Translation***

As in both Ottawa and Toronto, I'd be provided with the money I'd need and I would meet the right people at the right time. I'd always have a roof over my head and things would just fall into place as they already had. I knew wholeheartedly these things would happen because I knew God was great and He always looked after His own. I was doing all of this for Him. I had given my life to Him. I expected nothing in return, but I hoped deep down within me that heavenly rewards would eventually come.

I remember rolling down the window, as I turned from Spadina, and yelling aloud, "Set a table for me, God! Lots to get done, but keep a light on for me!" There was nobody there when I yelled it out, but I laugh as I remember that moment. I truly believed everything that was happening to me was for a reason, every single experience, every single coincidence and connection, all of it. I savoured the "what's around the next corner?" approach to my mission. It made things so exciting!

I drove through Toronto for twenty minutes or so, looking for the highway out, and when I found it, as I was about to enter, something mysterious happened with my car. It stalled, and I had to pull up to the side of the road. This had never happened before!

"What's going on?" I said, as I tried to start the car, again and again. I was now talking to my damned car. It was less than three years old!

"Stupid car!" I uttered, banging the steering wheel. I sat there for several minutes, and a few people who passed by gave suggestions, but nothing seemed to help. I got out of the car and stood there with the hood raised and looked up into the sky. One gentleman had even tried to boost my engine, but to no avail.

"This is ridiculous!" I sat there stunned, and then sat down on the curb for about fifteen minutes. "What is wrong with this dumb car?"

I stood up and put my hands on the roof. I watched cars exiting the city and going onto the highway. I should be there, I said to myself. I never thought this would happen!

Then, out of the blue, who showed up? Mark's cousin! I don't know how he found me but he did. I was nowhere near Marky's! He tried my car and he couldn't get it going. He then called Marky.

Marky came right away. He had a huge look of relief upon finding me.

"Wow, thank God we found you. I thought you'd be long gone by now!"

"Well, I would have, if it weren't for this pile of ...." I gave my car a kick.

"Chris, you can't go anyway. I'm so glad I caught you. I can't believe your car stalled here!" Mark said, pointing towards the highway. He was breathing heavily.

"Yah, and I can't believe I bumped into you!" his cousin exclaimed.

"I know. I'd been gone almost half an hour!"

Marky frantically interjected, "Chris, hear me out. I spoke with my pastor just after you took off. I told him about your story and he said he wanted to see you before you go forward with your mission. I mentioned you had left, but now ... will you please see him?"

"Why?" I asked puzzled, and a bit defiantly.

"He just wants to make sure you're doing the right thing," he said. "He's a bit worried and so am I."

"I don't want to see him!" I said, slamming my hand on the roof of my car. "Of course I'm doing the right thing. Besides, how would he know? God is showing me so many signs anyway, so I have my answer!"

"Please, just see what he has to say, Chris. Come on, for me? I'm really worried."

"Did you call my parents or something?"

"No, Chris, no strings attached."

I agreed to take Mark's advice. I really didn't want to do it, but he was a friend and I knew it would reassure him that I was doing the right thing.

"What about this piece of junk? What are we going to do about this?"

Mark got in the driver's seat. "Give me the key. Let me try."

"I tried it dozens of times. It won't start. Trust me!"

Lo and behold, Mark turned the key and the car started, just like that. I was amazed and puzzled, and started to be convinced that God didn't want me to leave: not yet. I later understood that this was another mini-miracle I had experienced during my high. Without that stall, who knows where I would have ended up? Who knows what I would have done or seen in New York, which was a hell of lot more dangerous than Toronto? No one would have known where I was. I concluded that for now, maybe God wanted me to do more here in Toronto. There had to be a reason for all of this.

I followed Mark to his church and spoke with his pastor that afternoon. The pastor convinced me that my fast was not called on by God. If it had been, I would have known for how long it would be and I would have had someone from the church endorse and direct it. He did, though, agree that I was on some sort of mission, but he prayed to God to point me in a different direction. He said it was time for me to go home and to, please, start eating! He also told me that my mission would not have consisted of running from anyone, as I'd been doing.

***"The most difficult phase of life is not when no one understands you; it is when you don't understand yourself."***

***Unknown***

I felt disappointed by his words, although they had been caring and kind. I really felt that I was heading in the right direction. Perhaps I was reading things wrong. Was everything a hoax? I felt sure it wasn't, but some things had to be changed, and some things had to be reconsidered. And they would be. Time would eventually tell me what those changes would be. It could not have been for nothing!

Heading back to Ottawa around suppertime, after eating my first meal in NINE days, I reflected on my time in Toronto. I had been indestructible there; nothing could hurt me. I really believed that, especially on the night I walked the streets. I remember feeling invincible and believing that nothing could harm me ... nothing at all. Again, as I said earlier, I truly believed that a bullet shot at me would redirect itself around my head; I believed this wholeheartedly! Now that's a scary thought. To really believe that you could survive anything. I knew God was with me, but it still makes me uneasy. How can the mind play tricks like these? What causes thoughts like these to surface? What would make one feel this way? In time, the truth would emerge.

My journey may have turned that day, but I believed that this was only the beginning of a mission that would eventually take me everywhere. It might be tomorrow or the next day, but it would come ... soon. New York couldn't have happened anyway. Why? You idiot! No passport! No insurance! As one can see, I was not an experienced traveller in any way. Being in this state of mind, I was a bit absent-minded and scatterbrained. Next time, though, I would be prepared.

My parents tell me that I rolled in at the stroke of midnight. I learned subsequently that my mother had called Mark that same morning. She had emphasized to him that he was "letting a good friend starve to death" by not persuading him to come home. It appears that Mark was then inspired to contact his pastor to convince me to eat and to go home. That is when he headed out to track me down. Thank God for my car stalling ... for the first time!

Mom had confided in my father that she believed that I would be home that day! My dad swore, that that morning, he had seen a flash of light whip through their bedroom TV screen! Had these been signs of my pending return home?

Mom and Dad were sitting in the kitchen waiting for me. Mark called in the late afternoon and told my mother that I was on my way home. The look in their eyes I will never forget. It reminded me of what true love is all about. They weren't upset. They weren't disappointed, either. They were overjoyed that I was home and that I was safe. There were tears in their eyes as they hugged me. I realized then how the prodigal son must have felt when he returned home to his father. It was nothing but selfless love from these people I cared so deeply for, and quite evidently, it was reciprocated. No judgment here.

We sat in the kitchen for hours, talking over tea and a donut. My parents couldn't believe how thin I looked and they pushed the donut on me. "Eat it!" I really was thin. Nine days will do that to anyone. None of us could sleep right away. We had all been impacted in a big way by the events of the past few days. My parents were beyond relieved that I was home and I was not hurt. They were very surprised to hear of my antics in Toronto. This terrified them, but for now they were just happy that I was back.

And it was good to be home, I had to admit, but I didn't share with them that night that I knew that this mission was not over. I had only just begun. And what about Mark? Had he been fooled? Had he and his fellow charismatics really believed that I was chosen for greatness? Other than a few questionable things I did, my being sick was probably the last thing they imagined to be true. None of us did.

***"He was lost, but now he is found!"***

***Luke 15:32 (NLT)***

# PART II

# THE MANY FACES OF MANIA

## CHAPTER 1
## ARE YOU THERE GOD? IT'S ME, CHRIS

"God is great and God is good", but boy, was I fooled during my mania and, to this day, I'm still paying. Things make more sense now that I've been through the wash but, at the time, it felt so real. In hindsight, it was complete nonsense. Others saw it, but not me. I was being fooled; I did not realize that I was very sick.

Spirituality, although not one of the main symptoms of mania, is often expressed or exaggerated by one who suffers from bipolar disorder. In my manic state, this was SO true. This is because those in mania usually indulge in deep, profound thinking. They are searching for answers, meaning and understanding as to why they are feeling and acting the way they are. I, for example, was looking for meaning in every little thing that was happening to me, and I could not figure it out, until after I crashed. Years of recovery and therapy allowed me to start.

In the early stages of mania, leading up to Christmas 2000, I released control of my life to God, to direct and guide me in everything I did. Where I would go, what I would do, who I would talk with, when I would leave any situation, how I would feel about most things. I found myself constantly reading into things and waiting for something spontaneous to happen in my life and, when it did, I would ride a wave of chain-reacting events that would take me somewhere new. *FROG* was my motto, "Fully Rely On God". I never knew where He would take me, but it was exciting to just let go and leave it to God! Needless to say, living this new way made for some late nights, but that was fine by me since I wasn't sleeping much anyway!

No offense to you, God, (none taken, Chris) but, in 2001, I went completely overboard when it came to faith. Alleluia, I went overboard big time! Since that high, my spiritual life and my fundamental beliefs have paid a hefty price. My spiritual views led to heavy-duty obsessions and subsequent anxiety.

Winter 2001, I was *attending new churches* weekly, two to three times a week. I was meeting with *priests and pastors* repeatedly to discuss spiritual concepts or ideas and ideals that I was contemplating. I was hanging out with *new "spiritual" friends* (my own friends had shied away from me—they couldn't understand me anymore and couldn't take the preaching!). I was *praying and singing* for hours a day, mostly at my roommate's home! I was saturating my mind with messages from *spiritual books* (I eventually got rid of over 100 books I had purchased during my high years ago), *spiritual music* and *religious TV programs*. Everything I did that winter involved God. I spoke to Him over everything, including what I ate! My Bible was attached to my hip 24/7 and I littered it inexhaustibly with highlights, stickers and notes. I was *preaching to people* all over town, believing in all my heart that God was giving me His Good Word directly. And, you know, it seemed SO normal to me at the time. I never felt more security in my life than that time but, in reality, I was probably the most insecure I'd ever been. I was so confused, seeking answers that just didn't come.

Looking back, I equate my spiritual journey that winter to hitting a brick wall. Here I was, as high as hell, experiencing full-blown mania, believing absolutely that the things happening to me were ordained for some reason or purpose. I awaited the moment when everything would come together, and then, BAM, I hit the wall. What had happened? Nothing … except falling into the most difficult time I have ever spent, when my very being was in jeopardy.

It was like watching an exciting movie, and having the ending cut off. What? What the hell is going on? What happens next? I was waiting for the big bang that never came. There was no conclusion, no grand finale to the craziness, and definitely no encore. Then, as I anticipated more fireworks, an unexpected sequel materialized. This sequel was incredibly awful. A terrible script, the worst actors, and no excitement whatsoever. Yep, that's depressing, er … depression.

Everything I did those months created a surreal plot for my life. My sickness made me believe I was doing everything the right way, and that became the only way. One can see how powerful the mind is, and the rollercoaster it can take you on when things are not balanced. Before delving into some situations I found myself in, one important thing about my faith at that time, was that there was no room for mistakes. My vision became hard-nosed and judgmental. Religiously, it was my way or the highway. This affected not only others but, more importantly, me. It still does.

I attended dozens of churches during that time, none of which were Catholic. From January to June, I might as well have moved into a church! I even spent time recruiting others to come and join in "the fun". That winter, I was committed to testing and experimenting with many different branches of Christianity. In addition to going to churches several times a week, I even took spiritual courses on the Bible and faith. Mania led me completely away from the church in which I was raised.

During mania, I thought that I was far too spiritual for the church I had known my whole life. Catholic churches would not satisfy my new spiritual needs. I needed a church where I could stand anytime I wanted, where I could sing whenever I wanted, and even dance if I chose to. I needed a church where I could hear people "speaking in tongues" and see women "birthing" the Holy Spirit. Where I could listen to someone preach extensively, not a measly fifteen minutes! A place where I could tithe hundreds of dollars, not just loonies and toonies. Yes, hundreds of dollars! I threw many a dollar away at so many churches because I felt assured the money would be used for good, particularly my own salvation.

I danced in the aisles at several churches, even lying on the floor flailing and shaking to the music! I must have looked pretty darned silly! Church folk believed that I was being "moved" by the Holy Spirit. I don't know about the Holy Spirit, but I was really in a nifty groove. Was I "in the spirit" or just caught up "in the moment"? Who knew? Maybe I was just being plain manic. Was I putting on a bit of a show? I did that sometimes. I will say, however, that I was moved to tears a few times that winter, when "prayed upon" or while praying on my own.

God, I even wrote a note to my family about the Rapture, a prediction made in *Revelation* about the world's end. I figured that I'd be taken to Heaven soon, while my family might not. My thinking and my behaviour were absurd. To think that my God-loving parents, who raised me to know Him, may not be going to Heaven.

On this manic journey, after learning so many new and exciting things, and experiencing all these spiritual revelations, I tried to rid myself of my Catholicity. I was actually embarrassed by it. Another branch of Christianity was now steering my life. They had taught me new ways and, what I thought, were better ways to praise the "Big Guy"! They also guided me to delve into other diverse concepts, the biggest: trying to avoid the place down under. No, not Australia, people, ... H-E-L-L! My mind went out to change everything I had learned growing up: to "relearn" everything spiritual.

I want you to remember that everything I thought and everything I did during my mania was construed and constructed by a very sick mind, unaware of its dangerous path; one that had no control of its destiny and was moving aimlessly to eventual destruction. My faith life took a huge turn for the worse, where I worshipped a false god, and spent countless hours praising it.

I'd begun to believe that Catholics and some branches of Christianity were going straight to hell, which included me if I didn't get my shit together and pray it all away! I believed they were doing things the wrong way, mostly because they were not "born again". One should only be baptized when old enough to make their own decision. One must believe in their heart that Christ is their Saviour.

My mind, under the influences of my chemicals and subsequent learning, led me to believe that, if I didn't change, the consequences would be dire. My warped mind made me feel that my life was off course. Everything was now up for debate. I took everything I heard literally. My state of mind propelled me to convince others of the same and to try to bring people back from eternal demise.

Who was this new god? He wasn't the God of my upbringing. For me, he was the iconic image of God sitting in the big hard concrete throne in the clouds, including the long white beard and white robe, a god not so loving, more to be feared. Few would make it to Heaven. The rest, that's right, damned to hell. Talk about fatherly love.

Eternal damnation began to drive me crazy, as if I wasn't already, and fear of going to hell caused me to say and do things I later regretted. If you were a father, would you close a door on most of your children forever? Is that why you created them? I had not rationalized this.

Possessing these views, I started to go everywhere sharing my faith and trying to convert people. This would happen anywhere: home, friends, schools, etc.. It didn't matter where I was, I spouted on about how great God was and all He was doing for me and all He could do for you. If you chose the other way, well then ... you go to hell. During my highest times, I even told my doctor that he and the nurses with him on the ward were all going to hell!

However, while I was trying to convert everyone to follow my way of thinking, things backfired. I actually ended up turning people off! Those who adopted my views simply adopted FEAR.

I got into heated discussions, to the point of yelling, with my parents, friends, and even strangers. Topics of conversation were always about being "saved", following Christ's footsteps and *Revelation*. In 2001, I was convinced that the end of the world was just around the corner, and that I had to save as many as possible. If I didn't, well, you know the answer. Hell became one of the driving forces of my faith and I feared it with all my heart. I prayed my own "prayer of salvation" thousands of times. I had to draw every person in, or I'd end up going to hell! One can see how fucked up I was! I went overboard with everything.

One night, during my high, at a local restaurant, I had a heated argument with a former colleague. It actually became a shouting match! He didn't know about my sickness. No one did then, including me. Our evening started off with simple chit-chat, and a beer and nachos. Then it started. Accusations were fired at me concerning the way I was teaching and preaching faith in the classroom while supply teaching. He was right but, at the time, I had to prove him wrong. Besides, I HAD to preach to the kids, because I felt it was the only way THEY'D get to Heaven! The consequences were just too severe, and I couldn't see my kids perish. We argued until we were blue in the face and nachos were flying all over! Actually, I was the one with the blue face and my nachos were on me. It got to a point where I was yelling, swearing, standing and pointing right into his face. "How dare you accuse me of that!" I would say. "I'll bring up God anytime I want to bring Him up, and you can't stop me! We work in the Catholic school system, for Christ's sake!" I really let him have it. By the end, he was exhausted and I was still firing on all cylinders. You might say I was "hit with the Holy Spirit", or some spirit, for sure!

During these months, those kinds of things happened more than you can imagine. I'm sorry my colleague had to be put through that. I hope he can better understand me now and where I was coming from. I'm certain he'll be reading this. So, sorry, good friend.

I was so obsessed with saving people, I got into a raging discussion at my parents' home with my sister about life after death. We ended up continuing on our street corner. She was meeting up with some friends that night for beer and wings, and I was telling her that we should try to cut out such pleasures in life and just focus on God. This would ensure entry to Heaven. Hate life, love God! I tried to convince her of this, along with re-baptism for her and my parents. I also felt the need to have each of them pray the "prayer of salvation" with me, fearing for their salvation. I was convincing, and they did one night! I thought I won the battle, but they probably did so just to shut me up!

Another time, one of many, I got worked up over something spiritual with strangers. I got into an argument with two Jehovah's Witnesses. I was at a Local Heroes restaurant on Bank Street and I was trying to sell a bunch of my movies to make some money to give away. I was selling a lot of things at the time. We got into expressing our beliefs and one thing led to another. It, too, led to a shouting match! Neither side parted on good terms. I was convinced I had to prove them wrong or else; what they were preaching was just bogus.

I was extreme and, yes, that included classrooms in which I taught. Was there anything wrong with that? This is how things panned out in numerous classrooms that winter and spring.

I had to save every kid before Christ made his return, I believed, by the summer of 2001. I sought to save all my students. I remember feeling such an urgency to save precious children from damnation. So, in every class, I had all the students pray with me the "prayer of salvation", with our heads bowed and our eyes closed (yes, I checked). Every class did this, even a gym class! The high school kids weren't overly responsive!

You may wonder what a "prayer of salvation" sounds like. The following is an example.

*"Dear God. You are wonderful and amazing. Your name is blessed, and Your love is pure. I come to You humbly, asking You to cleanse my heart and soul, to make me whole again: to be forgiven of my sins. I ask for Your pardon. Strengthen my trust in You. Christ, I invite You into my heart and ask You to change my ways. Please bless me with Your love. I ask all of this in the name of the Lord Jesus Christ. Amen."*

I must have prayed a variation of this prayer hundreds of times with kids that winter. I was obsessed over it. There I was at every school, praying prayers and spending at least 70% of the time preaching the Bible through neat and cool (I thought) lessons that I believed were being sent directly from God. I was even a spiritual mathematics teacher! Go "figure". I incorporated the Bible into all my teachings, and talked about faith and God way too much. I also left a "Get To Know God" booklet for their teacher, which would instruct a person on how to be saved. Crazy? It was, but I thought that I was so normal at the time, and that the world was full of unbelievers who needed to clean up their act or pay the eternal price. Talk about pressure!

That winter, I was actually kicked out of three schools in our board! One principal told me, "You're too happy and you're talking too much about Jesus! I don't want you in our school anymore!" I was flabbergasted after hearing that. It was a Catholic school! She actually cost me over a thousand dollars, taking nine days of work away from me that day. What's funny is that, I was feeling so full of energy, I remember kneeling in her office begging for pardon and laughing so hard I couldn't contain myself. She told me to get up and leave! Another elementary school and a high school banned me from going to their schools also. Screw them! I thought, at the time.

Late March, 2001. The air was warmer, the snow was melting and I was experiencing periods of extreme psychosis. Thoughts became completely abnormal and absurd. I was not only fanatical, I was also becoming delusional. I believed that I, Chris Nihmey, was actually Jesus Christ Himself, the Second Coming. Yes, I'm 100% serious! I believed it in ALL my heart, mind and soul.

Here's how it transpired. It was early morning, and I was driving in Orleans to a man's house in the country, to try and sell him into my Quixtar company (a pyramid company that you will read more about later). On the way over, as I was praying (the car was great for this because I could pray aloud and sing and not bother anyone), I had a HUGE revelation. My eyes were opened. Due to earlier enlightening experiences, I believed, at that moment, that I was actually becoming Jesus Christ! I believed that one day, in the very near future, I would miraculously transform into Christ Himself in front of the entire world, and it would happen very soon. People all over, whom I had met, thousands already, and soon to be millions, would see me, Chris Nihmey, on live TV! They would recognize me immediately and remember how I had changed their lives through our interactions. And then, on billions of TVs worldwide, maybe on *Oprah* or *CNN*, the world would witness my transformation into Jesus Christ. Right there, I would suddenly morph into the Jesus we all know: beard, robe, sandals and all. Not only that, but since the Bible says that Christ will return and come forth in the clouds, I figured I'd have live footage of myself descending in an airplane or balloon, approaching earth for all to see! I truly, honestly believed this completely! Isn't that wild? I believed it so much at that moment and the months to follow, that I was bounding with happiness in the car when this thought came to me. I pumped my Christian music up and could not believe the great gift God was bestowing me. I was His actual son! The Second Coming! Christ Himself ... ME! It was the highest I'd ever been.

At that moment, I wondered. Why would God have chosen me? How was I so much more special than everyone else? I felt I had a straight line to God, and I was completely blown away that I was His only son. God was going to do something beyond comprehension with little old me from South Ottawa. It wasn't until my depression that I realized that this was not the case. My depression opened my eyes to a whole new world. I still suffer from its ramifications.

That day, I drove along and prayed and played my spiritual tunes and I cried and cried some more. I was on cloud nine, sweating and breathing and bawling heavily. I couldn't wait to tell someone, anyone, but I felt that God wanted me to keep it a secret. He wanted it to be a surprise to all when it actually happened. So, although it was very difficult, I told no one about this until my deepest depression hit. I figured then that the deal was off. Not even my family knew about my grandiose delusions, which were part of my own thought fabrication; you might call them illusions. It was best I kept things under rap at the time, because I knew they'd only think I was crazy.

In the years that followed my mania, I would say that there is some irony, because my sickness, which affected my faith so much, eventually helped me to find a warm and loving God. I had to reshape my way of thinking entirely and search out the real God who loved me for me, and who did everything He could to show me His love. It has taken a lot of spiritual reflection to get where I am today, and I've had to make a lot of changes, but I think I can finally say that, today, as you read this, I have almost found the true loving God that we all long and dream for.

Would I erase what I went through? No, because it was part of my life I can't forget. To forget it would mean possibly going through it again. Hopefully, I won't have to because I have devised strategies to avoid walking this same path. Philosophically, I now look at things differently.

***"Trust in a loving God who will love you with all His heart ... no matter what."***

## CHAPTER 2
## MONEY MAKES THE WORLD GO ROUND

For thousands of others who have experienced the exhilarating highs of bipolar disorder, money becomes an issue; not making abundant amounts of money, but losing it big time! Let's face it, everyone needs money. Whether you're bipolar or not, we can all safely agree that money is very important to each of us. We like to spend our money, and if we aren't buying something, we are planning to buy it. And if we aren't planning to buy, we are probably dead. For people with bipolar, spending becomes contagious ... the more you spend, the more you want to spend! It's a vicious cycle.

***"When someone is on a manic high, they want to spend way too much, and in the end, they finish with very little."***

Billions of dollars are exchanged each and every day, as money is spent on everything one can possibly think of buying. Sometimes we have way too much or, like me, we don't have enough. For a manic depressant (defined today as a person suffering from bipolar disorder), it is almost always the case that they end up not having enough. Why? Because people on a manic high like to spend, spend and spend! They LOVE to spend their money on everything under the sun, and this also includes spending money they don't have. They are just so exhilarated that they want to spend not only on themselves, but on others!

Money is given away, credit cards are used, loans are made. That's where I stood in 2001 and, ten years since my high, I am still trying to recover. You're probably wondering what I could possibly have spent so much money on, since, for the longest time, I had no real estate, no fancy car, nor a preponderance of cash.

As I indicated, people with bipolar, in their manic state, love to spend. They love to buy, buy, buy and give, give, give. They buy everything! I was no different. Two of my best friends were Mastercard and VISA. Having credit cards made spending way too easy, along with my bank account, which also paid a hefty price.

I was so high during my mania, that I firmly believed in my heart of hearts that God was providing me with unlimited amounts of money, and that every time I headed to a bank machine, or went to use my credit cards, there would be plenty more for me to take. With every visit to a bank machine, I NEVER looked at my receipt because I knew God was providing. Because of this, I created the false sense that I had unlimited amounts in those accounts, kind of like a money tree, or an oasis of cash. I always seemed to have money, so I always found a way to spend it! I thanked God after every withdrawal with a look upward, and a big "Thank You, God!"

People have spent their entire savings, sold their cars, possessions and even their houses! They've taken trips on money that they didn't have, they've eaten in restaurants they couldn't afford, and they've bought things they couldn't eventually pay for. How do I know? I was there. In June of 2001, entering my major depression, my accounts were dry and my credit was gone. I had to borrow a lot of money from my folks just to survive. Thank God for Mom and Dad. They're helping me out to this day.

But what did I spend my money on? Not myself!

I liked to spend on people, and especially on people I was meeting for the first time. I don't know why. I seemed to like spending money on strangers. Maybe it was the thrill of seeing their reaction.

One March day, at East Side Mario's, I was with students from one of the high schools in Ottawa at which I was supply teaching. They had called me using a card for a business I had created *(Turtles Ministries)*. I had given it to them while supplying at their school (a whole other story, read on!) They wished to talk about God and spirituality because I had pounded it down their throats when I was at their school. I will say, I was convincing. Being with them was not a good idea to begin with, since I shouldn't have been with students outside of the school setting. Not smart but, at the time, it never even crossed my mind.

Anyway, we headed out for lunch on a Friday afternoon. I made sure they weren't skipping classes to see me, of course. When they arrived, I was feeling so high I was flying.

First of all, before they arrived, I ran around the restaurant meeting everyone, as I often did at the time, waiters and patrons. I finally sat with the students and talked our waiter's ear off as he was taking orders. I wouldn't order right away. I wanted to get to know our waiter really well. He laughed. He'd never seen someone acting quite this crazy before—I was burning up! I then asked the waiter a question.

"Ross, what's your favourite movie?"

"Umm," he thought for a moment. "I'd have to say *American Beauty*. Why?"

"Great. You three, I'll be right back!" I ran into the mall and went next door to the music store. I went to the movie section and I found *American Beauty*. And not only that! I bought several other movies, too, including the music store clerk's favourite movie, *Remember the Titans*. I paid for all and handed "Titans" right back to him. "Here you go!" He looked a little puzzled. Then, I ran to the pet store to buy some stuffed animals. I liked buying them at the time. After several minutes, I re-entered East Side's with arms full of gifts for my new friends!

I gave the movie to our waiter. He couldn't believe I'd do that for him. I gave out movies to the three students (movies with strong morals, of course!), and I gave a stuffed puppy to a little boy who was eating across from us and who'd been staring at us. He was so cute and his mom was grateful. I felt great, and this made me want to give even more. So, I went out to the bank machine to take out more money. My wallet was filled once again! Phew!

We chatted about all kinds of things, and especially about the girl who called me on my cell phone for advice. She had not been getting along with her parents. I counselled her with my intelligent(?) advice and gave her direction regarding her situation. If I could only hear me now! I don't think it was sound advice, but it felt like it at the time.

In our conversation, I was so into giving, that I remember telling one of the boys that he could have my car if he wanted! What, you're thinking? Well, at the time, I was actually leaving my keys in the ignition wherever I went. I did that for months! I believed that God would protect my car, so I would just leave the keys hanging there. I told the 16-year-old that he could take the car if he really wanted. "It's a black Civic." He laughed and scratched his head. Was this guy for real?

Then I told him that he'd probably feel a huge shock from God if he did, because I believed that God wanted me to keep my car for my impending mission. But I said, "Go ahead, try it," with a confident smirk. He never did. He was sure I was right, and I could see the fear in his eyes. That's how convincing I was.

Following the meal, I pulled out my wallet. The bill was nearly fifty dollars. I grabbed the bill before they could reach it and pulled out three twenties. "I got it, guys. It's on me. Your presence at my table has been an honour!" The waiter came by and I stood up and gave him a big hug. It was like I had known him forever. This was nuts, he thought. I could see it in his face as I stepped back.

"Thank you for your service." I handed him the cash and we stood up to leave.

"Uh, sir, you forgot your change," he uttered, as we were walking off.

"Keep the change, and don't forget to look under my plate!"

I walked out with the kids and said goodbye. I looked back inside. The waiter was scratching his head at my table. It was exciting to see his face when he found it. I had left three twenties under my plate! As I said before, I loved to spend on everything, mostly on others. I'd like to say that this was the only time this happened, but I'd be lying. Everywhere I went, whomever I was with, I was "Mr. Money Bags". And the people that I spent most on, particularly, were strangers! I did spend on friends and family, too, but I seemed to save my big expenditures on people I didn't really know.

I spent an evening in March at Local Heroes, a sports bar in Ottawa. I was meeting a friend I hadn't seen since high school. I had to get up several times from my seat to release excess energy. I told my friend I was making a trip to the washroom each time, but these trips don't usually take as long as I was taking. Some of my trips that night included meeting various groups of people, as I walked by table after table on these "so-called" washroom sojourns. I felt somewhat badly for my friend who had to sit by himself many times that night. I apologized; he just shrugged it off.

"Well, Chris, it's time I got going. It was really great to see you again. I'd feel bad leaving you here but you seem to know most of the bar anyway!" We laughed.

"Yah, I'm going to stay for a bit more. It was great seeing you too!"

We stood up and shook hands. I gave him a big hug. No one, and I mean, no one, during my mania, ever shook hands with me without getting a big hug after. Off he went. I made my way through that bar meeting everyone I could. I saw some familiar faces but, most of all, I met many new ones. I was talking a mile a minute, I was as friendly as hell and I just loved every second of it. WOOHOO!

I met almost every person in the restaurant that night, as usual. When I headed back to my table, I saw my bill lying there, along with half the meal I hadn't finished. My friend had paid for his bill and mine remained. I picked it up, ate a few cold fries, and looked at it.

"$17.45." I said under my breath. "Hmm ..."

I opened my wallet and flipped through my money. I scratched my head and looked over at the other side of the restaurant. It's really crowded, I thought to myself. I grabbed a twenty, then another, and another, and ... wrapped my fingers around six crisp twenty dollar bills and chuckled. Was this for real? Was I about to do this? Well, it was, and I did! I threw $120 on the table and put the check underneath. A $100 dollar tip! I lifted my plate and slid the money half under. I looked around the restaurant again. I felt like a thief trying to hide something, but I was doing just the opposite! Why did I feel like this? I don't know. People normally just don't do that. Who did what I was doing here? Who? I guess people just like me!

I put on my coat and slowly made my way to the front of the restaurant. You idiot, I thought. Anyone could take that money!

I stopped and looked back nervously at the table. The waitress, whom I had befriended (along with the whole freakin' bar!), was taking plates away from our table. Phew! And then I saw it. It was all I needed to see to assure me that what I was doing was maybe NOT so crazy. I saw a smile on her face and a look that I'll never forget. She looked around for me. I watched as she placed the money in her pouch and made her way over to talk to another waitress about this crazy tip. I had seen all I needed to see. I turned and walked away a very happy man. Giving could be so enjoyable. It was, and I was loving every minute of it! I would do the same at another restaurant a week later. It was just as satisfying, even though I didn't see the server's reaction that time. I felt assured both times that I had done the right thing, but was what I was doing really right? That's a whole other story.

On another occasion, on one particularly cold winter night, I was sitting at home and I decided to do something exciting. I didn't know what, but I wanted it to be "over the top". As I was sitting there, meditating on what I could do, a thought entered my head. I knew that we had some neighbours in our area that were not well off. I had led myself to believe that they suffered financially. So, with that, I established a plan of attack. First, I drove to the bank and withdrew some money. I hustled back home and grabbed two envelopes. I put a handful of $20's in each and sealed them. On the front of the envelopes, I wrote the words, "Jesus Loves You". Finally, I headed out, secretly placing the envelopes in their mailboxes. Then I headed back home. MAN that felt good! My reward came in the form of the feeling I had on my return. I had just given each household $200 dollars!

I don't know how much money came and went through my hands during my high, but I do know that it was in the thousands. How many thousands, I'm not sure. Being on a high is an amazing feeling, but your wallet takes a beating. To this day, as I said before, I am still trying to recover after more than ten years. You're probably wondering why my family or my friends didn't stop me from spending so much. It is because they did not know until it was too late. I was very secretive and, remember, I usually gave to strangers. I was not around home much in those days but, when I was, I was careful as to what to say when it came to money. I was on a mission for God, and they just wouldn't understand. If I kept this secret, I could keep going without interference. Meanwhile, I had depleted both my bank account and my RRSPs.

I was also into trying to raise more money for my mission. One night in April, while spending an evening at Friday's Roast Beef House, I came up with what, I thought, was the greatest way in the world to make money and turn it into a fortune. At least I thought so!

Friday's was quickly becoming my favourite place to hang out, that is, until I was actually kicked out. I entered the restaurant with my pouch around my waist and wearing my token *Ottawa Senators* jersey. I headed upstairs with my friends, and we sat down to listen to piano music. As we sat, a thought entered my head. "These are well-to-do people here at Friday's. Maybe I can make some money tonight? Then I could give it out to whoever." So, I took out a pad and pen and contrived a system that could make me some money. It was simple, and, on that night, it worked; pay a penny, receive two pennies. Pay a dollar, receive two ... and so on. Simple, right? Easy to do, but you needed to have the guts to do it, and I had plenty. I was high, for godsakes!

So, I started to tour one of the ritziest restaurants in Ottawa and tell the patrons about my "money-making" scheme. I told each person I approached that I could make them millions! And remember, at this time, I was very convincing. I could sell anything! I told them that whatever amount of money they gave me, I would double it and get it to them by leaving me their mailing address. Of the 50 or so who gave me money that evening, only seven wrote down their addresses.

Basically, it worked like this. I would say to a patron, while staring directly into their eyes, "Listen to me. I can make you a rich man (or a rich woman)." I solicited whoever I thought I could get a few bucks from. And since everyone was dressed to the "nines", I solicited everyone!

"You give me a certain amount of money now and, in one month, I will double your investment. Just like that. I promise." I snapped my fingers and said this in a very persuasive manner and sold it that way. "Any amount will be doubled, this I promise," I emphasized again, waving another customer's ten dollar bill in their face.

I had my system charted out on paper, and off I went touring the restaurant. I started off slowly, but with time, things really picked up. You wouldn't believe! I was actually getting people all over this place to give me money! My scheme was working! If they wanted their money doubled and returned to them, all they had to do was give me their address and I would mail their money directly to them. It was that simple. Amounts ranged from quarters, loonies and even five and ten dollar bills, all to the "Chris Nihmey Mission Fund". People were completely sure that they'd make some money with me, and I was too. I really thought this would work, and with my other grandiose financial plans, I felt assured that this would lead to big bucks. So, I toured around for over an hour before being told to leave! I had been a good and valued customer several nights previously, but I was now playing the fool.

All in all, I actually did make some money that night. Surprisingly, $89! But $89 didn't go as far as I had hoped! I had good intentions. I planned to use the money in my world mission. That night, I applied the scheme at two other restaurants. I was kicked out immediately! Although I considered using this scheme more following that night, I never used it again. Did I ever get money back to those who left their addresses? I actually did. I mailed small cheques to their homes. Remember, I'm an honest guy! "Money makes money," I had sworn to them, and I was true to my word.

During these months, I also paid to join some legal "pyramid-style" companies to earn money for my mission. I was willing to try any new idea, especially one that promised cash! One was a telephone shopping network, *Quixtar*, and another was a company that sold magnetic devices, *Nikken*, which was supposed to be great for the body. The idea was this; join the company, convince others to join and everyone makes money. Simple, eh? The more people you brought in, the more money would be made and the better the company would do. I was into these two companies for awhile, until my mission from God became clearer and I was headed towards much greater things (?). I even tried to get some of THEIR customers to join my business: *Turtles Ministries.*

## MY WORLD SUMMER MISSION

During that manic period, from January on, I believed that God had chosen me to perform a special mission. He was helping me to develop a plan of attack, and on one particular Sunday, late May, I believed my world mission was to begin. Finally, the plan would come into fruition. I remember being so pumped and excited when I felt His call, and I ran to the basement to plot out the steps of attack on the blackboard. I had a vision that could not fail. I was sure. My girlfriend, at that time, was visiting and I actually compelled her to listen to my plans, and remember, I was very convincing. She thought my ideas might just work. So did my parents, or so I thought.

This was the mission. I would travel the world and help entrepreneurs develop big businesses under my financial guidance and expertise. I had none, but I thought I did! I would carefully select different "bigwig" businessmen and women throughout North America (Europe was a plan for the fall!) who would then build complex businesses or organizations throughout their countries. Businesses would range from hospitals, schools, churches and high tech companies to industries, daycares, retail outlets and restaurants. You name it, I had a plan for it. My over-flowing binder held evidence of this.

These businesses would become *Turtles* brand companies and they would make billions under God's guidance, His hand on their shoulders. My goal was to invest the money given to me by God, and also from donors, which would also lead to the growth of millions for investors. Ultimately, this would make them, and me, rich. I would then pour back this money into these companies, thereby encouraging them to make donations for worthy causes worldwide. I hoped that this would lead to many more *Turtles* companies being established all over the globe. I was convinced that my partners would open these *Turtles* companies and they would thrive because God would make it happen. It was just as He desired.

***"If you give, you will receive." Luke 6:38 (NLT)***

The deals made with these business people comprised this; once they built their organizations with the money I provided, they would be trademarked with my *Turtles* logo and motto ... "*With Jesus moving at pace, all of us will win the race.*" All I would ask in return, other than the bestowed logo, was 10% of their earnings. Only 10%! Not a bad deal!

Then, in short order, these *Turtles* companies would begin popping up all over the world, each one providing me with 10%. I'd be rich and I knew it would happen most definitely, because I was chosen by God for greatness, with this ultimate goal: to bring the world to know and put their trust and faith in His hands. I would then appear before the world in God's greatness and bring salvation once I, as I've mentioned previously, transformed into Christ Himself. Seriously. I know it sounds way out there, and it was ... but I believed it with all my heart and soul. It would all come together very soon. I just knew it. This financial mission would merge perfectly with God's spiritual mission for me.

***"While friends were marrying, working high paying jobs, having kids, I was on a mission to save the world, and I had it all planned out."***

In early June, it was all moving forward. I wrote the many documents that would kick-start all of this. I was ready!

However ... it never did happen. Events in late June took precedence. I became preoccupied with another personal project. More about that later. And then, in July, money didn't matter anymore. Friends and family didn't matter, and even God didn't matter. A new chapter in my life set in, and the worst time of my life began.

## CHAPTER 3
## IT'S LIKE I KNEW WHAT WAS AROUND EVERY CORNER

Good God, am I seeing things? This was my reaction to a strange phenomenon that developed during my manic high. It began with one intense "got to sit down" coincidence that happened in early January, 2001. It was followed by a second mind boggling coincidence, which led me to believe that there had to be a reason behind these two happenings. They just couldn't possibly happen by accident. And then, things got really crazy!

It was like this. A multitude of coincidences began and continued right through months of mania. Each seemed to have a purpose and a connection to the previous one and the ones that followed. The odds were incalculable.

In my state of mind, I truly believed these to be God's way of communicating with me. I believed that each was a sign from God, and I dissected and deciphered each one so carefully. It was like trying to break a code, or search for lice ... well okay, break a code. I felt like a detective receiving clues and it was really exciting when they happened. I remember having to sit down often because they would "blow" my mind, and these experiences made me feel higher and higher. With each incident, I felt I was coming closer and closer to a direct pathway to the Almighty. Wasn't I? I had seen some weird shit before, but this was absolutely ridiculous!

I mean, sure, we've all experienced the odd coincidence here and there, right? But this was different; trust me ... this was really different! I was seeing and experiencing them ... ALL ... THE ... TIME! I truly believed that God was guiding me with these signs and was trying to show me things that others just didn't see. I was really the perfect vessel for Him at that time, ready to do whatever He asked, including, I hate to say it, giving up my life for Him. Suicide? Nah, He wasn't like that. And, thank you, God, I didn't feel you calling for my life. However, I was definitely ready for whatever situation came. I would have done anything for Him. Anything! Scary? Yes, very.

I remember being amazed, time after time, at some of the signs that were appearing. These signs completely took over my life. For instance, I would let things like my phone, my email and even my mail direct me to taking certain paths. I would be somewhere and a call would come and then, zoom, off I'd go to my next calling! I have to admit, it was exciting when it happened. Some examples:

We've all heard it before, more than once, maybe even hundreds of times! This phenomenon occurs when a freakish event takes place, making a person confirm that they were "in the right place at the right time". It is at this exact moment that they feel that everything has aligned, oh, so perfectly. It, too, is an astounding phenomenon, and it always leaves a WOW feeling for those involved. Things like this happened to me constantly during my mania.

It was Monday, February 26th. I had been in Toronto for three days during my manic high. My parents and my sister were frantically trying to convince me to come home, fearing that I would starve to death if I didn't start eating immediately. My mother, desperate to find something to motivate me to eat, grabbed the only thing that she felt could possibly change my mind: the Bible. On impulse, she opened to a random page. She then lowered my sister's head to a reading. It was a verse about God's directions against improper fasting! They couldn't believe it! They quickly telephoned me in Toronto and read the verse to me, and emphatically, Mom pleaded, "Chris, you should be eating and you must come home immediately!" I listened but ignored their advice.

Tuesday afternoon, due to Mark's advice, I visited his pastor. Mark was convinced to do so, thanks to my mom's urgent call concerning letting his best friend starve to death. To my astonishment, the pastor, without any encouragement or prompting, turned directly to this identical reading to convince me to reconsider my fast! This reading, out of a multitude of verses he could have chosen on fasting! On his suggestion, I returned home. I was completely convinced that this was a sign from God and, therefore, the right thing to do.

On my return home, I resumed supply teaching that week. At my first assignment, to my surprise, upon entering the staffroom to put my lunch away, I noticed a scripture written on the staff whiteboard. Guess what? You got it! The same passage! Coincidence? I don't think so.

This is what I experienced time after time those months of mania. Things do happen for a reason, and this is an example of why I believe that to be true. These situations are very unique when they happen and all parties are taken aback when experiencing them. They talk about the rare chance of the event happening and relish the joys of being "in the right place at the right time". Would it be that things are "meant to happen"?

I share these stories because they were of such impact on me during my mania. Sure, we notice the odd one in our day to day travels, but I can't stress this enough. These incidents were happening to me, over and over, day after day. My doctor attributed these occurrences to my "heightened awareness", part and parcel of my disorder. I can't help but wonder, though, if this was indicative of a greater phenomenon. Was I seeing things that other people did not see? Was there something more happening here?

I leave you with this. Life is a helluva lot more complex than we think, and answers are always popping up, but most of us are too preoccupied by everyday life to notice them. Maybe we need to open ourselves to a world that is filled with much more "reason" than we admit to. Maybe we need to raise our level of awareness, so that we don't miss the things that matter the most. I believe this heightened awareness at that time saved my life.

## THE TURTLE

A familiar theme that occurred hand in hand with many of my experiences was "the turtle". I don't know why, but during my manic high, I really felt that I'd been given this sign from God, something to reassure me that I was on the right path ... His path. I saw it as a way He was communicating with me.

You may have experienced this: you see something repeatedly over a prolonged period of time. For me, this was the turtle. It wasn't just seeing the odd turtle and saying, "Hmm, another turtle." This was about seeing the turtle in some way, shape or form, many times a day! Everywhere I went, or whatever I was doing, there was a freakin' turtle lying there! It drove me nuts and made me laugh over and over in amazement. I just couldn't believe what I was seeing!

Turtles in classrooms (on posters and as pets), on bumper stickers, t-shirts, students' jewellery, in movies, on TV commercials repeatedly, on books, in malls, even on a dog's handkerchief! Friends were amazed at the number of times I pointed out little turtles appearing in our path. It was freaky and funny at the same time. It was not like I was looking for them. They just seemed to pop up wherever I went. They just seemed to find me.

Turtles played SUCH an important role in my life, that when we published our first two children's books, we registered them under our own company which we called *Turtles Publishing.* I also founded a ministry which, as you know, I named *Turtles Ministries.* I repeatedly handed out *Turtles Ministries* business cards to people seeking spiritual guidance. I even established a prayer line. Funny thing was, I was actually the one who needed the guidance, but did I believe that? Never! Since extensive healing on my part, I'm not doing that ministry stuff anymore. You can now safely throw your *Turtles Ministries* cards away!

Contrary to what my doctor may feel, I can't help but still believe there are reasons for everything. Who knows the real answer? I've come to realize that life does have some kind of intricate plan, and that multitudes of connections are intertwined. You have to figure out what the occurrences mean in your life. Some of us figure it out and revel in the discovery; most of us just brush it off as merely a "coincidence". Next time you go to the bank or grocery store, try talking to that person in front of you. You will be surprised at the connections you share with them. God knows, I have done so, more than what is normal, of course, but I truly believe that these interactions are relevant and important to my life. Taking an elevator instead of climbing the stairs could change your life completely.

# PART III

# OTHER MANICDOTES

## CHAPTER 1
## A BLIND MAN TAUGHT ME HOW TO SEE

It was late on a Friday night in early March, 2001, sometime after 1:30 am. I remember that I wasn't tired at all, as was usual at the time. I was actually wired and was still barely sleeping at nights, maybe an hour or two at most. Nights were a lot longer when you weren't sleeping, and that was alright with me. I wanted to do so much!

It was a cool evening as I walked along Ottawa's Elgin Street strip. The bars were buzzing with party-goers, all trying to take in their last drinks of the night. The strip was busy; it usually was on a weekend night.

I had just spent another evening of entertainment with my friends at a bar on Elgin. I had recently befriended them, although I did know Pauline from high school. It was a really fun night, and the place was very entertaining, but actually, it wasn't only the place that was entertaining ... it was me! I remember dancing a storm and getting the crowd cheering and chanting several times. By the end of the night, no matter what age, they were whooping and hollering to the music. It was fantastic! Rick the DJ had kindly given me the microphone; it was something he quickly regretted. My voice sounded awful, and I had the microphone for only a second. Rick pried it from my hand, patted me on the head and pushed me aside.

My friends' night was ending, but because of my state of mind, my night was only just beginning. I bade them both farewell and headed off on my own for the rest of the night. I did that a lot at the time.

I met a panhandler outside the bar. "Can I have a loonie, man?" he asked me. I reached into my pocket and retrieved a ten.

"Here you go, sir," I said, flipping him the bill.

"Thanks, man," he said, lowering his head again. I smiled and saluted him and continued down the sidewalk. It was then that I bumped into Roger, a man that would play a prominent role in my life at that time.

I first saw him approaching me on the sidewalk ahead. I could hear a rude and obnoxious voice coming towards me, and I noticed a tall lanky figure making his way from bar to restaurant along the Elgin strip. He was loud and crude and he staggered down the sidewalk towards me. People were moving aside to let him pass. Not only was he loud, he smelled awful, which made the path clear even more!

"Come on, I'm only asking for a buck ... fuck!" Roger said to a young couple who quickly veered around him. As he came into my view, I noticed that he was staggering for a reason. He was holding a walking stick in his right hand. Roger, amazingly, was blind!

"Hey baby, how's about some lovin'?" Roger asked, as he put an arm around a pretty woman eating a hotdog. She slapped his arm away.

"Stupid bitch!" he laughed obnoxiously, as he walked past her.

As I watched him making his way towards me, I remember feeling sorry for him: a blind, lonely figure with grey curly hair. And to top this off, he wore a pair of huge (Elton John huge!) odd-shaped sunglasses. I later found out that they were just for show. He was really quite the character, animated and all.

I stopped for a moment and watched him as he continued to holler at passersby who made their way around him. I was entertained by his crassness and boldness.

"Somebody, somebody, please give a blind man a dollar!" he belted out, as he waved a baseball cap at people walking by. I reached into my pocket. I pulled out the last of my cash, a twenty. Should I do this? I thought. Of course. The man obviously needed it.

"Here you go," I said, and I handed him the money. I could really smell him and he did not smell like roses. He smelled of strong BO and urine. Yuck! I tried to ignore his smell and I struck up a conversation with him. We shook hands, I introduced myself and we chatted. He told me about his misfortune: how he had lost most of his sight from a car accident at age fifteen. He was now fifty-five. Five years off the big 6-0, a year he would be proud to reach. He said, "They said I'd never hit forty, but look at me now!"

I told him where I was from and a little bit about me and we had a few good laughs. He startled me when he reached out and touched my face. I was taken aback by this action, but he meant no harm. It was his way of saying I was okay.

"You're a handsome chap, aren't you?" he said smiling. I agreed I was! He reached both hands towards my shoulders. "You work out, don't you?" he said.

"I do exercise a bit," I said proudly, flexing my arm and shoulder muscles. I often did that when people touched my muscles. I think we all do! Come on! You know it!

"I better move on, kid," he told me. He said he had to get going, and so did I but, as always, I felt the need to "save the world", so I asked Roger if he wanted a ride. He told me that he lived in Hull, just over the river from downtown Ottawa.

"I'm heading right that way!" I told him, although I really wasn't. I just didn't want him to think that I was going out of my way. "Really, it's not a big deal. I can drop you off, and besides, I don't sleep that well anymore. I'm always up pretty late." He was put in my path, so I knew this was right.

"Are you sure it's not a problem?" he asked. "I can hitch a cab."

"No, it's not a problem at all," I said, "but please, take a shower first, man. You stink!" Okay, I didn't say that to him, but I definitely thought it. Poor guy.

We got in my car and headed over the bridge to Hull. On our way there, out of instinct, I tried to convince Roger to join my *Quixtar* shopping company. I was so gung-ho about getting him to join, that I almost got us into an accident. Money, money, money, give, give, give.

"Dumb driver," I said aloud, as I told him what had just happened. It was really my fault, but that's the bonus of being with a blind man ... he couldn't see what was really happening! I guess at the time, that company was so important that even driving took a backseat to making money. With a blind passenger, I could get away with anything! We arrived at his apartment. I pulled up to the front.

"There you go!"

"Thanks, Chris. Can you come up for a bit?"

"I don't know," I replied, wondering how I was going to get the smell out of my car. I looked at the time. It was nearing 2:30 am. "Okay," I said.

What was I thinking? As I'd done many times prior, I made a decision based on instinct. Spontaneity was my middle name. I rarely said no to anything in that state of mind. Everything I undertook had meaning to me, and I was convinced that every path I took was taken for a reason. I just followed along the path. I knew that God was showing me the doors to take, and whatever door I took was the right door for me.

We entered Roger's building. He ran his hands along the elevator panel, feeling for the numbers. He pushed the button, and we headed up to the twelfth floor. I was surprised he knew which button to press. He put his key in the door. Inside his apartment, I encountered the smelliest and dirtiest room I had ever seen! Garbage lay all over the floor, cans and boxes, along with rotting food; and the smell, the smell was unbearable! I felt like vomiting when I took in the air, staring at a countertop covered with coffee stains and littered with bread crumbs. A dirty knife lay in the sink beside some rotting meat and stale toast. I couldn't believe what I was seeing. Jesus, I thought to myself, please get me out of here!

"Have a seat," Roger offered. I sat in an empty patio chair in the middle of his living room. There were no other couches or chairs in the room. To my left was a computer-type machine that was plugged into the wall. At the time, I thought it was just a nifty computer, but I later found out that it was a machine he used for communicating. It was equipped with braille keys. I stood astonished as I gazed from one end of the apartment to the other. How could someone live in a state of poverty like this? I thought to myself. This was terrible.

"Can I get you something to eat?" he asked, grabbing some bread from the counter. He popped some into the toaster, and felt around for the refrigerator. Inside, he grabbed some mayonnaise and some mouldy cheese.

"I ... I ... I'm not that hungry, Roger, but you go ahead and eat."

"Come on, kid. Have a bite with me."

I gulped and grimaced. How could I say no? I thought of taking the food and placing it somewhere in the apartment, where he wouldn't find it. I would use his blindness as my ally. After thinking about this for a minute, I knew I couldn't. I would have to eat the food. I didn't want to be rude or make him feel bad.

The next few minutes seemed to slow right down as I heard the toaster pop.

With his filthy hands, Roger reached for the toast. He pulled it out of the toaster and threw it on the dirty counter. It landed in a pile of crumbs, hair, bugs and coffee stains. Just the look of it made me sick. He reached for the butter and that same dirty knife from the sink. He spread it on the bread, along with some mayo, and cut some cheese (no, not that cheese, although the room smelled like it!). He cut the sandwich in two, handing me my half.

"Cheers," he said, as he downed his. I knew he couldn't see me, but at the time, I wouldn't have been able to live with myself if I'd hid the sandwich somewhere. In my head, I pictured Roger finding that sandwich a year from then, rotting with maggots and flies. I couldn't bare it. I had to eat the sandwich, so with all my strength and resolve, I did. It was disgusting, but I'm still alive, thank God. But man, was it gross! It tasted as bad as it looked!

"So, Roger, you'll be happy with this company I'm a part of," I said to him, spitting out a stale piece of toast. "It's a fantastic company! You really have to check it out. It's huge, tons of money to be made! Just tons!" At the time, I was SO convinced that this company would make me rich, so much so that I spent a whole evening trying to convince a blind man that he should drop everything in his life, trust me and take an unlikely path to security and financial freedom.

"This is all I have right now. I can't join your company but this might help," he said, handing me a $50 cheque! A week later, it bounced. And then he continued, "I have a friend who might be interested. He's a priest in Toronto! He's helped me out a lot in the past. Here's his number," he said, as he handed me a card. "Give him a call!"

"But it's 3 am, Roger! I can't call him now!"

"Sure you can. He's always up!"

"Okay," I said, scratching my head. It WAS money! So I did. At 3 am, on a Saturday morning, I dialled this stranger priest from Toronto. Who would have thought?

He answered, and so there I was, talking fervently to Roger's friend on the phone, trying to convince him to join my money-making scheme. We talked for several minutes and, he being a priest, we got into some spiritual talk, of course. Being so deep in conversation, I'd actually forgotten about Roger. And then it happened ... all of a sudden, something completely screwy happened. It was something I never saw coming.

First, I felt a hand gently rubbing my back, Roger's hand. What in God's name? I thought to myself. I brushed his hand away without taking my eyes off the phone. He took his hand off my back. I felt weird. Anyone would. What the hell was he doing?

I continued talking with his friend, when, once again, the strangest of things happened. It wasn't a hand this time. It was Roger! I turned my head around, only to find him saddling my chair, trying to hump my back! I couldn't believe what was happening! Here I was, deep in negotiation, making every effort to lure a new member to the elite club of my money-making scheme, and a blind man I had just met was trying to ride me! I didn't know what to do! You can imagine!

"Roger!" I yelled in disdain. Trying to make the best of both situations, I quickly leaned forward and fell to the floor to avoid him, while making every effort to remain in conversation with the priest. There was no way I would lose this call! At the time, getting Roger's friend to join my company meant everything!

In a stooped-over position, I looked at the phone cord. It was definitely too short for me to step away without losing the connection, so I crouched down to the floor to avoid Roger and kept on talking. Ingenious, I thought. But Roger, for some reason, had not yet received the message. He continued trying to gyrate his body along my back. I then swooped my free arm back to pry him off me, carefully cradling the phone in my other hand. I finally yelled, "STOP! What in God's name are you DOING?" I stood up and stared angrily at him. I took a deep breath to cool down, and it was then that I got my biggest surprise.

Roger wasn't the same shabbily dressed "man" I had met earlier that night. Roger, for some unbelievable reason, was now, get this, dressed in purple leotards, with makeup and ribbons in his hair! It was at that moment that I realized something else about him. Roger was a transvestite ... a blind transvestite! Everything became crystal-clear at that exact moment!

Looking back at him in disgust and shock, in complete and utter surprise and fear, I slammed the phone down, letting go of my big money grab and stepped way back. "What the hell?" I gasped, pointing at him. He stood with an embarrassed grin and stared up at the ceiling. "Uh ... I'm sorry," he said, flustered.

I was not happy at all and was very repulsed. Here I was, 3:30 in the morning, on a Saturday, standing in a dirty, smelly, sickening apartment, face-to-face with a man dressed in ladies' tights! It was typical of this night, I guess, but definitely an unpleasant surprise. I have to shake my head at that crazy night, one of many that followed. My evening with the blind transvestite was only part of a much bigger picture that would eventually unfold. Who knew what was next? I'll tell you what.

We spent the next few hours sitting in the lobby, Roger playing guitar, and both of us singing at the top of our lungs. Most people would have left. Not me. I didn't want to hurt his feelings.

At around 6 am, Roger put on a new dress and some much needed eye make-up, and we went to a restaurant for breakfast. You had to see everyone's eyes when they saw Roger. They couldn't believe what they were seeing! I couldn't believe it either, as he entered in high heels. The funniest thing of all was when he started being loud and boisterous to the patrons and waitresses. "Hey baby, come sit on my lap!" He had that same loud and obnoxious laugh, and with his smoker's cough, it was rather entertaining. He would yell at the waitress loudly and comment on other people, when he couldn't even see them! It was quite embarrassing, but funny too. God love him. I wonder where he's at now? I wonder if he knew he'd ever be in a book! Gheesh, I even panhandled with him on Rideau Street with my harmonica one day!

Add to that, on another night in late April, I accompanied him to ritzy Friday's. While I strolled the place pleading for people to join one of my pyramid companies, Roger hobbled around the dining room reaching for whatever female he could find for a thrill that night. I didn't realize that this was happening because I wasn't there long enough to see it. I had already been kicked out by the manager for bothering customers!

As I sat on the steps outside, the doors flung open again, and out came Roger, flying, literally. "Fuck you! I'll take my services elsewhere! Fuck you all to hell!" We both had a good chuckle over our escapades that night, sitting there looking stupidly at each other. That was the last night I saw

Roger. He vanished away ... I have since wondered where he is now. I hope he's doing well.

How did a blind man teach me how to see? He was a person who had nothing. No friends, no family, no one. He lived in a dirty apartment with no furniture. He was blind, unclean, unshaven, yet he had a small flame within him that was evident in the way he carried himself. He knew he had very little, but that didn't stop him from living, even in his difficult state. He wasn't one to give up, even when life had handed him a handicap. He would persevere somehow, some way, and I realized this that night. I will never forget the lesson he taught me. Never give up. I haven't.

## CHAPTER 2
## COMING OUT OF THE CLOSET

On an early April evening, a night downtown with my friends came to an end. They were ready to call it a night, but was I? Never! I knew that my evening had only just begun. I waved goodbye to my friends and headed off. This, they noticed, had become a pattern. "Chris is at it again!" They didn't understand what the hell was up with me, so they just let me be. They just saw it as a phase or something.

Where to? I thought, as I wandered the Market. "It's almost 1 am and last call. Where do I go now? My night's only starting!"

Suddenly, a cabbie saw me standing at the side of the road. He pulled up and rolled down the window. He yelled out, "Cab tonight, sir? Sir? Cab? Sir?"

"Nope, not for me, thanks," I responded. The cabbie waved his hand in disappointment and moved a little further up. Three boisterous and liquored-up guys jumped in. They were loud and a bit obnoxious. I heard one of them yell out to the driver, "Somerset!" The others laughed and yelled the same. "Yah, Somerset! Woohoo!"

I couldn't help but be fascinated by their enthusiasm. They obviously wanted to continue their drunken frolics. Just before the driver started to move, I hustled over to the car and talked to the guys in the back.

"What's up, guys? What's going on?" I asked. Feeling the way I was, I always had to find out what was happening. "What's on Somerset?"

One of the guys had an angry streak and yelled out, "Mind your own business!" The other two laughed and another one yelled out, "Somerset is on Somerset!" He trailed off and they all laughed ... obviously enjoying the effects of their alcoholic debauchery.

Looking for something crazy myself, I asked them if a party was going on down there. The third guy, the drunkest, yelled out, "Yah, come on!"

I smiled and laughed. The other two complained but I didn't care.

The cab pulled out of the Market and headed towards Somerset. We finally pulled onto Somerset and got out. The three guys immediately ran into a bar on the corner.

"So long!" I yelled, waving at them. Like they really cared!

I stood and looked around. Things WERE really happening here. Down the street, there were a number of house parties going on. I thought strongly about crashing one, but for some reason, the bar my friends went into was calling out to me.

I forget the name of the bar, but I remember hearing heavy bass music and watching people trickling in and out. What's going to happen tonight? I thought to myself. It was always a mystery, and so exciting. I checked my wallet. I had enough to do it, so here goes!

I walked in. The man at the front carded me. I'm 27 years old, for godsakes, I felt like saying! I walked past the counter and checked my wallet again. I only had a ten left, but that would do. I ordered a Malibu rum and pineapple. It was my drink of choice that spring. I turned around and scoped the scene. It was busy for 1 am.

There were people spread out all over and loud music pounded from below. There must be a band down there, I thought. Looking around for a minute more, I started to feel a little bit queasy when I noticed something happening in the corner of the bar. I thought I might be seeing things, but God, no ... no, man! It looked like two men kissing! It was then that I noticed a couple of other sets of guys hanging out in the room. I noticed that there was one thing in common among the patrons here. They were all freakin' men! I was in a darned gay bar!

I looked around the whole room.

OH MY GOD!!! There were men everywhere! Not a woman in sight! It was at that exact moment that they all seemed to come out of the woodwork. Some were talking, some hugging, and yes, several were kissing! *Not that there's anything wrong with that*, I laughed to myself. I thought about it for a moment, but in my state of mind, nothing really mattered. Things fell into place and fate had brought me here! So what if they're gay? I thought. That's not going to stop me from enjoying myself!

I decided to start talking to some of the men at the bar.

"Hi, I'm Chris!"

"Hiiiii there ...," one of the men said, in a very effeminate way.

I smiled and said, "And you ... are?"

"I'm Rob; this is Kevin. You new here, sugar?" he said, as he put a hand on my shoulder. Feeling uncomfortable, I backed up and bumped into another pair who smiled and waved. I turned to them again and smiled. We talked and I found out that one of them actually knew a friend of mine! I then had an interesting conversation with Kevin. We started to talk about nature and nurture, putting all the cards on the table. When I asked him about this theory, all he said to me was this, "Would anyone CHOOSE to be hated?" It really made me think about things. I still don't have a stand, but it hit me. Gay? Straight? Why? I guess it's not really up to me to decide ... this was God's job!

As the night progressed and the music got louder, I found myself making my way downstairs with my two new friends. We entered a packed room. Yes, all were male, with one exception.

A band was playing on a small stage and, surprising to me, the lead singer was a girl, the only female in the room. She was rocking the place out and the men were cheering and dancing to the music. I noticed a keyboard on the stage. DING!

"A keyboard?" I questioned, as I looked at Rob.

"Why? Do you play?" he asked.

"Awww ... no, I mean, yes, but not much," which was a bit of a lie. I could play ... quite well.

Rob was about to egg me on to play, but I had already made up my mind. I left the two of them and moved my way through the crowd. She was singing, and loud, but good. At the end of her song, I yelled up to her.

"Can I play?" I said, pointing to the keyboard.

She smiled and reached for my hand. I hopped onto the stage and the keyboardist moved aside. You'd think I'd have been nervous, but I wasn't at all. I was excited! This was going to be another story, another night, another chapter of my new and crazy life.

Being on my high, as I did many times that winter and spring, I always had the urge to do something outlandish. So, when I went up to the front and told her that I'd play, I was not surprised by my actions. Nothing, and I mean nothing, surprised me at the time. With God guiding me, anything was possible!

The set ended and the lead singer asked me what I wanted to play.

"We got to keep this party rockin'," she said, as she awaited my song choice.

Rocking, I thought. Rocking ... what could I play that was rocking? And then it hit me ... there is no better "rockin" song than this. I looked at her and said, "I'll play the theme song to *Titanic*. Do you know it?"

She nearly fell over.

"In here? Honey, I don't know whether that will satisfy this crowd. I do know the lyrics, but look, honey. Look behind you."

I turned back to face the boisterous crowd, who seemed to like my presence on the stage. Whistling and chants filled the air.

So, as high as a kite, I put my arms up in the air like I was about to body surf and I yelled out to everyone, "My name is Chris, and it's time I rocked the boat, baby! You'll love this one!"

And so I played ... the theme to ... *Titanic*. It was a LOT different than the rocker crap she was playing, but that didn't seem to matter to the crowd at all. It quieted down for only a moment, but once they saw me play, they went absolutely nuts! I couldn't believe what I was hearing! I was in absolute shock as I heard a repeated chant going on in the room! It sounded like this:

"Chris ... Chris ... CHRIS ... CHRIS!" They were all pumping their arms in the air. A few of them had taken off their shirts and were whipping them around and around and beating their chests. It was like a freakin' zoo!

The men hollered and they chanted and they cheered me on as my fingers dazzled the keyboard, and their chanting gave me even more energy, making me feel higher and higher. The lead singer was amazed at the crowd's reaction and she did her best rendition of the words to "My Heart Will Go On", by Celine Dion. Needless to say, even though she sang beautifully, I appeared to be the main attraction! There was a whole lot of affection going on down there, and I knew I'd have to head out soon, or else!

We actually sounded great up there! When the song ended, I stood up from the keyboard and gave the singer a hug. She thanked me for a great memory. I thanked her, also. I knew I had another tale to tell, I wild one at that. It was great, really; something neither of us had expected. As I stepped off the stage, the crowd called out for an encore, but that was it for me. I waved and received my applause graciously and then made my way to the back of the room. As I walked through the crowd of ravenous men, I couldn't believe how many high-fived me, or patted my back, or patted my … yep, that happened too!

You can't imagine the number of drinks that came my way over the next hour, as I chatted and laughed with several patrons. Sure, I had a few. I was being treated like a king. I mean, there was Billy, and some guy named Matt, and a Butch was there, just to name a few. It all ended with just the drinks. Oh, and also, drinks weren't all I got that night. I also got a few phone numbers!

## CHAPTER 3
## STICK'EM UP PARTNER!

Friday's Roast Beef House, as you've read, was one of the ritziest restaurants in Ottawa: a place of very high class and elegance. Located in downtown Ottawa, it entertained hundreds of clients weekly for dinner and dancing. People would head there for an evening of *mambo* or *jitterbug* or *can-can*, or *cha-cha* ... whatever one fancied.

On a Friday night in April, after being high for several months, I and some friends decided to pop in. We'd been there before, but we heard that tonight was a special night and we wanted to see what all the hype was about. At 10 pm, we made our way through the tall metal doors and entered. I was sporting an *Ottawa Senators* jersey with pride, as our team had just won a playoff game. GO SENS GO!

We climbed a dark stairwell that led to the restaurant's dining hall. Three gentlemen passed us in the stairwell. I looked at what they were wearing, and right away, we realized we looked out of place. They were dressed up in rich suit jackets and snazzy ties. I looked back at my friends. They looked concerned, but not me. We entered the dining hall.

All eyes were fixed on us as we stepped slowly into the room. We found a table along the back wall and settled quietly into our seats. "I'll get us something to drink. What'll you have, Chris?"

We looked around the room. Men in their finest were accompanied by beautiful women in smashing dresses. I remember looking down at my jersey and snickering. But then, I reminded myself, none of that mattered. Who really cares? I thought. Jersey or no jersey, we were going to have a damned good time, dressed up or not dressed up!

My friend returned with some drinks and our focus turned to a piano man who was entertaining. We listened, enjoyed, and sat silently minding our own business. I looked around the room. Looking with precision, from table to table, I noticed that people were not really interacting with each other ... at all. This is boring, I thought. And in my mind came five ... key ... words. WHAT CAN I DO HERE?

My mind started to race again. And as the hamster ran around upstairs, I did it. I came up with one of my outrageous ideas, one that I knew my friends would just love!

"Chris?" my friend said, looking over worriedly. "What's up? What are you thinking about?" They were used to seeing that look in my eyes and they knew I couldn't sit still anymore. Having spent a lot of time with me during my mania, they knew quite simply that I needed to move when I needed to move!

I reached for the pouch around my waist and opened it. The first thing I saw was my harmonica, but I didn't think that would go well ... maybe later. Below it were hundreds of stickers ... hundreds! I'd ordered these only a year ago and, to me, they were priceless. I had been using them while supply teaching and kids just loved them.

Each sticker had an animal on it, along with a fun comment like "You're Incredible!" or "You're Number 1!" For example, the one I was holding was a kangaroo jumping, and it read, "Top of the Pack!" There was one with a bear that read "Here's a Bear Hug!" They were all really cute, like the "I'll Squeeze You!" snake, or the "Fat Pig!" pig. Okay, there was no fat pig one, but you get the point. "Fat Pig!" wouldn't have impressed my students' parents!

So, this is what I came up with. Although my friends wouldn't help me, they knew I was going to do something crazy no matter what. They shook their heads every time and turned their attention elsewhere. And so, off I went!

You should realize that none of us really knew where this craziness was coming from. They just knew that lately I'd been hyper, very hyper, and very animated in everything I did. Charismatic also. No one, friends or family, knew I was sick. They just thought that I was having fun, being my crazy self, on some type of kick or something.

First thing, I started to hop around the dining hall as the music played, and placed stickers on men and women in the room. The mission, which had started in Toronto, was continuing in a different way now, and I still felt the need to meet as many people as possible.

"You're Amazing!" I said, as I placed a sticker on a gentlemen's suit jacket.

"Thanks," he smiled, as I pinned a "Pretty Snazzy!" on his lady friend, dolled up in a beautiful red dress. "Thank you!" she said, as she grabbed a sticker from my pouch.

"You Hairy Ape!" she laughed, putting it on my jersey. I smiled and continued placing stickers and meeting person after person, including the singer and his piano player. I even handed out handfuls of stickers to some people, so that they could go around and "sticker" others. Slowly, but surely, in that room of about 200, every single person was sporting a funny and wacky sticker on their expensive clothing!

And then, the craziest thing happened. People were actually walking up to complete strangers bantering about their respective stickers. For example, I saw one lady walk up to a man and point to his sticker. "You're Incredible!" she said, and he replied, "You're Beautiful!" Her sticker had actually said, "You Rock!", but "You're Beautiful!" really was better. His quick thinking, along with my nifty sticker idea, probably got him action that night!

When I sat down with my friends after touring, we surveyed the room. The energy was electric and people were now interacting with each other, something that otherwise would not have happened if it hadn't been for my stickers. Yes, I was proud, and all in only twenty minutes! It was amazing how such a trivial idea could spark so much enthusiasm from a bunch of well-to-do women and men, who ordinarily would have kept to themselves. They were having a grand ole time!

Suddenly, the tempo of the music changed and two women grabbed me and put their hands on my waist. "Conga!" one of them yelled, as the three of us started to make a line around the piano. People joined and it got longer and longer. Meanwhile, people kept coming up to me and pointing to their stickers. I looked around the room again. I was right. Everyone, and I mean everyone, was wearing a freakin' sticker! I didn't notice anyone without one, and it pleased me, and it was so. Even the bartender and hostesses were wearing them!

At the end of the night I sat back and chuckled to myself. Let's think about what I had achieved. I'd taken a ritzy, elegant, posh, exquisite, stuck up, snobby crowd, at Friday's Roast Beef House, and with one idea, simple stickers, turned a whole building of rich folk into a complete dancing frenzy.

It was really amazing and, as we left, we really had a good sticker about it. I mean, snicker! What a fun night for all, but especially my friends. They had sure seen a lot of crazy things that winter and spring. I was really loving life, and I suspected nothing of sickness at all. Oh to feel so good! Did it have to end? I hoped not.

## CHAPTER 4
## THE CONCERT OF ALL CONCERTS

Being on a high can have its benefits. In the middle of May, my friend (co-writer of my children's series, *A Quarter Past Three*) and I went to U2's *Elevation Tour.* It was a worldwide tour, and they had come to Montreal. Originally, tickets were sold out everywhere, but a few days before the concert, we found some tickets on-line. They were $150 apiece! That didn't matter to me whatsoever. Money was nothing. We jumped on them because it was U2. Nothing was bigger.

We got there early. We brought a copy of our book's manuscript to review and edit while we were waiting. Our book would come out that June. We went to a local pub to have a drink and to chat. While there, I had another great(?) idea. I was still quite high and continued to have wild and crazy ideas. My friend thought it was weird, but he went along with it. Most of my friends were resigned to my wild ways. He didn't know the reasons why I did the things I did, but he let me do my own thing. He had no idea that I was sick, either.

We walked over to a dollar store down the street. We looked around for the sticker section and, finding it, we were pleasantly surprised to find stickers in the shape of glittering hearts. I grabbed 30 or so pages of stickers. Why? Well, the *Elevation Tour* was all about the heart and love. U2 was promoting the heart for their tour. These were perfect!

We cut the stickers into groups of three or four so that they could fit in my pouch. Time was ticking and we had to line up right away to get a good seat. We got to the stadium and got in line when it started to rain. We didn't have umbrellas, so I ran to get one for us. "I'll be right back," I told my friend. Thankfully, because of the rain, many people had left the line. It got us right up to the front!

I arrived back in the line after only minutes, with umbrellas, and lots of them, ten bucks a pop! I had at least five or six, and passed them out to others behind us in line. This puzzled my friend. "Well, you know ... I felt for them. What's ten bucks?"

"You mean ... sixty?"

While we were talking with others in the line, one of the guys mentioned the stage setting.

"Man, I can't wait to get in there. I hear the stage is amazing! It's in the form of a heart! The top part of the heart is the main stage, and the two sides of the heart down to the bottom part are catwalks that Bono will actually sing from!"

"Really?" I was intrigued, as I thought about my "heart" stickers. Hmm, happening for a reason?

He continued, "And the great thing is this. The first 200 to 300 people get to watch the concert from the centre of the heart! Man, looking at things the way they are, we're going to get in there! It'll be like a "hot tub" full of fans with us in it!"

I looked at my friend and smiled. "That's amazing!" We were both so excited.

After many hours, the line started moving. As it did, I started to pass out the hearts to the people around us. People were telling me the hearts were such a great idea. They placed them on their faces, shirts and pants. My friend and I covered ourselves with the hearts all over our bodies.

Inside, we entered the centre of the heart-shaped stage. We had made it! We would be watching the biggest band in the world, right in front of the stage! We continued to hand out hearts to everyone, including those outside the heart, just to reach as many people as we could. We even now had dedicated helpers. Thousands of stickers circulated the floor.

We returned to the "heart hot tub" and got ready for the main attraction. The opening band was finishing. Just before U2 came out, I took a look at the crowd. Almost every person had hearts on their bodies: red, glittering hearts. It was amazing to see what we had accomplished. Men and women had them on their cheeks, shoulders, arms, chests and butts!

Finally, U2 came onto the stage, and the crowd erupted! They opened with their hit, "Elevation", and the whole crowd started jumping. Me 2! The place was rocking; I could see the hearts all around me. They were glittering brightly on and off in the glow of the flashing lights. I smiled and wondered if the band could see the hearts? Of course they could … everyone could! The things were everywhere!

And then, the most wild of things happened. As everyone was dancing, and floating and singing to the music, the second song went into the third. Suddenly, someone pulled my arm and screamed, "LOOK! Look up there!"

I looked up, and there it was. Bono, from the biggest band in the world, who had toured the universe, had one of MY hearts that I had bought with my OWN money, on HIS forehead! Bono, freakin' Bono!!! I couldn't believe what I was seeing! It was incredible! I had to slap my face a few times.

I grabbed my camera, and click! I took the picture. I remember a week or so following the concert how excited I was to see these pictures. I flipped through them and, yes, there it was! It was better than I'd hoped. It was a clear picture of Bono singing and, smack-dab on his forehead, there it was ... a shiny glittering heart!

The idea of the hearts went off with a bang. It brought everyone together that night. I heard people talking about the hearts, even after the concert. They wondered where these hearts had come from. How do you unite a gathering of 25,000 screaming fans together as one? U2 ... oh, and some stickers!

# PART IV

# BIPOLAR DISORDER

# CHAPTER 1
# WHO ARE WE?

We are teachers,

We are lawyers,

We are doctors,

We are construction workers and civil engineers.

We are dentists,

We are technical workers,

We are biologists and professional athletes.

We are carpenters,

We are store owners and clerks,

We are artists, chemists and accountants.

And we are so much more.

What do each of us have in common? Can you guess? You can close your eyes for this one; you can't see it no matter how much you try.

We each suffer from a mental illness. It doesn't matter who you are, what age, where you come from or what you do in life, mental illness can hit you at any time, but often during adolescence and young adulthood. It has no favourites and makes no preference. Its goal is to destroy. Mental illnesses are biologically-based disorders of the mind. They cannot be overcome through "will power" and are not related to a person's disposition or level of intelligence. They are very complex, a combination of many factors. These include genetic, biological, personality and environmental factors.

**What does that mean?**

**That they affect the individual as a whole person ... in every single way.**

## CHAPTER 2
## WHAT THE HELL IS BIPOLAR DISORDER ANYWAY?!!

*From NIMH and American Psychiatric Association*

A lot of things happen in a manic episode, also termed ***mania***. We call it "being on a high", because that's what it is. For six months, none of us knew I was sick, although many questioned my actions. It did, however, take six months for me to be diagnosed, and what a six months it was! ***Bipolar Disorder*** **(BD)** is a severe mental illness, a chemical imbalance affecting the neurotransmitters of the brain. It results in momentum-building mood swings that can range from the high peaks of mania, to the lowest of depressions. The mood changes are not day to day. They are gradual waves that build up, becoming more and more intense and severe for the sufferer who is not medicated. Highs, though they are exhilarating, are life-threatening. Lows are at the other end of the spectrum. They are deflating, depressing and debilitating, and they can be even more life-threatening. All in all, bipolar packs a very dangerous weapon. Without support, continued therapy and proper medications, it will squeeze the life out of its victim.

First off, your ***energy level is elevated***. I was a ball of energy; I wanted to explode! I couldn't sit still, couldn't wait for morning, wanting to do anything and everything at that same moment. My mind was racing, my body couldn't keep up. When I had ideas, I was so eager to make them happen, as outrageous as some were. I would hang onto thoughts so intently. My ideals, which were "way out there", I tried to make happen. What if people tried to stand in my way? I would either ignore them, or try to convince them that I was sensible. Nothing could stop me.

During mania, ***you feel overly good,*** euphoric. You feel "on top of the world"! Nothing could bring me down, and nothing did, until my chemicals shifted.

***Irritability*** becomes prevalent. You are feeling so sure of yourself that you want everyone else to feel the same way you do about things. But they can't. They are in a completely different state of mind. The things you love, they may not. The things you enjoy may bore others or mystify them. This is very hard to accept when you are in mania and, therefore, you become agitated with others. For me, this pertained to expressing my philosophies of life and faith to others, and being told that what I was saying and doing was not reasonable or rational.

Your ***thoughts race*** and your talking does its best to keep up with your thinking. I tried to say everything that was on my mind. I was under the notion that I didn't have enough time to say it all. I would get very restless. I wanted to talk, I wanted to be heard. At a restaurant, I would be so anxious to talk that I would start walking around talking to anyone.

You ***can't concentrate and are easily distracted***. My mind was racing in every direction. I would change topics repeatedly. I might be talking about a movie and, all of a sudden, start talking about the new shaver I bought. And then, why dogs should be allowed in apartments, and then ... well, you get the point. This caused a lot of frustration for friends and family who didn't even know that I was sick.

You are ***never tired***. I wanted to live and play 24 hours a day! I needed very little sleep. I remember being up very late. Most nights, I would sleep less than an hour and half!

You have an ***unrealistic belief of your abilities*** *or* ***powers with grandiose delusions and invincibility***. This psychosis convinced me that I could avoid death, that I possessed super powers, that I would one day lead a multi-billion dollar industry that would change the world. I even thought that I was the Second Coming of Christ!

You ***use poor judgment*** many times over. I assumed that others were thinking the same way as me. For example, my cousin had to convince me how dangerous it was to leave my keys in my car's ignition. I was convinced that my car would be safe and that God would not let anyone take it. He rationalized that a drunk could have driven away with it, causing a fatality which would have made me liable. We argued "tooth and nail". Fortunately, his opinion won out.

You ***spend and give money carelessly***. During my high, I spent thousands of dollars erratically. I was convinced that my bank account was being replenished by God.

***Sexual arousal is heightened***. Because of my morals and obsession with hell, I may not have been having sex, but I was definitely sexually active in other ways. I was very aroused and wanted to be with my girlfriend all the time. And then, after being with one of the most amazing women I could ever want to be with, I ended our relationship. I did so because I couldn't give of myself completely. Most of all, though, I needed to meet other women. Within two weeks, I had at least four other encounters.

You may partake in ***aggressive behavior***. This happened when I tried to express opinions or ideas. When people disagreed with me, I became annoyed and discussions would become heated.

You ***deny that anything is wrong***. This was totally me! I remember sitting with my parents who had Julie's psychology book out to show me the section on bipolar disorder. I slammed it shut quickly. I was fine, I told them. Worry no more. There was nothing wrong with me! Nothing! I was the new me! God's way!

***NOW WHAT ABOUT THE OTHER SIDE OF BIPOLAR DISORDER? IT NEEDS NO EXPLANATION ... DEPRESSION!***

# PART V

# INTO THE DEEP

## CHAPTER 1
## I GOT THE JOB!

I had never, up to that day, felt the way I had the weekend before starting my first teaching job. Something was not right. Let me begin by quickly taking you back two months prior to the shit hitting the fan.

*[I got the call at the beginning of July, 1998. She hired me right over the phone. I was thrilled. She knew my credentials and had many recommendations and knew I'd be a perfect fit for her staff. I would actually be the first full-time male teacher the school had ever had! I was a newbie, a rookie about to play his first game in two months. I was hired to teach two grade four classes with the Catholic School Board, in Ottawa.*

*After hanging up the phone, I was beaming. I remember grabbing the Ontario curriculum documents and racing over to Staples to make copies. I got back home and zoomed downstairs two steps at a time. My mind was in a fury! I would be the best teacher in the Board; I just knew it!*

*"Chris, are you hungry?"*

*"No, Dad, talk later!"*

*I began to cut and tape documents all over the chalkboard and surrounding wall. I had documents everywhere, a wall mural of paper. I littered the floor with all kinds of teaching books I had collected from my practice teaching, along with several that I bought at Staples. I was on my knees turning pages and tearing pages and writing notes so furiously that my hands were actually shaking, which made it hard to write. I was highlighting expectations and drawing lines and arrows all over the documents, cutting out specific expectations and linking them together. I would be the best damn teacher in Ottawa!*

*I began to put themes together and I even remember having the phone on my shoulder, calling other teacher friends to tell them the news and to ask for any cool ideas. My mind was working at an all-time high. The hamster would not sleep tonight! I was full of an energy which I had felt several times in high school and university. This time, however, it did come on like a tidal wave.*

*My parents had to laugh, at first, at how fast I was talking and how crazy I was acting, but they thought I was just overexcited. A couple of weeks later, when this persisted, they remember telling me to slow down and breathe. They didn't suspect that I might be sick.*

*"One thing at a time, son."*

*"Sure, Dad! Sure, Mom!"*

*I admit I was jumping from one thing to the next, never really finishing up on things, but that didn't seem to matter then. The same thing applied to my whole first teaching year, where I would not really finish up anything unless it was due the next day. Because of this, I would end up leaving school very late every night, often around 10 pm. Was that really a problem? I was never convinced it was, even when experienced teachers told me that I shouldn't stay so late and that I needed to slow down. I would have nothing to do with this type of advice. I was fine; besides, the things I was producing were "state of the art". I thought they really were. In my mind, everything would have to be as good as could be.*

*The summer moved on and I worked away at "over-preparing" myself for my first year. But, early in August, something changed. My over-excitement and zest for the job were replaced by anxieties and fears, and my work slowed. I remember saying to my parents, "I just don't feel right," and, by the last week in August, I was starting to doubt whether I could even handle the job. I couldn't sleep well or focus, and my thoughts were getting the best of me.*

*And that is when the Labour Day weekend hit. Something happened. None of us understood why.*]

On the Sunday morning before school began, I stood downstairs staring at all I had done that summer. I looked at my books spread out over the floor, I looked at the chalkboard and the wall and I remember scratching my head. What the fuck was I doing? I was feeling really shitty; my mind was no longer on the workload before me, but on to awful and terrible thoughts. My stomach felt uneasy and I started to sweat. I was so anxious, and although I tried to stop thinking about work and stuff, I couldn't, and it started to drive me crazy. I couldn't get my mind off things. Incidents of that sort occurred in university, but not with such intensity or of such duration.

I ran upstairs, past the kitchen and out the door. My folks were out and I was on my own. I got in the car and I was breathing heavily and sweating profusely. I felt awful and I didn't know why. I raced down the street and headed out to a place where I could escape. I had to take this to meditation ... to God. I needed to get away from everything. This had happened several times before, but this was much greater.

I headed into the countryside. I found a secluded gravelled off-road that led to a forest. I drove deep into the brush and parked my car. I found a large rock to sit on. I remember pondering much as I sat there talking to God. "What's going on?" I asked Him. "What the heck is this?"

I talked to Him, but most of my time was spent just looking up at the clouds through the trees for answers that never came. On the way home, I popped into a local pub and ordered a coffee. The room was empty, and I remember speaking to the waitress for a whole hour about my anxieties towards teaching. I told her that I wasn't sure that this vocation was for me. She tried to ease my mind, but to no avail.

I returned home that afternoon very sombre and despondent and spoke with my parents. I was worried, as were they. I didn't care about the job anymore. I only cared about how I had been feeling for the last couple of weeks. It was not good.

On Monday afternoon, the day before school, my dad and I headed to a clinic to meet with a doctor, a friend of my dad's. I told him my story, and we talked about the last few months and years, where I experienced similar symptoms. He concurred that there was a problem. He said to me, "Chris, this is depression." He knew it. My dad knew it. They believed it, but I didn't. I took a prescription anyway and, for the first time in my life, I swallowed a couple of pills. Little did I know that this would be the start of something that would last a lifetime.

I wish I could say that these were magic pills and that I was okay by the morning, but I'd be lying. That first day was one of the hardest days I'd ever experienced in my entire life. I was depressed, anxious and obsessed. Life isn't fixed automatically by a few pills. In fact, in two years of teaching, the pills would not actually solve the problem. The diagnosis was not complete. We never imagined it was part of something much bigger.

***"In the middle of the journey of my life, I found myself in a dark wood, for I had lost the right path."***

***The poet Dante***

## CHAPTER 2
## ICEBERG ... STRAIGHT AHEAD!

June 23rd, 2001, marked one of the most exciting days of my life, but also the beginning of a steep decline into the worst days I'd ever experience. On this day, my co-writer and I launched our very first children's adventure novel titled, *A Quarter Past Three* – "Medieval Madness". We released it to over six hundred people at a local elementary school, which happened to be the school we had both attended as young farts.

For months before, we'd been preparing for the big day, and June fell on us faster than expected. This had been a project of one and a half years. This had left us with much to do. We decided that we wanted to do things up big since, at the time, this was our brand new baby—our first novel!

Still in mania, I was overly excited about the book's release. With an increased energy level, sleepless nights, racing thoughts and an unrealistic belief that we'd be instant millionaires worldwide, I was able to work around the clock to ensure that we had everything ready for our big day. With all the hype, my mania was not as evident, and I had come down from the extreme highs to a degree. Any mention of odd or unusual behaviour on my part, I quickly dismissed. "What, I'm just excited, that's all!"

In order to make the day successful, there was much to be done. First, we had to finish our book. We had to complete the editing to the last letter. Since we were self-publishing, we also had to get an artist to create our cover and a graphic designer to finish it. We then had to get it printed, and we did, big time. 10,000 copies, under a company that we called *Turtles Publishing*. Yes, turtles. As you read earlier, you know I was crazy about turtles, my symbol from God. My co-writer agreed it was a good name, but mainly because I was so adamant about using the damn turtle!

We had taken a big chance, spending more than $20,000 dollars to get it printed, but once we started, we would not look back. We borrowed heavily. By May, I was still spending freely, so $20,000 plus didn't scare me whatsoever, but it scared the shit out of my writing buddy!

Our story? It is about a young boy named Tommy, who one day finds himself lost in the medieval time period. Alone and scared, he begins a journey to find his way back home. On his travels, he meets many people, some wise, some friendly, and yet others with evil intentions. He also meets a friendly wizard named Percival (I had a tough time with that one ... tell you more later), who vows to help him get home. *"Tommy, to get back home, you must find a magical door which will appear for one minute, at exactly "A Quarter Past Three". After that minute, should you miss the door, it will disappear and you will be lost in time forever!"* I know, it's catchy and friggin exciting! Want to know more? Buy the book!

Over those few years, we published two books under the *A Quarter Past Three* umbrella: "Medieval Madness" and "Treasures of Times".

Now, where was I? Oh, yes, the launch. With the book nearly completed in late April, we went about planning our launch. We knew it was going to be big, and with my added energy and enthusiasm, it was! May began with a bang. I started, by myself, touring over 35 elementary schools in the Ottawa area, giving each child (some gyms full of five to six hundred kids!) a newsletter about our big day. I loved doing it and had so much fun speaking to the kids. With my liveliness, I really got caught up in the moment and the kids responded with just as much excitement.

Then we hit the press. We were on TV at least five times in May and June and we had several articles about our book and launch in local newspapers.

For our big day, we booked two local mascots, we had popcorn and cotton candy machines, we had horses giving rides and medieval wear for kids. We even had a barbecue going, and, oh, a face painter too! It was really the perfect day with the perfect results.

That day, in only four hours, we sold over 1000 books! This was completely unheard of for two local boys releasing a self-published title. The book became an overnight success in Ottawa. Bookstores were calling, media was reaching out for us and we were becoming instant celebrities; on a small scale, yes, but we felt that Oprah would be knocking soon! Kids just loved us, parents adored us and my damn wrist was so sore from signing books all day, 1000 big ones!

With bells and whistles going off all around us, you'd think I would have been on cloud nine but, for some reason, that wasn't the case. In the days following the launch, I remember feeling the exact opposite. I wasn't as happy as I should have been. I was very uneasy. Something was not right and I knew it; I could feel it, although I tried to ignore it. Something was beginning to take over my mind and my body. And so, while my co-writer was enjoying all the instant gratification that came with publishing and releasing one's first book, I was actually being hit hard by a punch that would eventually knock me over, launching me into my worst nightmare.

I remember the exact day when my thoughts began to turn. It was when I was working that summer as a lifeguard. I remember standing starry-eyed at the bottom of the baby pool, during one of my shifts in early July. I knew something was really wrong with me, as tears filled my eyes underneath my sunglasses. It just wasn't right to feel what I was feeling. Behind all the glitz and glamour of publishing, at a time when I should have been celebrating, I was being shrouded by something far greater, something I just couldn't understand.

On July 17$^{th}$, a Tuesday, my parents were at their cottage enjoying their second week in the sun. They had been going for over 20 years, Cuddy's Pine Cove Camp, mine and my sister's favourite childhood summer getaway. Julie and I, older now, would visit one weekend every summer to see friends we had made years before. This particular year, however, things changed dramatically for me.

I had just come home from seeing the doctor, recounting to him all that had happened over the last number of months. I had avoided seeing him throughout the winter and spring since I felt so good. So good, in fact, that the prior February, I had actually thrown all my medication away: after almost two years! On that particular visit, I was told something that no one ever wants to hear.

"Chris, you're suffering from ***manic depression***."

NOOOOO! I had been diagnosed with bipolar disorder. I had heard about it before, but it was pretty much foreign to me. I didn't take the news well and I sped home to my apartment on Elgin. I remember sitting with my head in my hands on the couch. I could hear people walking outside, and trucks and buses buzzing by, but nothing mattered. They were living and I was dying. I was bipolar! I sat there, and tears started to cloud my eyes. The doctor had given the verdict, and I took it very hard. I felt that I was no longer myself. I was now "Chris Nihmey, The Bipolar". I would wear the "label" on my sleeve from now on. I would be ostracized, rejected and, in time, removed from the lives of all.

Did this mean that everything I had experienced over the last six months was a sham? Did it all mean nothing? Was God toying with me? I was the Second Coming, for godsakes! All these thoughts flooded in as I sat alone in my apartment.

I wiped away the tears and looked at the phone. I knew my parents were away, but my sister was at work. Should I call her? I thought. I really needed to talk to someone and a friend would not do at this time. I picked up the phone and dialled the daycare where my sister worked.

"Hello, Children's Daycare, Donna speaking."

I cleared my throat and asked to speak with my sister.

"One moment," she said.

"Hello?" Julie asked.

"Hi, it's me ... I, I had to call."

She became alarmed when she heard my voice. "Are you okay?"

"No ... not really. I can't say."

"Are you sure you can't talk about it with me?"

"No, I can't talk over the phone." I was a bit annoyed.

"I'm done at 5:00. I'll come by right after work. Will you be okay?" I could hear worry in her voice. I knew she'd wonder and worry at the same time.

"Okay. I'll be here. Bye." I hung up without waiting for her to say goodbye. I felt terrible. Nothing mattered right now except the fact that I was now a "sicko". I lay back on my bed and cried some more. Again, I heard the buzz outside my window. I was living on one of the busiest streets in Ottawa. During my high, being so impetuous, I had leased this apartment whimsically paying no attention to where I chose to live. Cars were passing, horns were honking, people were walking, people were running. All of this was happening while I lay still behind the curtains doing absolutely nothing. I closed my eyes and tried to shut out the noise. Life was happening around me. I felt like I was in a dream, where I couldn't move and couldn't change anything. It was mystical;

yet it was horrible. It was a nightmare that I could not wake from. It wouldn't get any better. Only worse.

I started to grunt and groan and I stood up and began to pace the room, slamming my fist in the palm of my hand.

"WHY? WHY? WHY?" I yelled. I didn't care who heard me. My neighbours could fuck themselves for all I cared. I started to pound my bed again. I walked to the window and opened my curtains slightly. I looked across the road and saw a mother walking with her young child. The mother was swinging her child's arm as they strolled down the street. I looked at the child, smiling at her mom and looking around at everything new. I couldn't help but be angry at them for feeling happy and safe. I couldn't even remember when life was that simple. What had happened? Where had the joy gone, a tumultuous joy I felt a month ago? It was gone and was replaced with this incredibly awful feeling of dread and despair. I longed for the good old days, but they were clearly gone.

An hour or so later, there was a knock at my door. I stood up and unlocked the chain. It was Julie.

"I got off early. What's wrong?"

I looked at the wall and then the ceiling. I didn't think I was going to be able to say it.

"I ... I ... went to see the doctor this morning." I looked away. "I ... sniff. He told me that ... I'm ... I have bipolar disorder." I looked away again and the tears began to pour. "He told me I have a mental disorder, for god-sakes!"

She stood up. I told her to sit back down. I didn't need sympathy. I was more pissed than sad. I looked at her and uttered, "What are people gonna think? They're going to think I'm a loony! What about a job, a family? I'll never have a family! No one would ever marry me! And what about all the shit that happened over the last few months? All the signs, all the strange happenings ... were they for nothing? Fuck!"

I looked up and yelled out crying, "God, were you ever fucking there?"

My sister tried to reassure me, "God is there, and no one will care, and no one needs to know!"

"They'll find out. They'll all find out! FUCK! SHIT!" I slammed my fist down hard on the coffee table.

"I know it's hard to hear but you can get help!" she exclaimed.

"Fuck the help!" I yelled. "God, you pulled a good one on me! Pulled the sheet right over my eyes! I never saw it coming. Why, God? WHY?"

The two of us sat together in my living room talking. I shed a lot of tears, and so did she. I was so thankful that she was there. At the same time, I wanted, I needed, to be alone. We talked for awhile. It was difficult for both of us: more so for me. I was now labelled. I would not be simply Chris Nihmey anymore. I now had a disorder attached to me, an arch-enemy named Bipolar Disorder. Others would call it by its former name: manic depression. Both damaged its victims, both mentally and physically, and definitely, socially. In time, it would mean so little to others who would never experience it, but it would mean everything to me. Because now I had to live with it forever! It was hard to believe. How could Chris Nihmey, a strong, confident and charismatic person be bipolar? Impossible! But it happened; a mystery to me and I saw no good from it. This thought would stay with me for a long, long time.

I agonized over the diagnosis, and tried to collect my thoughts. I called to cancel work for two days, very uncharacteristic of me. I never missed work. I told them I was sick with a fever and flu. That would buy me some time. Little did I know then that I'd be using the "I'm sick" excuse over and over the next number of years. Mental illness just didn't cut it when it came to excuses. That would only mean you were "crazy"! And those who did not understand would hold it against me.

You might say that I was now rolling down a hill at a very fast rate, but it was more like falling down a waterfall. I was feeling worse and worse, awful, terrible, falling into a dark abyss. A major depression emerged and I was slipping quickly. Julie, worried sick, made an emergency call to my parents at the cottage to tell them what was happening. They were stunned and also very worried. They came home immediately.

Later that afternoon, my father picked me up. He found me lying in bed staring at the ceiling. I spent the night at their place. In the morning, we headed to emergency at the Ottawa Civic Hospital. In spite of not wanting to face anyone, I was fortunate to meet with Dr. Boyles, who, I never imagined, would become my trusted psychiatrist. I must say that we didn't hit it off initially. It actually took time for that, mostly because I had such an aversion to seeing anyone who thought that something might be wrong with me. During my manic high, I actually had met Dr. Boyles for the first time, when my parents made me see someone to reassure them that nothing was wrong with the way I was acting. That meeting, I'll never forget.

[*Two months after returning from Toronto, my parents convinced me, rather forced me, to go to the Civic Hospital's Emergency Ward, due to my erratic behaviour the last few months.*

*I was accompanied by my father and met with a resident psychiatrist who conducted a question session with me. He diagnosed me as "hypomanic". He then referred the diagnosis to Dr. Boyles, the senior psychiatrist at the Civic. Prior to this, a neighbour, a psychiatric nurse, remarkably, gave my parents Dr. Boyles' name as one of the top psychiatric physicians in the City of Ottawa. We then met Dr. Boyles for the first time. I remember it clearly, and so does my dad. Dr. Boyles looked at me with an intense stare and said in a slow, low, monotone, "Chris, we've diagnosed you as hypomanic. On a scale of 1 to 10, where would you put yourself?" I replied that I was about a seven. He then handed me a sample pill bottle which turned out to be Xyprexa. He said, "Chris, I want you to take two of these at bedtime." I looked at him, nodded and simply smiled.*

*"Okay … sure," but what I really wanted to say was, screw you and leave me the fuck alone. I was infuriated with my dad for bringing me to see a doctor, when I knew, without a doubt, that I was fine. There was nothing wrong with me, and no doctor or anyone was going to convince me of anything different. I remember grabbing that pill bottle, standing up, and saying thank you in a nonchalant manner. I walked out waving goodbye to everyone. Dr. Boyles, he revealed to me years later, said to himself, "I'll see you again sometime soon."*

*That day, Dr. Boyles had not made a final assessment, but he led me to believe that something was not right, whatever that was. I, however, would have nothing to do with that assessment. After all, I was Special, I was Chosen, and this doctor could kiss my ass for all I cared. I was fine just the way I was! What an arrogant prick! I thought to myself at that time.*

*We left the hospital and went to lunch. On the way, I, very manipulative, which is characteristic of a bipolar person, convinced my father that, if I managed to bring myself down over the weekend, could I not have to take the medication. This was another common characteristic of a newly diagnosed mental patient—aversion to taking medication.*

*That bottle remained unopened in my parents' medicine cabinet until two years later, when my father threw it away. He told me recently it was to protect me from others finding out about my illness. This was due to the stigma of mental illness, which still persists everywhere. Subsequent to that day, I have learned that* ***hypomania*** *is a stage in mania. I had actually come down from full-blown mania!*]

I sat there with my dad waiting to see the doctor on that dismal July morning. I felt so shitty in contrast to how I had felt only a few months prior. Dr. Boyles came in. My dad stepped out and I now sat face to face with a man I clearly disliked. His walk into the room felt like he was strutting in slow motion. He looked at me with, what I interpreted was, an "I told you so" smirk on his face. I was sitting slumped as low as possible in a chair, staring at the wall behind him, and also at the ceiling. I wouldn't look him in the eyes. I couldn't look him in the eyes. He knew everything, and I knew shit.

I had nothing to say. He diagnosed me definitively, that day, with bipolar disorder. He gave my dad a prescription for a drug that I would learn to accept as a lifelong friend. It was Lithium and, although I fought to avoid medication the first time, this time I accepted it wholeheartedly. I felt outright awful.

***"Day by day, month by month, time after time, measuring life not by the hourglass but rather by the pill bottle."***

It was a bitter pill to swallow that day, and it would start a chain reaction, an uncomfortable daily routine that would last a lifetime. And through the years, I'd meet several of its friends, each with their own evil side … their "other" side. This included annoying tremors, which led to many excuses ("oh, it's just something I was born with"), to daily sweats and dry mouth that thankfully lay hidden under my arms and tongue. Add to that, many frustrating moments sitting on the can, to enemy number one ... next to no sexual drive.

I would become a slave, a victim to a vicious gang of thugs that for a long time dragged my self-esteem and confidence down. Its members included the infamous Lithium (my chemical stabilizer for bipolar chemical imbalance), Effexor, Xyprexa, Clomipramine, Lamictal and Ativan (for depression, OCD and GAD), at times swallowing up to 14 pills a day! Each would attempt to balance my moods, attack my unrealistic thoughts, decrease my anxiety and curtail my compulsive actions. On that unfortunate day, when the cycle would begin, and for years that would follow, I would feel beaten down and defeated. Little did I know that, in time, these many thugs would become my allies ... my saving grace.

With sickness comes a lot of things that bring us to our knees, wondering, questioning, praying for answers that often never come to light. We are lost, walking down a path that we have no directions for, without any clue of how to get there. But with sickness also comes something greater, something absolutely necessary. It is called responsibility, the need to survive and eventually conquer your greatest demons, your greatest fears. Those who have this instinct can move forward and heal. Those without it will wither away. I chose to take responsibility and found the discipline and desire to strive forward, through a yearning to become human once again. I capitalized on decisive moments like the following, early in my battle. Situations like these made me realize just how important those "little pills" were in helping me to get my life back.

[*It was 2004. I arrived at my parent's cottage for a weekend visit that I made each summer, until sickness kept me at bay. After a two-hour drive, I pulled up. I stepped out and gave my parents a hug, grabbed my bags and started to bring a few things in. And then ... "Oh shit!" My mom turned and asked me what was wrong. I smacked my forehead, "I forgot my stupid medication!" What was I going to do? Well, for me, the answer was simple. I hopped back into my car and drove the two hours back to Ottawa to get what I needed.*

*I knew it was my lifeline, and a decision that would prove wise in the future. I would never make that mistake again. I returned early the next morning having lost some valuable cottage time. This required discipline and dedication: a desire to get better, to live again no matter the cost. It was an example of the careful decisions one must make in these difficult times of hardship and sickness. These precious decisions will slowly add up, eventually leading you to times of triumph, times when you can pat yourself on the back and say, "I did it." These decisions are crucial. They are paramount. This is YOUR life and you have to want it back. Without smart decisions like these, you are all but lost, as the poet Dante wrote, in a dark wood.*]

It would take a long time to feel anything close to normal; this was only the beginning. Dr. Boyles had known this all along and I had not trusted him. It took depression for me to finally listen. My dad brought me to their home. Thus my major depression began. I could no longer function on my own.

# CHAPTER 3
# DEPRESSION: A LOG

## DAY 1

*At one in the afternoon, the sun was bright; my head was not. It felt like I was being punched in the face every five seconds, a good hard punch to the face, jerking my neck back every time. After the visit to Dr. Boyles, I stormed from the car and darted right into my parent's place, heading straight for the basement. Stomping down the steps, I entered "the hole". What had been my bedroom upstairs was now an office. But that didn't really matter. What mattered was the darkness the basement would provide. What mattered was trying to derail my terrible and unwanted thoughts. What mattered was the complete isolation I would get downstairs, from anything and anyone. I would have all that in the basement, lit only by small cracks of light in the window wells above, each covered by an arrangement of thick plants and vines. Very little light crept in, and that was what was so important to me. Important because I needed to hide from the world. I hadn't even said boo to my mom who sat in the kitchen in dismay.*

*I yanked the bed out from the couch and landed knees first onto the mattress. I heard the springs creak as I sprawled out face down. After only a minute, I rolled onto my back. I stared up at the ceiling and yelled into the darkness, "Oh God! Why? WHY?" Really though, I actually called out to the air, because I knew God wasn't listening. Why the hell would He care? He'd left me already; I was sure of that. I was alone. Had I always been alone? It felt like He had been with me over the last number of months. All the way, kiddo, He had said to me. Bullshit! Just plain old bullshit! The reality was, I was only subject to my own voice, and my own thoughts and that was how it was going to be from now on.*

*Were my last six months a damned farce? I didn't know what to believe anymore, or where I could turn. I had given my whole life to Him just a few months ago and now, here I was, in the dark, battered by sickness and utterly alone!*

*"GOD! Where are you? Godammit, where are you now?" I moaned and groaned. I was really loud and I kept slamming my fists into the mattress.*

*I remember asking myself these questions over and over, and it felt unbelievably awful. I shed dry tears: many. It was like I had lost a parent, only worse. I had lost God. My relationship with my creator was swirling down the toilet. I had put all my trust in Him and where did I end up? Here, in the dark, alone.*

*My thoughts began to twirl as I lay there. Why would God let this happen when I had given Him my life completely? As far as I was concerned now, God was gone from my life. God had pulled the stool right out from under me. What a fucking fool I was! I would learn a valuable lesson that morning. You can't trust anyone or anything, no matter how great you think they are or how strongly you feel about them.*

*As I lay there immersed in negative thoughts, I couldn't help but feel the metal rungs of the mattress stabbing into my back. "Stupid bed!" I grunted, rather growled, and I pounded the mattress again several times. I jumped up and pulled the damned thing straight off the couch onto the floor. I heard tearing as I ripped the mattress fasteners from their holds. And then I lay there on the mattress, just like that. I would lie there from now on, on the floor on top of a very thin, old and shabby mattress. I wasn't looking for comfort, just some sort of peace which I felt sure wouldn't come for a very long time. Maybe never.*

***"Time became meaningless in this state of mind. Mornings would blend into afternoons, which would then blend into evenings. Tick after tick of the clock, minute after minute. At times, slow as molasses; at other times, swift as a rocket."***

*Other than breakfast before my trip to the doctor, there would be no food that day, only tap water from the washroom for the pills prescribed by him. Yes, dreaded pills, four little unwanted capsules! Did they really matter? I had fought as much as I could not to have to take them, but to no avail. These would become my newest companions within the sick world I would now inhabit. I was a damned "sicko", a mental patient, a corpse ... dead to the world.*

*My parents brought me food, but I never ate it. It just piled up beside me: apples, crackers, peanut butter, soup. I realized quickly that depression did not have an appetite.*

## DAY 2

*Not knowing when the day ended and the next began, I continued to lie one more day in the dampness and the darkness of my parent's basement. I was amazed today, as I was yesterday, at how dark it really was down there, and I was thankful for my hiding place. I felt like a piece of shit, and I could feel my thoughts spiralling down ... down ... down.*

*As I lay there, not regarding the time, I could hear someone coming quietly down the stairs. My sister? My dad? My mom? My mom. At the bottom of the steps, she whispered quietly, "Chris ... Chris?"*

*"WHAT?" I replied, loud and frustrated, as I turned onto my other side to hide my face.*

*"Did you want something to eat ... for breakfast? It's 10:30."*

*"NOOO!" I barked at her. "Just leave me alone! Fuck! I don't want ANYTHING! And take this food back up too!"*

*"Okay, okay, you should eat something, though," she replied disheartened. "Here are your pills, Chris. I'll leave them right here on the table from now on." Then I heard her walk slowly back up the stairs. I could sense fear and worry in her voice as she talked with my dad upstairs. I couldn't hear them clearly, but it wasn't cheerful. I could tell they were really worried but, really, I didn't care because I felt so low. At that moment, there wasn't anything that I could possibly want, and my medication was the LAST thing I cared about. But, for some reason, against my will, I would take the fucking little pills as prescribed at bedtime. Man, I felt shittier this morning. I stared at the pill bottle. Fuck, if only these pills worked immediately ... like magic, I thought.*

*I lay back on my side facing the stairwell. I could see some light reflecting in the hallway, but only faintly. It was still very dark. My shoulders were becoming quite sore so I moved back and forth from side to side, hour after hour. Because of the thin mattress, and being on the floor, I was not getting any support, but who the fuck cared? I didn't!*

*I felt even worse today than I did yesterday, a lot worse. My head was hurting, I had developed a migraine, and my mind was racing with more and more negative thoughts. "Fuck," I said, as I stared up at the dark ceiling. I felt SO shitty! I shook my head and I could feel worry for the hundredth time over the last day. I was really concerned. I had never ever felt anything like this before. I'd been so lively and full of energy only months ago. This wasn't me! This wasn't Chris Nihmey! I rolled back and forth, trying to fall asleep. It was my only escape from these terrible, destructive thoughts: the thoughts that pounded my head over and over ... thoughts that I would be subject to for so long, not only in the basement, but thereafter. I equated these thoughts to Chinese torture experiments, where a drop of water falls on your forehead every thirty seconds, repeatedly, until you go crazy and die. I'll never forget it. Never.*

## DAY 3

*Without knowing it at the time, I was also suffering from something other than bipolar disorder, which I will delve into later. A second mental illness, an awful debilitating disease was also invading my mind that summer. Something we just didn't understand. Although it was always there, we never saw it fully develop until my major depression of 2001, where it all but took over my mind. Daily, my thoughts that summer took on a whole new meaning. The medical expression for these unwanted thoughts was "obsessions". These thoughts drastically caused the chaos which took over my mind, and would for so many years following. In hindsight, I had experienced these obsessions for years before.*

*So, with that, lying in the dark basement, my mind started to fixate on certain "subjects" that I deemed as the most important things in my life. That morning, although there were several different thoughts coming in, one particularly awful obsession started. I'd obsessed about it many times prior, but in this depressive state of mind, it took on a whole new meaning ... completely destructive.*

*My parents and sister heard it over and over again throughout my days in the basement. From downstairs, I sounded like a broken record day after day, repeating the same things. There were slurs, and there was swearing and dry tears.*

*The Wizard. "Why God, why? Why did we put that stupid damn wizard in our book? Why? I knew it was wrong, I knew it all along! (moan, groan, slam!) Mom! Dad! I'm going to go straight to hell for this! I KNOW IT!!! Straight to hell! Ahhh ... man! (slam!) I knew it was damn immoral to put that fucking thing in our book but we did it, we did! I knew it went against you, God, but I kept that stupid thing in the book, just to have a more "interesting" plot, even when I knew it was wrong! I knew it! NO! (moan, groan, slam!) I'm going to go to hell for sure; there is not a shred of doubt in my mind!"*

*So, even though I had had many obsessions that summer, I'd have to say that none of my thoughts were more destructive than these: the wizard and, more intensely, hell.*

***I was convinced I was going straight to hell when I died because my co-writer and I had written a friendly wizard into our children's book series. I was influencing every child who read my book to become immersed in the occult.***

*That was the thought, and it literally took me through "hell on earth". I was half of the way there, godammit!*

*You may wonder why "this" particular thought? Why did this fester so much in my head during my depression? Let me explain. There is a reason, not that it's really a valid one.*

*As mentioned already, spirituality is a theme often induced by a chemical shift into mania. One might attend different churches (yep), read monotonous spiritual material (yep), pray incessantly (yep), adopt new faith practices (yep), meet new spiritual friends (yep), and donate insurmountable amounts of money (yep, that too).*

*That was me only months before. You remember my antics. Now the question was this. What were the terrible repercussions of the journey I had taken only months before?*

*I had acquired something from that manic journey, something that took hold of my mind and rocked me. It seemed to never let go. It was a thought that I truly believed deep within my heart and soul. From the array of churches, spiritual hotlines, spiritual books, and on and on, no spiritual concept was greater than the horrific subject of "hell", and ending up there eternally because of making poor choices.*

*This was the worst thought I could ever have! Can any thought be worse than going to hell, the thought of being separated from God for all eternity? The answer has got to be a resounding NO! You might lose a loved one in your life, you might be in a serious accident and subject to a bed or wheelchair for life. You might lose the best job you ever had, or even go bankrupt. But I assure you ... they all pale in comparison to going to hell. Nothing in life is as severe as the consequence of eternal damnation and my mind accepted this in a profound way.*

*During my mania, books and churches and church folk were constantly reminding me of this horrific place. Many of these spiritual experts (as I had seen them at the time) had talked constantly about many things that God would never condone and would point His condemning finger at. One of the topics that continued to come to the surface during my journey was the subject of witches and wizardry. These books and church folk had all stated ...*

***"A man also or woman that hath a familiar spirit, or that is a wizard, shall surely be put to death ...." Leviticus 20:27***

***King James Version***

*This stood alongside numerous other spiritual assertions. Add to that a "God guilt" that I developed as I grew into my teens. These thoughts led to one fucked-up individual. Then add the chemical imbalance of bipolar disorder to the mix. That'll fuck you up big time, and it did ... big time!*

*So, in the depressive state I was in, I conjured in my mind quite simply that God would NEVER let me in through Heaven's gates. I would surely be condemned to a life of eternal suffering. Despite speaking with a priest and a pastor about this issue before we published, and both having given me the go ahead, I still felt this immense anxiety. I would continue to lament the decision to put the wizard in our book. How could we have done that?*

*This hell thinking was not new to me, but in my state of mind that summer it really affected me. I had had a fear of hell growing up, but as a twenty-six-year-old suffering from mental illness, hell took on a whole new meaning. What was causing me to transfix myself on this completely destructive obsession?*

*Although I sat there asking myself these questions, I learned later that the answer lay deep within my mania. I was deeply affected by these thoughts about the afterlife. Only months before, I was on a one way trip to the "pearly gates"! But now?*

*Eventually, I did fall asleep late in the afternoon. My sleep was uneasy, and I remember having horrible and intense dreams. This became a pattern. I woke up often in huge sweats. I was panting and my forehead was hot and wet. All my negative thoughts were getting the best of me, even in my sleep. Good God, what was next? I thought.*

*My dad came down the stairs close to suppertime and asked, "Will you have some soup, Chris?"*

*"NO."*

*"Just a little?"*

*"NO!" I said louder and with more conviction this time.*

*"It will be right here," he said, as he placed the bowl on the table and headed upstairs. No food for me, I said to myself, but I could smell the soup. It was tomato. Maybe a little wouldn't hurt. I rolled over to the table and took two spoonfuls. It was nothing special and, like yesterday, my appetite was still gone, so I ate very little. I spent the rest of the day alone quietly in the darkness of the basement. My sister came down to talk, but I refused to, like yesterday. I preferred to be alone.*

## DAY 4

*"RING ... RING ... RING!"*

*"OH GOD, my damn cell phone again!" I rolled over to face the phone. It was the fourth time, at least, that it had rung since I'd come down here, but like the other times, there was NO FREAKIN' way I was answering! I didn't want to speak to ANYONE at all. I actually remember that I had a fear of speaking to anyone because of how terrible I felt. I would have been lost for words, speechless. What would I say? What would they say?*

*"RING ... RING ... RING!"*

*It rang again and again. I finally reached for the stupid phone and looked at the screen. GOD! It was work again, my lifeguarding job at the RA Centre. Just great! I can't answer it! I feel so shitty ... man, what do I do? What do I do? What DO I do? I can't lifeguard right now! Think Chris think. Finally the phone stopped ringing. It obviously went to my voicemail. What the hell do they want? Oh my God, was I supposed to be at work? I looked at my phone. It was Tuesday. I didn't work Tuesdays, thank goodness. There was no way I could handle anything right now! I had already changed a shift yesterday to avoid going in. Actually, my dad had made the call. I just couldn't do it. I couldn't speak to anyone. Now work was aware I wasn't feeling well. How long could I hold them off? Time would tell. All these thoughts were rummaging through this confused head of mine.*

*I picked up the phone and dialled into my voicemail to see what work wanted. I had done this a few times already.*

*"You have one message. First message ..."*

*I listened. It was my pool boss, Chuck. He was wondering if I could come in for an afternoon shift. They were short a lifeguard and he asked if I was feeling better and could get back to them, ASAP. I listened again and again and hung the phone up. Work? Man, I couldn't even imagine it! What would I say? What would they think? I didn't have the energy, let alone confidence, to say that I couldn't work. I yelled upstairs in desperation.*

*"DAD! DAD!!!"*

*My dad hurried down the stairs. With my hand on my forehead, and propped up on my elbow, I looked up at him and told him my predicament. Fear and worry rested on my face and filled my voice.*

*"I'll make the call, Chris. Don't worry. You sit back."*

*"BUT, BUT ...," I said anxiously, "they're going to think ... they're going to think ... oh my God! I can't, I can't, you can't call again! I gotta go in, Dad!" I began to whine and moan, not for the first time. My dad reassured me that they would think nothing of the sort.*

*"People get sick ... and you're sick." He told me to trust him, and I did, and what was done was done.*

*Man, I was feeling worse and worse as days continued. I felt myself falling lower and lower into an abyss of depression. Could I feel any worse than I do now? Little did I know that this was only the beginning of a long and uncomfortable journey.*

## DAY 5

*Over the next few days, and the many that followed, there was a lot of moaning and groaning going on. My head would throb and I would moan and groan aloud and, at times, I would be loud ... very loud. It disturbed everyone in the house, but I just didn't care. My life had become a sham and I felt so damned awful about everything. I guess I just wanted to let my family know how bad I felt. I wanted them to know how bad it was, so they didn't think that I was faking. Then again, how could they? I mean, why would anyone ever fake something like this?*

*"OHHHH! WHHHHYYYYY? WHHYYY?"*

*I remember many times that my parents had to run downstairs just to see if I was okay, because I was so loud. They became so fearful and frustrated. I would yell out exactly how I felt and where my life was heading: going nowhere fast and wanting to end everything. It was very hard for them to see and hear me like this. I was their son, a grown man, with skills and training, with a vibrant mind. Yet here I was, stuck in their basement with no hope of ever making it back into the world again. I was a lost soul, with nowhere to go but down.*

*That morning, and into afternoon, I continued my downward slide towards a living hell. That's what it really was: a living hell. Little did I know that, on this particular day, I was not near the brink; I still had a long way to go. As I did, from these days on, I ended my night by downing a handful of pills prescribed by the doctor. For some reason, even though I didn't want to, I continued to take them. What good were they doing? I thought. At the time, NOTHING. That's how it felt.*

*As night approached, my dad came downstairs. He made his way through the darkness and sat in one of the reclining chairs beside me. Only a bit of light came from the stairwell upstairs. The windows were pitched- black now, as night was upon us.*

*"Chris?" my dad whispered quietly. "I want to read you something."*

*I rolled over to my other side and cupped my ears. I didn't want to hear anything he had to say.*

*"It's just something I think you'll find useful,"*

*"What? What is it?" I asked, wishing he'd go away.*

*"It's just a prayer that mom had. I thought I might read it with you."*

*"NO!" I barked out loud at him, "Just go away! I don't want to hear anything! Nothing. Take it the fuck away! Christ!"*

*"It is not very long," my dad coaxed. I felt nothing but negative feelings towards things such as prayer ... besides, I was downright angry at God for letting this happen to me. I didn't want to talk to Him anymore, not for a long time, maybe never. He led me down this path and I would never forgive Him. Here I was, dying in the dark while He sat up there watching in His damned white chair. It took a while before I was ready to let God seep back into my life. My dad gave up trying, wished me goodnight and crept quietly up the stairs.*

## DAY 6

*By now, I was getting accustomed to living in the dark. With a washroom downstairs, where I had finally taken my first shower in the dark, I needn't ever go up. And that sat well with me. I remember feeling the stubble on my face, but I did not have the strength to shave, nor did I really care.*

*I could see fairly clearly around me, a couch, a chair, a table and TV, OFF! I lay flat on my back on a thin mattress in the centre of the room. The covers that I had over me were kicked to the base of the mattress. I wore only a pair of boxers and t-shirt, but I remember being hot and sweaty, kind of like having a high fever. I had to splash some water on my face, at times, but I never turned the washroom light on. I avoided looking at myself in the mirror. I didn't want to see what "shit" looked like, because I definitely felt like it.*

*Even though the air conditioner was in full mode, I still experienced the "sweats" and found out later that this was one of the many side effects of the pills I was taking. I didn't even know what they were at the time. The pills were there to get me going again, but I doubted their results right from the start. Nothing was going to help me. Nothing. No doctor, no medication, nothing would help me anymore.*

*I was now feeling worse than before. It felt like I was getting sicker, rather than improving. Was the medication doing anything? It didn't feel like it was. I felt like a lost soul, trying to find his way back to the light, surrounded by nothing but darkness.*

*I could faintly hear my parents and my sister upstairs on her visits, living life how one ought to live: meeting friends, sitting on the computer, talking on the phone, watching TV. Yah, watching TV. Many would think, "Oh, he's feeling sick; at least he can lie down and sleep and watch TV." Well, I did none of the sort. First off, I barely slept because my mind wouldn't rest. My thoughts were spinning and taking me all over the place; negative and obsessive thoughts pounded me down. Secondly, I never watched TV. For almost a whole month, I never turned the damned thing on. I despised it, and hated hearing it on upstairs. At the time, TV, to me, meant people were alive and living their lives and doing things and feeling happy. I wanted nothing of that because of how I felt. It would take a long while before the "on" button of the remote was pushed. Little did I know, or care, that my family was not living "the grand life" upstairs. They weren't feeling what I was feeling, but they weren't feeling good either.*

***"... though I walk through the valley of the shadow of death ...." Psalms 23:4 (KJV)***

## DAY 7

*It took more than six days for me to actually start eating a decent meal. Over the last few days, my mother had tried to "force-feed" me by providing me with food, but I didn't finish it; sometimes I didn't touch any. I felt too damn awful, and I just wasn't into eating anything. Soup and crackers seemed to be the only thing that would go down.*

*I lay on my side staring at one of the basement walls. In the dark, I could faintly see pictures and plaques on the wall—many years of great achievements— swimming ribbons, football certificates and plaques, along with dozens of pictures of a life that I once knew. But things were different now. Both family and friends would no longer see me the same. I had morphed into something that was hard to get a handle on, and I wondered if anyone would ever truly understand me anymore. I doubted it that morning, as I glanced at the far wall. A tear trickled its way down my cheek when I noticed something very precious hanging on the wall. It was the first poignant thought I had experienced since the day I'd found out about my new condition. A tear holds so much inside it. At least mine did.*

*On the wall, I could make out a happy memory from my past. A circular clay frame hung between many great family achievements. And although I couldn't see it clearly, I knew what it was. I had seen it countless times from being down here, but always in a different light. What hung there was a clay imprint of a four-year-old's hand, moulded many years before, during this child's first year of school: a healthy child who was ready to take on the world. It was a much simpler and happier time for that child: a time of innocence, a time of passion for life, a time of exploration. It was a child with a whole world ahead of him, new and exciting. He had a verve for life. And, yes, that child was me.*

*It definitely had been a much happier time. We were now all suffering.*

*I rolled over and shut my eyes.*

## DAY 8

*I was suffering horribly. This was very obvious. I mean, for God's sake, here I was lying here, refusing to go anywhere, in the middle of a pitched-black room, in a mental state consisting of agony, defeat and depression. Mentally, I was completely shot, but I was also experiencing physical discomfort. My body was starting to ache from lying on the thin mattress. I found myself having to change positions over and over to relieve the strain on my body. Horror stories of bed rash in hospital rooms kept me moving periodically from side to side and front to back. The mattress wasn't giving me any cushioning. It was so fucking thin!*

*Each day, I hurt more and more and this caused me grief; physical discomfort affected my mental state. It seemed that the deeper I fell into depression, the more pain and suffering I was enduring, both mentally and physically. However, I must say that nothing outweighed the mental pain. Nothing ever did. I could deal with the physical for as long as I had to, and I did. But it was the mental anguish that kicked my ass day in and day out.*

*After returning from the cottage, my parents faced another dilemma. They did not want others to know that I had fallen into a depression. They had to keep things hushed from those who knew that they had had to leave. They didn't want anyone to know, including mine and their friends, in order to protect me from the stigma surrounding mental illness. They pretended that they were still at the cottage and laid low until the time of their scheduled return. I was thankful they did. I didn't want to talk to anyone or listen to anyone, or see anyone. Although they made all efforts to ensure my privacy, it was difficult when people did call the house, or even visited. This was challenging for them. They often had to peer through the window blinds to see who was at the door. It may have looked silly, but it was vital to keep things "under wraps", and we all did for a long while.*

*That day, as I did every day, I continued to experience an over-abundance of thoughts concerning the wizard and hell. Also, many other obsessions began to fester and fill my mind. Fears of going to hell forever played havoc on my thoughts and took me on a teeter-totter ride between being safe in God's hands, to being a ball recklessly bobbing in an ocean of fire. Thoughts pierced my mind over and over. It was like being shot with dozens of arrows, not enough to kill one instantly, but enough to leave you hanging on for dear life, in ceaseless pain, and hoping to survive another day.*

***"Superman's not brave. You can't be brave if you're indestructible. It's everyday people, like you and me, that are brave knowing we could easily be defeated but still continue forward."***

***Unknown***

*By night time, I was exhausted. I had no idea where I was heading or what would happen tomorrow. I cared less about tomorrow, though. I was just relieved to have barely survived another day of all this shit.*

## DAY 9

*At about this time, I was starting to realize that I had been in the basement far too long. But you know what? I just didn't care. I needed my own space and my own time and I didn't want to do anything or see anyone ... ever. I couldn't bear to face the days, so I stayed right where I was. I needed night, twenty-four hours a day. Besides, I had everything I needed down there—a washroom and my food brought to me. My clothes were sprawled out all over one section of the basement. My parents continued to bring me fresh clothing, but that didn't really matter. Most of the clothes just ended up piling up beside me. I changed sometimes, but mainly I was comfortable in what I was wearing at the time. I just didn't care.*

*I spent a lot of my time under the covers. I would often throw the heavy blanket over my head to turn everything completely off—no light from the window sills, no light from the stairwell and no sound underneath. It was my way of escaping it all. Hiding under the covers became normal for me that summer, and especially came in handy when the odd person did come by to visit my folks. This persisted intermittently for years after in times of depression. Because my parents were "technically" back from the cottage now, people were visiting and the regular flow of phone calls was flooding in. I didn't like it one bit. I would hear stomping in the kitchen above and I would hear voices and laughter that I just couldn't stand. They were happy and joyful while I lay in shit and shambles. My parents tried to keep my situation quiet; most still assumed that I was at the place on Elgin.*

*My cell phone continued to ring. My friends were calling, wondering where I was. Work continued to call to see when I'd be returning. Dad was doing a bang-up job returning my calls. My friends were worried because I usually called them right back. This was way out of the ordinary. How long could this go on? Little did I know that it would go on ... and on ... for a long time. Thankfully, my work was to end in August. Little did they know, at the time, that I would not return again.*

## DAY 10

*On this day, I actually had my first glimmer of hope ... small ... and I mean, small. I had been in my parents' basement for nine days ... now ten, ugh. I had avoided the light of day since my last doctor's visit a few days prior. My parents found out the hard way that getting me out to these weekly visits was difficult, and always ended in a battle. So, other than these visits to the hospital, my time had been spent in the dark basement.*

*For the first time since I'd gone downstairs, I actually made my way up, slow step by slow step, under my own will. I was following the doctor's directions. He told me to try and go into the light, even if it was for only one minute a day. He had told me this the day I went into emergency, and it took until DAY 10 to do so! I did it, but I felt that I had failed. It was all of a minute or so, maybe less, but it was dreaded. I slowly crept up the stairs and surprised my parents when I walked into the kitchen. I looked at them, they looked at me, I felt nauseous and right away I knew I had to get back downstairs. Life was scary up there, so I turned around and quickly made my way back. I threw the covers over my head and stayed under them for the rest of the afternoon, coming up only for air. I also remember screaming into the blanket again, as I had that morning. This happened often over that time.*

*Although I ended up back where I initially started, the trip upstairs was not for nothing. In retrospect, we looked at it as a defining moment in my recovery from depression. Dr. Boyles had given me a simple list of progressive steps I should take each day of the week. Each step, he said, would bring me closer to joining the world again. When he gave me the plan, I was so averse to following these steps, I ended up fighting against them. A fear of going back into the world feeling lost, confused and angry, made re-entering difficult. Because of this, I became stubborn and didn't want to follow his advice. Because of the depression, I was afraid to do anything. My confidence was shot.*

*Following are the steps he laid out for me. They were what he termed, "Baby Steps". It was almost like learning how to walk again.*

***PROGRESSIVE EXERCISES FOR COMING OUT OF DEPRESSION:***

1. *Take sheets off the head, open your eyes.*
2. *Take a shower each day. (Lights off, then eventually on)*
3. *Seek daylight by walking upstairs to sit in the kitchen.*
4. *Step into the backyard, 5 minutes per day.*
5. *Sit outside in the backyard for 15 minutes per day.*
6. *Go for a 5 minute walk around the neighbourhood.*

*To give you an idea of how long it took me to achieve these goals, I didn't reach Step 4 until August. It took me that long to stay in the light for that brief a period of time. Depression was that excruciating. Every day was a fight that I felt I just couldn't win. I didn't really start any of these steps until late July. Before that, I was basically hibernating in the basement. I just didn't care.*

## DAY 11

*Early this morning, I got up to go to the washroom. I usually did this in the dark but, for some reason, I turned on the light. I surprised myself, and my eyes surprised me; they adjusted relatively quickly to the light, considering the fact that they had become so used to the dark. As I stood there, I looked at myself in the mirror. God, I looked terrible, but what did I expect? I was living the life of a hermit. I stared at myself, my hair in disarray, my skin pale, my face unshaven. I looked like a real horror show. I looked terrible, and seeing myself only made me feel worse.*

*As I stared in the mirror, I suddenly caught myself reminiscing. I remembered something that affected my life in a profound way, a negative stepping stone to the distraught life I would live for years following. It was an earlier episode of depression.*

*It was 1998. I was teaching at a Catholic elementary school, my first job as a full-time teacher. I was young and vibrant, eager to learn and gifted to teach, but something was not right.*

[*The lunch bell rings at 11:15. You leave your class for lunch. You're not really hungry, but you have to eat something. You walk down the hallway with a smile on your face. To everyone else, you look amazing. You are Mr. Nihmey, the rookie, the hero, the dependable.*

*"Hi, Mr. Nihmey!" the kids and teachers shout out, as you walk down the hall.*

*"Hey there!" you respond, with that big smile of yours, the one that helped get you to where you are.*

*You look strong and confident on the outside, but deep inside, you carry a dark secret. Inside you feel nothing but fear, shame, loneliness and despair.*

*You head quickly downstairs and take your lunch out of the staffroom fridge. You quickly gobble down the "cold" items in your lunch, because you can't carry them back up. You're trying everything to avoid seeing anyone else. You do bump into the odd teacher, but you are great at deflecting your emotions. They see nothing different in you at all. You're good at hiding things. It would become life's ritual from this time forward.*

*You finish up some of your lunch, grab your bag and head back upstairs just as the kids are heading outside. It's 11:35. You hear the doors at the back open up as the students flood outside. It happens the same way every day, Monday to Friday. Quickly, you enter the quiet upper hallway of the school. The last few kids are trickling out. You can see them running now. They are late and the lunchtime fun has begun. Kids hate to miss any part of recess!*

*Finally, the coast is clear, so you head to the only place you can to avoid seeing anyone, anyone at all. You head to the staff washroom.*

*You enter and lock the door behind you. Click. You turn on the light first and stare into the mirror. You see a worthless, no good, piece of shit standing there. What good are you? You're going to fail miserably. Why go on? Give up now!*

*You flit with your tie a little bit, and you look away and turn off the lights. You check again to make sure the door is locked. It is. You are safe ... for now. You then lie down on the floor on your back with your head at the base of the toilet. Your body is lying flat. You don't have to go to the washroom, but you need to lie down. You feel weak, tired, and have no energy.*

*While the other teachers are laughing and enjoying their lunch in the staffroom, you need to escape from your thoughts and your fears, so, for 40 minutes, almost every day, you do this for months and months. Others think you have stepped out, or that you are in your classroom. Little do they know. Even though you are in the dark, you close your eyes to escape the voices inside your head. You listen as teachers walk by, oblivious to what is happening inside. The odd person tries the locked door—occupied, they realize, and walk on. You can hear voices and you see shadows pass by, but you remain quiet and still. Nothing. No noise, you are barely breathing. And, worst of all, is the complete despair you feel, the thought that the world has beaten you down, and you can't ever get up. You are alone. Even God has turned His back on you.*

*For the next forty minutes, you will feel these thoughts. You will try to fight them, but they always win. You can't win this battle. You can't. They are too strong and you are too weak.*

*At 12:13, the same warning bell startles you: every time. The kids will be coming inside in only two minutes. Quickly, you stand up and turn the light on. Your eyes slowly adjust. You look in the mirror once again and you still see that same worthless loser in front of you. You fix your tie and you tuck your shirt in your pants. You dust off your shirt and pants, splash some water on your face, check your hair, your teeth and your shoes. You slowly open the door. Thank God, no one is around. Where am I, you wonder? Oh, I'm here.*

*You feel safe for the moment, until you bump into the first person you see. What will they say? Will they find out about your secret? On the inside you feel like shit and, at the time, little did you know that there would be times far worse than this. But for now, you must teach, you must laugh, and most importantly, you must smile. It is your only saving grace—your beautiful smile. You are living behind a lie and no teacher or student you taught, ever knew. Until now.*]

***"For anyone suffering from mental illness, a mirror is a dangerous place. It exposes your weaknesses, your deepest fears, reminding you just how infinitely small you really are. You are truly alone. The mountain is yours to climb and no one else's. The decision to begin healing must be yours and yours alone."***

*That morning, I thought about this and the many difficult moments of my first two years teaching, where depression was frequent, and mania peeked its vicarious head out. I remember staying at school most nights until 10 pm, working frantically and obsessively in my classroom, and returning the next morning at 7 am, before the custodian! I would return the next day to a room in disarray, only to realize that I had nothing ready for that teaching day.*

*[One day, I pretended to faint in class, just to be able to leave school to get to a safer place. I was off for a whole week, most of the time lying in bed, depressed. I even missed my sister's university graduation in Nova Scotia. People wondered what happened that week. Thankfully, few asked, but who knew what they assumed? That same year, many mornings, I would cry on the phone to my dad from the photocopy room, where I would simply say, "I'm not going to make it, Dad."*

*It was from another grade four class the following year that I would actually leave in December, resigning from the job. It was a class I loved with amazing kids, but what could one do? It would take much courage to face my principal in December, 1999, to be able to tell her and the staff and students that I was leaving teaching to pursue my writing career. Thank God I had writing to hide behind. Writing was never the real reason. It was just an excuse. As I've said, I was* ***living a lie****, and would for years after.*

*It would be a grade five/six class that would bring me back to permanent teaching in the next school year, this time, only to resign once again, in December 2000. "I am going to travel and write." In reality, my mind couldn't cope with its thoughts, and depression was destroying me. This was the reason that I would cry silently in the supply room every morning, staring out the window at birds flying so free and wishing I was one of them. Tears would fill my eyes, as I heard the kids making their way down the hall towards our classroom. And with a quick wipe and a silent prayer, I received them with open arms.*]

*God help me! Here I am again ...*

***"Inside my heart is breaking***
***My make-up may be flaking***
***But my smile still stays on."***

***THE SHOW MUST GO ON – Queen***

**DAY 12**

*I refused prayers early on in my depression. I would have nothing to do with them. I hated them. I hated God for letting me down. I wanted nothing to do with Him. How could I trust Him anymore?*

*I remember my dad or my mom coming down each night into the basement to try and pray with me, hoping to breathe some life back into me.*

*"Get out of here!" I would constantly yell. "Leave me alone! Go back up!"*

*I detested even the thought of prayer. It made me sick. Prayer sucked and it took a long time for prayer of any kind to become part of my life again.*

*I felt that God had been toying with my life all along. He definitely knew something that I didn't and He'd taken me for a wild ride. God was everything only months before. I had put my entire trust in Him. Nothing else mattered. I felt, for the first time in my life, truly alone. Sure, I had my family, but my God had turned His back on me and left me in the darkness. At times, I even questioned His existence.*

*I held this position over the many days I spent downstairs. With much coaxing from my parents, I finally let my dad downstairs to pray for me, but NOT with me. That would not happen for a long time. And even when I did allow him to pray, my heart and my thoughts were a great distance away. His voice was somewhat soothing, but the meaning behind the words was lost.*

*My dad would pray one simple prayer and then he would leave. He started to do this every night. He read it so many times that summer that eventually it became ingrained in my mind. At the time, it was like a headache and I tried to filter it out. Now, it means much, much more to me.*

***JESUS HELP ME***

***In every need let me come to you with humble trust saying, Jesus Help Me!***

***In all my doubts, perplexities and temptations, Jesus Help Me!***

***In hours of loneliness, weariness and trials, Jesus Help Me!***

***In the failure of my plans and hopes, in disappointments, troubles and sorrows, Jesus Help Me!***

***When others fail me and Thy grace alone can assist me, Jesus Help Me!***

***When I throw myself on Thy tender love as a Father and Saviour, Jesus Help Me!***
***When my heart is cast down by failure at seeing no good come from my efforts, Jesus Help Me!***

***When I feel impatient and my cross irritates me, Jesus Help Me!***

***When I am ill and my head and hands cannot work and I am lonely, Jesus Help Me!***

***Always, always, in spite of weakness, falls and shortcomings of every kind, Jesus Help Me! and never forsake me.***

***Dear Lord I pray, Thy Hand to take my body broken now for Thee. Accept the sacrifice I make Oh! Body broken once for me!***

***AMEN***

*My parents recited this prayer repeatedly until I started to recover. Most often, my ears shut out their words of hope.*

## DAY 13

*Depression continued to beat the crap out of me in that basement, as did my obsessions with hell. My thoughts and my feelings were still so negative, and I continued to feel myself spiralling downwards to who knows where. Where would it take me? I wondered. I hoped that I would never have to find out. I feared where I would land. I hoped that I could avoid falling into it. That would only mean a point of no return. Yes, suicide. I did think about it ... often.*

*My thoughts were horribly negative, my dreams equally awful. I had terrible nightmares, making me sick to my stomach. I've not talked about them until now. You may be aware of a dream in which you are running towards a door and you never quite reach it. In my dreams, I would reach and reach for a life I once had, only to find out that life would never be the same again. I had changed forever.*

*In one particular dream, I was reaching for someone's arm as I began to fall. I reached and reached, but to no avail, and tumbled towards the ground below. But, like all dreams, I would wake up before landing. Some people say that if one dies in a dream, they literally die. You can't imagine how many times in that basement I hoped I would hit the bottom and die. But that didn't happen. The hole seemed bottomless and I kept dropping and dropping, falling further and further towards a dark hell below. I quickly realized that death was not my biggest fear; it was being alone ... forever. Maybe that's really what hell is about—being alone.*

## DAY 14

*Two weeks. I still hadn't watched any television. It took me a long time to watch the tube again. I would have nothing to do with it. I'd stare at the blank box and hate the thought of even turning it on and hearing those voices: voices of people who were living their lives, happy and fulfilling. These sounds represented life; I felt mine was lost. My life was gone, and I hated anything that reminded me of my former life.*

*Upstairs, life continued. My sister, who attempted several visits downstairs to be there for me, was constantly being told to leave.*

*"Get out of here!" I would yell. "LEAVE ME ALONE ... FUCK!" Mom and Dad got that same treatment often, also.*

*Julie tried her best, but I would have nothing to do with her or anyone. Mom and Dad would continue to bring food, and I made my way up occasionally, but I still persisted in hibernating much of the time in that dark basement.*

*On this particular day, I remember waking up early in the morning and slowly creeping up the stairs. It was still quite dark in the house. I sat at the table and ate some cereal. I was surprised with myself. This was a first positive step. However, within minutes, I heard my dad coming downstairs. Mom followed. I stood up in a panic to go down. I didn't want to see them. But it was too late. They came into the kitchen and caught me trying to escape.*

*"Hi," my dad said in surprise. "Did you eat?"*

*"I had some cereal," I said. "I'm going down," I replied abruptly.*

*My mom asked me to stay for a bit. I sat back down. We looked at each other and I lay my head on the table. I really just wanted to go back down. Mom and Dad tried to make conversation. And then, something happened that was completely beyond my control. It came as a big surprise to all of us, because it was something I had not done. I started to cry. This was the first time I had done so in front of them. I cried really hard about everything that had happened. I cried, sobbing about the condition of my life and how awful I felt and how life had changed forever. I was finally realizing that I was about to live a new life, one that, according to me, made me less of a person. I was now going to live a life that would be so different from others. And I could not share this with anyone outside of my parents' home. Mom and Dad did their best to assure me that things would work out, but their words fell short. At that moment, nothing would change my thinking. They didn't help much at the time ... nothing really did, but their presence there while I cried was what I needed.*

*I wiped away my tears and headed back downstairs to hide. I threw the covers over my head and lay there for as long as I could. Then I turned onto my side and tucked the blanket into my neck. I put the blanket under my feet and, as I did, I closed my eyes and began to fall into another dream I'd regret having. And that's how life took its toll on DAY 14. I stayed put for the better part of day in the basement. Mom visited, so did*

*Dad, but I wasn't a good host for either of them. Each of their visits ended with quiet steps back upstairs. Once again, I lay alone, and that's exactly what I wanted.*

***"... it was then that I carried you."***

***Footprints In The Sand,***
***Mary Stevenson***

## DAY 15

*Into the third week of my depression, I was starting to think that I would be stuck downstairs for a long time. Things did not seem to be looking up. I had no hope in anything I was experiencing, and when there was a small spark, I simply dismissed it. There was only fear, doom and gloom in that head of mine, which led to thoughts of suicide. I had been suicidal several times already while dealing with depression, and as I lay down there in the basement, I started to think about it often, especially when obsessions of hell got the best of me.*

*ESCAPE! Would I slit my wrists, overdose? Would the future see me steering dangerously off the road in my car (that was, oh, too familiar)? Feeling so down in the dumps, these were the thoughts that sprung to life the longer I lay there. At the time, I kept these thoughts to myself in fear of scaring my family.*

*When I was first diagnosed with bipolar, I actually lay in bed and visualized myself taking a kitchen knife and slitting my wrists. It was a terrible thought, and one that I almost followed through. I even put the knife directly to my wrist, but I couldn't do it. Something kept me from doing it. As I write this today, I thank God HUGELY that I didn't. I've come to realize that I do have a purpose here and that God has a plan for me. Part of that plan was writing this story, and so I have.*

## DAY 16

*"Oh man, I feel like shit! This is ridiculous! How can I feel so goddamn shitty?"*

*I would repeat these thoughts over and over daily (just ask my folks), which was not a good thing. I would yell it from the basement, and the worse I felt, the more terrible the things I said. And as I said these things, I felt even worse. It was really like a double-edged sword and I continued to stab it into my head and my heart. I hated life, I hated it, I hated it ... I hated myself. I was just a useless piece of shit and I vowed to never come out of that basement. Ever! I didn't want to face the world. I would be down there the rest of my life, I was sure, and it's exactly where I wanted to be.*

*I must say, that my family was amazing during my time in the basement. They would make my calls, make my meals, motivate me enough to take a shower every few days, to shave, to dress, and did their best to give me mini pep-talks. I hated that, but I heard them, and I believe that they helped me in my recovery. Any caregiver can parent a healthy child, but the true measure of parenting is exemplified when they take care of a child who is sick, especially when they are a full-grown adult. Their love becomes a lifeline, a beacon of hope, and an instrument of healing.*

*On this particular morning, I took a shower. After soaping off, I stood with my arms up against the far wall. I stood there letting the water run down my back. As the water flowed, I closed my eyes and started to think of better days, but it didn't last. All that stayed in my head were the terrible thoughts I'd been having. I opened my eyes and looked around the shower stall. I started to move my feet quickly on the base of the stall, hoping that I'd trip and fall and hurt myself bad. Self-punishment was filling my mind. I agreed that if I couldn't successfully kill myself, I would definitely try to hurt myself. I failed this day, but I planned to attempt it again in different ways.*

***"No one sees the secrets, the lies, the ugly truth, the deep dark places—not family, friends, spouse, kids ... only you."***

## DAY 17

*"Who's that? Who's there?"*

*I stare into the darkness around me.*

*"Leave me alone!"*

*I stare deeper into the darkness.*

*"Are you still here? I said, leave me alone!"*

*I blink and rub my eyes. Is it still there?*

*"I just want to be by myself! Please! For godsakes!"*

*I roll over to my other side. It's still there. It won't leave me. It's unbelievable!*

*"Go away! Leave me the fuck alone!"*

*I close my eyes to escape the horror, but it slaps me again.*

*"Please, no, please, please! NO!"*

*I lie on my back and stare above into the darkness.*

*"Oh, you're up there too! Jesus, man!"*

*I grab a pillow and throw it into the dark. I slam another one down.*

*"You NEVER leave! Get the fuck out of here, NOW!"*

*I moan and groan and complain. I turn and toss.*

*"Why won't you leave???!!! Why?"*

*I put the covers over my head. Is it still there?*

*"Holy shit! I want to die!" I slowly pull the blanket down.*

*"You ARE still here! Oh my God. Holy shit!"*

*I stand up and carefully walk around the room in the dark. I fall back onto the mattress, and again throw the covers over my head. I close my eyes.*

*"Hello?" I ask. "Are you gone?"*

*I open my eyes.*

***YOU NEVER LEFT.***

*My mind was playing tricks on me. This was a conversation I had many times over with depression, or what I called at the time, "death". My thoughts were scattered and my mind was racing with negativity. And through all of this, I ended up back where I started— depressed in the dark basement. That's the tragic thing about being depressed. You hate it, but you accept it as normal because you see no other way and you can't see over the mountain that's right in front of you.*

## DAY 18

[*Earlier, I noted some of the baby steps I had to take to regain control of my life. Needless to say, the rehabilitation from the depths of depression was very slow, taking many months ... long months. In my progression from death to life, I had made only a few steps to heal until this day, and even those were minimal. Sure, I had made it up a few times to eat, and out for a weekly doctor's appointment that I was impelled to attend but, other than that, my time was spent in the dark.*]

*First and foremost, my doctor had recommended my going outside in daylight by myself and, by this day, I finally started to do so of my own volition. He had instructed me to do so three weeks prior and it was one of the hardest things I remember ever having to do. Up to now, I had done so only under escort. I would do anything to stay out of the light. Even going to the washroom was a struggle for me, but it had to be done and, this too, I often did in the dark. There were no bed pans down there, and I wasn't about to sit in my own filth, although I entertained that thought at times—yuk. That's how low I was!*

*It took a long while to follow my doctor's instructions. At first, he wanted me to go outside for at least five minutes. That was all he asked. That's it, that's all, but for me it was a huge struggle. I remember fighting so hard to step into the backyard on my own for the first time, to get the so-called "light" that he prescribed. I hated him SO MUCH for it! My first time outside seemed like hours, but it was only a measly minute. I stayed bent down to avoid anyone seeing me. I then darted back downstairs into the safety of the basement. It happened like this during the second and third week downstairs. I HATED the goddamn light!!!*

*But I persisted.*

## DAY 19

*By this day, I was finally moving on to "brighter" things. I was now able to sit in a room with a low light, but even that was tough. The darkness had become my ally, my friend, and I retreated to it as soon as possible. I had to relearn living in the "light" and make it part of my life again. My folks continued to turn lights on, despite my objections, until I was able to sit in a low-lit basement. This did not occur until today ... almost three weeks!*

*By now, I was finally starting to get out of bed of my own will. This had also been prescribed by my doctor, weeks before. All I wanted to do was sleep, sleep and sleep. This is a major symptom of depression. In reality, I didn't really sleep much at all. Though it looked like it, I would often just lie there in the dark and be restless, moving from side to side. I really wanted to sleep to get away from everything, but pain in my muscles often woke me out of dreamland, as I tossed and turned on the thin mattress.*

*I continued to obsess over many things, but especially the wizard that would be my ticket into the hot place. Why had I done it? I dreaded the answer. Going to hell was the ultimate price I would pay for this mistake. God is a God of forgiveness. Would he forgive me? I hoped so, but I doubted it.*

*I was now eating very small meals. At first, I didn't want to eat anything. If I had been staying on my own, I might have starved. During this time, I lost more than 15 pounds! The only time I had ever fallen that much was when I fasted the 9 days during mania. To me, food represented health and happiness, and I wanted nothing to do with it. Besides, feeling as shitty as I was, food had lost its appeal. Even a pizza, a burger or fries, which I formerly loved, were not appetizing. Blah!*

*And friends? It took me a helluva LONG time to even talk to my friends on the phone. However, by this week, my doctor urged me to start. My friends were very supportive and had much concern, but I didn't want to see or talk to them at all. I abhorred their lifestyles. They were successful and happy, while I struggled so much. I could not have what they had. Seeing them move forward while I was going in the opposite direction really sucked.*

*Prayer still took a back seat in my recovery. I didn't even want to think about God. Ironically, my faith eventually did lift me out, but for a long time, prayer was something I avoided. I had had way too much of it during my mania, and it was not kind to me. My dad continued to read his prayer to me nightly, but inside I blocked out his words.*

## DAY 20

*My phone did continue to ring periodically; this would drive me crazy. Still, against my parents' advice, I refused to turn it off out of a fear of missing calls ... like that really mattered!*

*Truthfully, I think the phone gave me some sense, maybe a false sense, that I was still alive. Sad to think, but I saw the phone as my only connection with the outside world. Funny though, I never answered the fucking thing! Voicemail became a huge saving grace. My dad would either take my calls or reply to people that called me. Work now knew that I was really sick and had given up calling. They were concerned, but my dad kept things hush-hush. As for my friends, he only told them that I was not feeling well, but he could only save my face for so long. Eventually, they got curious and began to wonder what the hell was up. My having not spoken to them in almost a month was very unusual.*

*I would not only receive calls from friends or work, but from bookstores and libraries and prospective customers for my new novel. Fuck, the last thing I wanted to do was talk to anyone about my book, but calls kept pouring in as the world continued to spin. Since the book had just been released a month earlier, the demand for it was high. Sales were popping up all over and our services were being solicited. Although I was in the dumps, my dad again became a saviour in helping to keep our adventure alive, delivering books for us.*

*It took several weeks before I could actually join him. When I was finally able to spend a little time in the daylight, he dragged me along with him—it was miserable. He thought it would be therapeutic, but I hated those fucking rides. We took books throughout Ottawa, and neighbouring towns. I detested every minute of those trips!*

*I would close my eyes tightly and lean over against the window, my head bumping lightly against the glass. I wouldn't open my eyes until we stopped, and even then, I'd close them right up again. And because I felt so shitty, my dad would actually make the deliveries to the stores. I stayed put to watch the car, because it needed watching? Someone had to do it! As I said, these were awful trips, not really the father-son bonding my dad had hoped for.*

## DAY 21

*Today, I had a mini-breakthrough. Prior to this, as I had mentioned earlier, television was something I strenuously avoided. I just didn't want to see anyone or hear anyone, see anyone who was happy, or see anyone who was living a life I only dreamed of living. A life I felt I could never live again.*

*I remember rolling over and reaching onto the table for some Kleenex. By mistake, I actually knocked the remote off the table and onto the floor. The room was dark and I started to fret, thinking I had broken it. Finding it, I pressed the power button. Prior to this, the only voices I had heard were those of my family and the hum of the kitchen TV. I often put pillows around both ears to drown that out.*

*The television slowly lit up and voices began and I diverted my attention back to the remote. As I fumbled for the power button, something happened. For some reason, I did not push the "off" button. Was I doing this for real? I wondered. Was I ready for this? A talk show was the first thing to come up. I forget which one, but I remember hearing them talking about relationships. This was an indication that the channel needed to be changed! The last thing I wanted to hear!*

*I skipped quickly through the channels. My parents would have been beyond thrilled to see me doing this. Click, click, click ... I scrolled from talk shows, to sports shows, to soap operas, to game shows. You name it, I saw it, and I hated it! I felt so lousy about my life. How the hell could all these people be living such great fun lives, while I sat down here in the dumps? Screw them all!*

*And then, my channel changing stopped. I arrived at a show that I had adored growing up. It was a rerun, and as I listened to the voices and watched the faces on the screen, I was stunned. I could not change the channel! Although the show was a comedy, I could not laugh. However, the voices and the characters were soothing to me, a comfort. As the cast conversed, I reminisced about a better time, a happier time, a life free from sickness and free from doubt. It was a show I had loved growing up, and I had seen the reruns countless times. Jack, Janet, Chrissy.*

*For those who may not have seen the show, its premise revolved around a bachelor named Jack Tripper (played by the late John Ritter), who was living with two young and attractive women in a two-bedroom apartment in Los Angeles. The building was managed by an outlandish landlord who believed that Jack was gay. Quite the contrary, Jack adored women and had to hide the fact that he was not gay; otherwise all three of them would be evicted. Each episode took the actors on a journey of bloopers and blunders, as they tried everything to avoid being kicked out by their loony landlord, Mr. Roper. It was none other than the sitcom, Three's Company.*

*Anyway, that's a quick summary for you and that's exactly what I saw as I suddenly stopped flipping the channels. It was an episode I had seen many times before. I leaned my head back to watch. In only minutes, my mind became distracted, and a bit entertained. It was a good feeling. I watched, but I never laughed. I just didn't feel like laughing. I did, however, derive comfort. It was a reminder of a time I was free from illness, a time of good health and good cheer. For the first time in weeks, I was feeling something positive. I could only hope to bottle up those moments that morning. But you know what? Life doesn't work that way. Life happens and things are forgotten and people get sick and people die and it's those things that seem to keep the world spinning. We don't always like it, but that's life, I guess.*

## DAY 22

*By now, I was finally finding the strength I needed to get off the mattress and make it upstairs into the land of the living. I looked like shit and I felt like shit, but at least I was tolerating the light of day. I was required to experience sunlight more and more each day, but it was hard—I can't stress this enough. You know the feeling you get when you step into the bright sun after being stuck in a dark room for hours? You step out but you can't see anything. You squeeze your eyes tightly to avoid letting any light in. My first attempts at coming upstairs had failed miserably, but now I was starting to do it, hating every minute of it, but doing it nonetheless.*

*My doctor was laying out a plan of attack, with the goal of getting me back on my feet again. I still felt like a truck had hit me, but I was now taking the steps I needed to take. Mornings were still very hard, but I was now making my way upstairs to eat.*

*"Will you eat something, Bob?"*

[*I guess you're scratching your head wondering who the hell Bob is? I never mentioned it before, but my mom had called me Bob for years. Bob this, Bob that! She may have derived it from what my dad called me using an Arabic expression for father, "Ba". She may have derived it from the name, Jim Bob. Either way, I heard it early on in my life, and we just went with it. I would be Bob from that day forward. I didn't mind it. What's even weirder is that my dad calls me "Dad". He has for years. His dad had called him "Dad"; so my dad calls me "Dad"! It's a Lebanese thing!*]

*"Here's the cereal. Do you want some coffee?"*

*"No, no ... just cereal," I said, without looking up, reaching for the box. Mom poured my milk. Although I*

*felt uncomfortable being so needy, I didn't care. I took help whenever possible.*

*I still wasn't eating much. Mom would make meals, but I ate little. Cereal and toast became my staple foods. Oh, and peanut butter. I grew up liking that. Mom and Dad insisted on fruit and vegetables, but I didn't want them, much to my mother's chagrin. She wanted badly for me to get better, and quick. None of us knew how long that would take.*

## DAY 23

*Today I took my first walk outside. It only lasted a few minutes as I walked from the front of the house to the back. However, considering I hadn't walked outside in weeks, my parents were thrilled. I wasn't. I hated those walks outside. I felt so useless. I felt like a fool. Look at me! Look at me! I'm walking from front to the fucking back! The walks didn't get longer for awhile. It would take many more walks before I would do so without incessant complaining. I also did everything I could to avoid seeing anyone I knew. I would reverse or retreat if I did. Although I wore sunglasses and a hat, I had a few close calls! I didn't want anyone knowing anything about what had been happening to me that summer.*

*By this time, I was tolerating my dad reading the prayer with me. After several weeks and some steps forward in my healing, I allowed him to pray with me. Well, okay, I didn't pray, but he did. I would lie on the couch with my eyes closed and he would recite the Jesus Help Me prayer. This seemed to be "our" prayer, my dad's and mine. His voice was always both soothing and sincere. I hung onto his words, but still never thought much of the meaning behind what he was quoting. I was just comforted by his voice. Hearing my dad saying those prayers meant so much to me and I know they were vital in my healing that summer. I may have wanted him to shut up a lot at times, but there was a small part of me that knew deep down that I probably needed God. I just didn't know in what capacity I would allow Him back into my life. For the first time in my life, I was a skeptic. Was God really there? Many nights I would ask myself this question. I didn't expect to ask it for as long as I did, but that's where I was at. After trusting so deeply and then having your life turned upside down, boy, did your faith ever take a beating!*

*So, with all that had happened, I just didn't know which way to turn when my dad started reading. I decided not to turn at all. I just lay there, and every night at the same time, I would hear my dad's footsteps coming downstairs. And then, with my eyes closed, I would attempt to let God squeeze back into my life again, kind of like a mouse trying to enter a hole that is too small for its body.*

## DAY 24

*The twenty-fourth day of my depression, I had yet to speak to anyone, other than my parents, my sister and my doctor. I thought I'd have to learn to talk to people again! I wasn't able to man my own ship, so my family stepped up to the plate and did everything for me. Jesus, I felt in my heart of hearts, that I would never do anything independently again.*

*My thoughts continued to be so negative. I still never thought I'd make it back into the real world. I was convinced I'd be downstairs until I died.*

*That morning, my dad came downstairs.*

*"What are you watching, son?"*

*My dad sat beside me. I was flipping channels and my dad was pleased to see it. He knew that even channel surfing was a sign I was starting to heal, as little as it seemed at the time.*

*"Nothing ... nothing," I replied, as I turned a shoulder.*

*"Can I turn this light on?"*

*"NO! No, Dad. Please, I'm watching!" Although, I really wasn't.*

*Instead of trying to coax the conversation along, my dad said no more. All he did was sit there, I don't remember for how long, but he sat there as I lay, eyes on the screen. I told him I wanted to be alone, but I don't think that was the truth. His presence was comforting. He sat and he said not a word, but really, deep down, he left much unstated: strength, hope and love. I don't think either of my parents or my sister ever realized how much their support meant at the time. It was what I remembered as a child growing up, when I was reliant on them for everything. However, this time, I was a twenty-six-year-old and two things were vastly different. First, I was no longer a kid, I was a man. Secondly, and most importantly, I was sick. And that's what hurt the most. And it would be this way from now on.*

## DAY 25

*We all suffered. I may have been the one directly handicapped by the illnesses, but my mom, dad and sister were also feeling the heavy burdens of a sick son and brother. It was terrible seeing me on the doorstep to hell. Every day that I awoke moaning and groaning in mental anguish, was every day that my family suffered beyond belief.*

*Imagine. Imagine that your only son, a young and vibrant individual, charismatic and genuine, cannot make his way out of the darkness: his personality, beaten and battered by pain one cannot see, pain only he can feel, pain that no one can truly understand.*

*Even today, I can still hear those footsteps to the basement, and the countless times my family asked me the simplest of questions. Are you hungry? Are you warm enough? Do you need anything else? How are you feeling today? These were questions that no one should ever have to ask a grown man. I was a grown man, godammit, but one who could no longer feed himself, barely clothe and clean himself or simply take care of himself.*

*Wow, was I actually there? It's really hard to believe, but I was. As I sit here today, I have to say that I pray for every soul who has to go there, especially without the support I had. Mental illness sucks. I pray for everyone that has to sit on the same doorstep to hell that I sat on. For that high school kid who trudges the halls every morning and sees a climb rather than a simple walk.*

*Today I moved forward some, but it wasn't as productive as I'd hoped. I stayed downstairs, watching a bit of TV. What followed? Hopefully what my parents prayed for ... "just one day better than the last". If each day could be just a little bit better, we would chalk it up as a success.*

## DAY 26

*Shit, I think I'm going crazy!*

*And I was, I really was! I had been in the basement for too many days and thoughts were now getting the best of me. I felt like a failure. I felt from that day forward, I would fail at everything I would ever do. My confidence was shot! I would never teach or write or be in a relationship again. I just knew it. My books would stop selling and I would never be able to continue the series. I would stay sick and shut in here for the rest of my life. It was overwhelming to think all these negative thoughts, and although my family was a great support for me, I still felt like I was a ship going down.*

*Days rolled into nights, and my dad continued to read his Jesus prayer. All I could do was let the words roll off his tongue, through my head and then out. I'm not sure if I believed those words. I was still so angry at God for striking me down with this awful disease. I would have preferred cancer. It would have killed me quickly or I could have been cured. Instead, I would be stuck with these illnesses my entire life. I wasn't sure if I'd find faith in God again. What had He done for me? Oh yah, He made me sick!*

## DAY 27

*I woke up early and turned on the TV. Three's Company wasn't on, but I searched for it. I didn't think it would be on at 6 am, but I longed to hear John Ritter's goofy voice. On channel 15, I stopped at a morning talk show. I watched for a minute or so, but had to turn from it quickly because I felt sick to my stomach. How could they all be so fucking happy and bright? As REM sang, "... shiny happy people holding hands!!!" Yah, right! Shiny, my ass!*

*I rolled over and sat up on my elbows. On channel 3, a cartoon appeared. Quickly flipping through from 3 to 70, I watched our world transpire before my very eyes. Talk shows, comedies, game shows, soap operas, suspense; there was life and there was death. And as I flipped, I noticed something. While life had changed so much for me in such a profound way, the world around me had not. Little had seemed to change. People were still crying, lying, deceiving, stealing and dying. It was sad to see that, and it kind of ruined my morning. That's TV for you! Feel shitty, watch TV, feel shittier. I realized then that for me, TV was definitely a depressant!*

*The morning wasn't great, but I did manage to turn my day into an okay one. My accomplishments that day were few; some of them were firsts. It was the best that I'd had up to now.*

*I walked to my parent's car to get something: my first big trip away from the house, the parking lot, without being accompanied.*

*I read the mail. Well, flipped through a catalogue, if that counts!*

*I ate lunch in the kitchen. Okay, just some toast.*

*I watched some TV sitting up. Okay, up for 5 minutes, down for 30.*

*I talked with my sister about her work. Okay, mostly about my own problems!*

*I finally spoke to a friend on the phone. Well, my grandma ... isn't she a friend?*

*I didn't moan or groan all day. I just screamed. Kidding!*

*So I did okay. I was proud of myself. So were my parents. We saw today as a stepping stone towards better things.*

***"If the next step or step after is not the pinnacle, at least you will be two steps closer and that's what matters."***

## DAY 28-35

*About this time, I began to take walks around the block of my parents' neighbourhood. My parents were happy with that, and I tried to go out once a day ... only once, though. I have to admit that I didn't see the benefit of these walks, but as I look back, there were benefits. I realize now, that they were monumental in my journey out of depression.*

*With every step I took, I continued to agonize and feel the mental strain. There was, however, a small glint of hope that began to emerge without me even being aware. Bullshit to this, I would say to myself! Could it be true? How could a simple, lacklustre action be so important for me? It was. It really was. These small walks were huge steps towards me making my way back into the world again.*

*One day, this fifth week, my dad and I headed out to do some book stuff. I balked and argued and fought it, but ended up in the car anyway. My dad was still helping me out, taking books to stores and libraries. I still would not go into the stores, but I wasn't banging my head on the car window anymore. I was able to sit up and have a normal conversation with my dad, mostly about why I didn't want to go into any store or library!*

*I was beginning to eat more each of these days. I wasn't always hungry but Mom made every attempt to provide a good meal for me. "You're way too thin." And I was. Over the last number of months, from my spiritual fast to major depression, I had lost many pounds.*

*An entirely different basement had emerged. My lair had finally begun to change. I would now sit upright in a lounge chair and flip channels. Three's Company was a major staple, but one could only watch it so much. I now watched Oprah and The Price Is Right, oh, and Jeopardy (I could only answer the odd question, but I would watch it anyway). I still wasn't laughing at the comedies, but I was calmer and more relaxed.*

## DAY 36 THROUGH 40

*After being in the basement for close to a month and a half now, my parents and I finally decided that it was time to let my friends in on my "big" secret. I felt I had to let them know. These were guys I had known all my life! I hadn't spoken to any of them since I became cooped up in the basement, and I knew they were curious as hell to find out what was going on. They had called several times and left message after message that summer. In mid-July, my dad had thought it was best to contact them and tell them that I was not feeling well, but that I was taken care of. I knew that made them feel better, and they refrained from asking uncomfortable questions. They knew something was up: something more than a bad cold or fever, but they kept their thoughts to themselves. My dad told me these were quick conversations, and each had wished me well. So, with that, we were able to bide some time. I knew, however, that in very short order, they would come knocking again. Thank God none felt the need to visit. I would have died. I wanted to see no one, and much of the time, that included my family. I feared seeing them, but it was now time to face those fears head on.*

*My doctor and my folks felt that this would be a big step in my healing process. Sitting with my dad and Dr. Boyles at the hospital, I was totally against the idea at first, but finally I gave in. One might say it was "doctor's orders". So, one by one, we contacted each of my friends and set up times for them to visit.*

*We also planned a meeting with the girlfriend I dated during the months of my mania. Boy, had I screwed her mind up for four long months! She didn't know whether I was coming or going; and usually, I was going! I had ended things with her in mid-April, wanting to pursue other women, a classic symptom of someone with BD. I couldn't sit still and I wouldn't settle down with one girl anymore. I needed to roam, and I did. I met several different women that spring, but none of these flings lasted more than a few weeks. I spent very little time with them. It was all a bit of a blur, and each girl I met or "picked up" never satisfied my romantic hunger. Was I happy about this? I don't know, can't really say, but I just knew I had to keep on moving.*

*God, she had to have been so confused, being subject to so many of my manic antics: my extreme spiritualism, my gallivanting, my repeated sleeplessness, my exuberant spending, my "new friends". I became sure that she needed to know the truth behind my antics, and I was finally ready to give her some answers. She was a great person and I took her for granted without really knowing why. She would have been the perfect partner. However, sickness won out. My frantic behaviour must have caused her turmoil. I hadn't seen her since we ended things and I only hoped that I hadn't hurt her for good. Some answers were definitely in order.*

*That afternoon, I lay on the couch downstairs. My nerves were getting the best of me. A small lamp was on, illuminating one corner of the basement. I was now spending my days in low light, sometimes upstairs. My parents were pleased to see me turning the lights on now, and were equally pleased to see that I was no longer a hermit in the basement. I was now watching TV, eating three meals a day and putting weight back on. I still wasn't going out much, except to visit Dr. Boyles, take small walks around the block or deliver books to stores, accompanied by my dad. After a month and a half, surprisingly, I hadn't been out with anyone other than my family! A new chapter was ready to begin that morning.*

*"Chris. He's here!" my mom called down. Someone had arrived.*

*"Okay," I replied, as I sat up on the couch and folded my blanket. I sat in the beige chair by the TV and closed my eyes. Under my breath, I told myself, "This is it." This was where the truth would finally be revealed.*

*I took a deep breath. I could hear chairs moving and feet walking above. I opened my eyes and, man, was I ever nervous! I could feel sweat breaking out on my forehead. I wiped my brow and took another deep breath. This wasn't going to be easy.*

*I would embark on a difficult journey of sharing with my friends and ex-girlfriend, something that would undeniably change our relationships forever. I would begin to tell them about something horrible, something life altering, something that would from here on change the way they would see me as a person. From this day forward, without even knowing they were doing it, my friends would treat me differently. I would now live with a label attached to my name. As scholars list their qualifications following their names, I would henceforth be Christopher Nihmey, BA, BEd, BD. Hopefully my friends would see beyond this. I would know, in moments, who my true friends were. I hoped for at least one.*

*I heard a voice and, for a moment, drew a blank. Who was that? I tried to clue in on the voice. I had forgotten who was visiting? Who the hell was it?*

*He descended slowly. It was my long time friend, and roommate. I had known him since elementary school. Yes, you've heard of him before. I lived at his place during the peak of my mania. You'll recall me encountering him the morning I left for Toronto. Boy, he'd experienced a lot that winter!*

*"Hey," I said with an apprehensive grin.*

*"Hey. How are you?" he asked. He took a seat on the couch. He didn't know whether to hug me or not, so he just sat.*

*"I'm okay. Been better. Thanks for coming."*

*"Of course. I've missed you, man. We all have."*

*"Yah, things haven't been great. My dad say anything?"*

*"No, he called a while back to say you weren't feeling well, and the other day he called to invite me over. That's it."*

*"That's good. I wanted to talk to you first, before you heard things elsewhere."*

*I took a deep breath again, and looked up at the ceiling. This really was IT. We were sitting together alone and I was about to spill my guts on the table. God, could I do this? I had to. I had to. My doctor and my parents agreed that now was the time to share and, hopefully, start healing.*

*"So," I said with a wry smile. "I guess you have questions. I don't know where to begin, so maybe you can ask me some. I'm really afraid. I don't think I've ever been this scared."*

*"It's okay, Chris. It's okay."*

*And with those words, I began to tell him what was up. He asked me questions. I gave him answers. Halfway through our conversation, my biggest fear came up. The label. The fucking label! I had to say it. I didn't want to, but I had to. And I did.*

*"Well, there's a reason all these crazy things have happened. I've been diagnosed with bipolar disorder ... I'm bipolar." For the first time, I accepted the condition of my being mentally ill. There it was! I'd finally broken it wide open, and I felt a huge relief. Those few words started the process of breaking the chains that had been holding me since I was diagnosed.*

*"I've heard of it, but I don't know much about it. Can I ask you more?" he questioned. I nodded, and we started to talk about what bipolar was. I taught him about its other name, manic depression, and how that was not used anymore because it wasn't an apt description of the disorder and its effects. These two words put a negative spin on the illness. Words can hurt.*

*He asked me a lot that afternoon. He was so shocked to hear my stories and antics, and we actually laughed a little bit too. I had done some crazy things over the winter and spring. Really crazy! But you know what? It now started to make sense. He finally got answers to his concerns. He also gained an understanding of what I was dealing with. I gave him a lot but, in turn, he gave me much: his trust, his support and, most importantly, his friendship. He assured me that he would always be there for me, and that I could count on him anytime. This meant everything, and I needed to hear it that day. The relief didn't last that long because it was replaced by a harsh reality. My friends would take large strides ahead of me in life, accomplishing what I could only dream of.*

*That week, I met each of my closest friends. My roommate's visit had made me the most anxious. He was the first I spoke with, and he had been subject to so many strange behaviours during my stay at his house. He had seen the weirdest things. I knew that I had had to do some explaining.*

*Each friend that week told me that they were there for me. They repeated the same words of encouragement that one would say to someone who is sick. There was, however, one thing they couldn't tell me, which was probably the most important thing I needed. It was this: "Chris, give it to me! I'll take it away from you!" None could say that, and neither could my parents or sister. What I'm getting at is this. They would leave that day reassuring me of much better days and all the support they'd give me, but when they were gone, I would be left to live a life that would change me forever. I would carry this label the rest of my life. Sure, friends and family would support me, but that wouldn't make the bad things go away. That wouldn't make things the way they used to be.*

*Dammit, couldn't they make things all better? The answer was a resounding NO and I knew it. They couldn't take this shit away! NOBODY COULD! I was stuck with it. I was the disorder and I was alone. Did I really have anything to live for? At the time, I did not see beyond that.*

***"Why come out and tell. It only hurts. I don't want to be labelled weird, strange or not normal, a sick person, a "sicko"."***

## DAY 41

*Today ended up being one of the most difficult. This day, I would have a visit from my ex-girlfriend. She had seen the shit really hit the fan. In the midst of my mania, I'd been with her every day. I would eat with her, pray with her, sleep with her (beside her). I would go with her everywhere. I would do everything with her and, boy, was I ever high! High as a freakin' kite! She had seen a lot of wild things, and we both had been oblivious to what was going on. We hadn't seen past the love that we shared for each other. We had even discussed marriage! I had emailed my whole contact list of over 200, to tell them that I had met THE ONE, and she was soon to be my wife! Little did we know that we'd be the farthest from marriage only months later. It had been the most intense relationship either of us had ever had. It was wonderful, but obscure in so many ways. Her visit, therefore, was the most important. She needed answers NOW and I was finally ready to talk.*

*I heard her speaking with my parents, and my dad told her, "He's downstairs." I could hear her light steps coming down.*

*"Hi Chris," she said. She had a concerned look on her face, but I still found her comforting.*

*"Come here," she said, as she gave me a hug. It was warm and sincere. It was really good to see her. We had so much to talk about.*

*"Have a seat," I said, pointing to the couch.*

*"How've you been?" she asked.*

*"Okay," I responded.*

*With that, we moved from the normal pleasantries and got down to business. That afternoon, we covered everything, answering her many questions. I had never heard a person say "Oh" so much, and nod her head as much in one sitting. We talked and talked. Telling her about my disorder just seemed right. I didn't hide anything. She was warm and kind-hearted and made me feel good inside. I felt a genuine care and compassion in her voice. I was relieved to have finally answered her many questions. She, too, was relieved that I was now living with my family. It was where I needed to be.*

*She stood up and gave me another hug. She had heard everything she had waited months to hear. We both experienced a victory this day. We were ready to begin anew, living our own separate lives. We finally had the closure we both needed.*

*"Take care, Chris, take care." And she was gone for the rest of my life.*

*[And that is typically how relationships went for me through those years. I would lose Brenda, the summer before, with the obsessive thought, unjustifiably, that her thighs were too big. I obsessed and obsessed about her thighs, the whole time I was with her. Beautiful in every way, successful, and a wonderful person, who wanted a future, but I couldn't get her damn legs out of my head! Day after day, every time I met up with her, it slipped into my mind and the negative thought spiralled around and around, driving me completely crazy, as obsessions always did. I remember the day clearly when I ended things, very abruptly, tears in her eyes as I held her hands and said my goodbyes.*

*Like many relationships, prior to my being diagnosed, I did not feel right. Using the "I'm the problem" excuse always seemed to save me and hopefully free them without hard feelings. But did it really save anyone's face? What did they truly think of me? Who was I really hurting? I'd have to honestly say ... it was me. Without being fully aware of the dangerous path I was marching down, sickness continued to creep into every aspect of my life. Without having yet been diagnosed with it, a terrible obsession with perfection had raised its ugly head. As it had for years, it ended what could have been a long-lasting friendship, or more importantly a significant lasting relationship.*

*Things seemed to reverse in 2003 when I met Kaitlyn while supply teaching at her school. She was a pretty, successful and outgoing person who actually found the courage to ask ME out. I'll never forget our first date at a local Kelsey's, where I immediately brought up the fact that I had bipolar disorder. I vowed later that it was not something I would do again, that quickly. She seemed to accept this about me and we hit it off. We were boyfriend and girlfriend, yes, but I didn't realize that, in telling her my secret so early, I had opened quite a can of worms. Our relationship would find many holes in it. We shared the next bumpy year and a half together, as sickness came in waves and got the best of me at times ... many times. During this time, I had also been diagnosed with both* ***Obsessive-Compulsive Disorder*** *(OCD) and* ***Generalized Anxiety Disorder*** *(GAD), two illnesses that were already tearing things apart. With my bipolar firing up and down over the months, and these other treacherous heads popping out, it made for some very difficult times. She had become a "pseudo-therapist" for me which, according to my doctor, was dangerous. A trip in April to Toronto to see The Lion King was a prime example. I was obsessing about something prior to the show and we got into a huge argument in the middle of a busy street, as she attempted to solve it. We did reconcile, but only after the show, which made things very uncomfortable as we sat next to each other in the opera house ... not sharing a word.*

*In July of 2004, out of the blue, without warning, Kaitlyn dropped me like a rock; I was devastated. Our year and a half relationship was over, as I lay on a mattress in her basement bawling. She could no longer see beyond my ailments, and claimed that they would always be a hindrance for us going forward. Not to mention, the obsession I had for so many years about staying a virgin, because I thought I'd go to hell. For a woman of twenty-three, this had become a big problem. Sickness would once again destroy a special relationship. But her fears were not the only issue. Her parents, from whom she hid me for almost a year into our relationship, had their impact on us. Her parents never felt comfortable with my sickness, which put a lot of stress on her. I always felt her stress and their lack of sympathy when it came to my illnesses. They were scrupulous, like detectives, always looking, always searching. I, also, never felt comfortable around them, and always wondered what they were thinking. I knew that they would not see beyond my illnesses, and this affected Kaitlyn greatly. Perhaps if I had had a curable disease, would we still be together? As great as I was as a person, the stigma of mental illness took a front seat, and me ... I took a back one ... or the trunk? A spooked family, stigmatization, ostracizing, you name it. I prefer to use the word "alone".*

*In 2004, I met Lana. She would be my last serious relationship to date. I was in love with her. She had actually attended my high school. We hit things off immediately, and I quickly became an interim father to her cute little two-year-old daughter. I loved that kid and had accepted both of them wholeheartedly into my life. We were close. We were very close, until sick times set in once again and I began to fall into a deep depression. I knew there was a definite problem when I got very little enjoyment out of Bill Cosby's visit to the National Art Centre (NAC). Not to mention my anxiety and obsessions which were also knocking the shit out of me.*

*Out of nowhere, on an early January night following Christmas, she dropped yet another bomb into my life, ending our wonderful relationship. She claimed that her ex-husband was wanting back into the picture. I do think, however, the reality of the situation was right there in front of our faces. She wasn't ready to accept an "up and down" type of relationship that she felt would eventually sink. I was heartbroken once again, for months, and endured a long battle with depression that winter. I never saw her again. A trip to Mexico in March to visit my sister alleviated some of my difficult feelings, but she was on my mind constantly. Although my sister did her best to comfort and console me, I still clearly remember the day I arrived, where I spent almost two hours sitting by the ocean, watching the waves flow in and over a large rock on the shore below me. The water would rise over the rock, and then the current would pull back, revealing the top of the rock once again. I looked at it as analogous of my life thus far. I always felt I was bobbing for air.*]

*Since this last relationship, I have lost confidence, my sex drive (due to both medications and sickness) and the desire to be in a relationship; the fear of revealing my illnesses has been renewed (I have not told one person since—I continued to hide, until now). Sickness has always deterred me from moving forward, mainly for the above stated reasons. Who wants a husband who's sick? How could a family survive that sickness?*

[*Sickness has destroyed so much of my life ... so much of me. It has sabotaged everything about me, but I have not given up. Since those many relationships, and over the years that have followed, I have worked harder than I've ever worked before. It has been excruciating. High school was tough, university was challenging, work was very trying, but nothing could prepare me for the battle I have endured. I have learned to respect my illnesses, but more importantly, myself—whom I had lost for so many years. I have struggled, but persevered, and I can now safely say that I am finally getting "me" back.*]

## DAY 42 THROUGH 50

*By the end of August, each of my closest friends had visited. I trusted them to keep my secret (tell NO ONE!). Telling them everything was extremely difficult, and hard for them to hear. But I did it. I felt a huge relief. That summer, my parents also spoke to my grandmother about my illnesses. Mom needed to confide in someone outside our immediate family. In her nineties, a woman of much perseverance and strength, I was thankful we confided in her. Her continued prayers have made a difference. Granny has always been close to us and, like all my friends, she was sworn to secrecy. We trusted her.*

*I remember lying on the couch the morning following another visit. I was flicking channels with a glassy look on my face, one that could only mean I was obsessing. I was thinking of the many things I had shared with my friends. I shook my head when I thought of some of my stories. I wished I could have taken some back. God, they really were stories for the ages. They were humourous, embarrassing (lots of those kind), shocking, and all three combined into amazing. But the biggest realization that seemed to emanate from my stories was the fact that I was still alive. It was a blessing that, in over six long months, I had survived, even after doing all the things no one should ever do. My life had been at risk time and time again those winter months.*

## DAY 51

*All my friends' support that summer was so appreciated, but something was missing, and actually missing for quite some time. This day marked another critical day in my healing. It was the return of someone whom I had known all my life. I trusted him wholeheartedly.*

*He set foot in Ottawa at the end of August, returning from Europe, where he had spent the last two years of his life. He was like a brother to me, and when news reached him concerning the strange stories that winter, he knew something was not right with me. Even when we had spoken on the phone, he questioned my many antics and my new-found fanatical faith. So finally, after almost two years, he would be able to confront me and try to figure out what was going on.*

*Prior to his return, I remember lying in the basement getting some rest. I started recalling the times we had shared over so many years. God knows there were many of them. We had grown up next door to each other. He and I grew up together like two little weeds and we grew into two big weeds. We would call each other several times a day, and our conversations would take place just like this:*

*"Hey?"*

*"Hey?"*

*"What are you doing?"*

*"I don't know, what are you doing?"*

*"I don't know, what are you doing?"*

*"I don't know. Want to play?"*

*"I don't know, do you want to play?"*

*"What do you want to do?"*

*"I don't know, what do you want to do?"*

*"I don't know."*

*It would end with one of our parents yelling, "Just go next door!" It happened just like this every time, and I wouldn't have changed any of it.*

*We shared many experiences together: snow football in the yard, community football, haunted houses and horror movies, video game nights, weightlifting and boxing. They were special times and great memories of a time when I was not wracked with sickness. Many of these memories were now suppressed by illness.*

*I heard the doorbell. My folks spoke with him for a few minutes. He came down.*

*"Hey."*

*"Hey."*

*It was all we said. We hugged each other. I was ready to open up and share everything. I trusted him.*

*"Where do I start?" I said, as I sat in a recliner. He was sitting across the room. "I just don't know where to start."*

*He smiled and said, "It's so great to finally see you again."*

*"I know. It is great. I missed you. I almost forgot what you looked like!"*

*We both smiled and things just took their course. I started to tell him, face to face, what had transpired over the last number of months. He had questions; I had answers. He couldn't believe the stories! We laughed. We saw each situation as a way to understand what this awful disorder was and how to cope with it.*

*He saw a vision I could not appreciate. I was masked with depression, sickness and pessimism. Hell, I found it hard to be optimistic. He was hopeful and I was thankful. Our team was back on the field together again. I knew that his arrival would only make things better. At least I hoped so.*

## DAY 52 THROUGH 56

*It was early September. I wasn't having a good day. I felt like shit. I didn't know why I was feeling so lousy, especially since I'd shared my story with my friends. It was here that I realized that depression, no matter how good things may seem to be, will continue to rear its ugly head. I guess I was feeling a little bit of an emotional hangover from the many visits. And that's when something happened, reminding me of good friendship.*

*One of my close friends came by. Dad told him I wasn't feeling well. He came downstairs, stood in the stairwell and waved.*

*"Come on. Let's go."*

*"What do you mean? I'm not going anywhere. I just want to be alone."*

*"Well, that'll have to wait. Come on!"*

*Hesitantly, I followed him up the stairs and asked what was going on. He continued to the front door.*

*"We're going for a walk."*

*"A walk? No. No, I don't want to! I hate walks!"*

*"We are!"*

*My dad piped in, "It would be good for you, son. Go for a walk. Then you can come with me and we'll go to the drugstore to get your meds. Here, put this in your pocket for later." My dad handed me a prescription for my medications. Yes, I was on more than one drug. A shitload actually!*

*We went outside. I really felt shitty, but I took their advice and went. Up until now, I'd only walked around the block alone, but my friend had other plans. We actually ended up walking to the pharmacy three kilometres away! Three! I couldn't believe it! How are we going to get home? I thought. Well, we walked back! It turned out to be another critical step in my healing. When we got home, I quickly reminded myself that, only a month ago, I wasn't even going outside! Those days were big for healing and those steps were crucial, but the journey was just beginning.*

## DAY 57

*About this time, I seemed to be getting back on my feet again: however, never the same. I was not completely out of depression, after over two months!*

*To top that off, my confidence and my self-esteem were shot. I felt terrible about myself and negativity shrouded me. I had a sickness that would be with me for life. Things didn't bode well for the future and there was nothing I could do. I felt so small and insignificant in a society and world that was so large, moving so fast, was so complicated and so judgemental. I was obsessed with guilt, fear of failure, even fear of success and, yes, still a huge fear of hell that would stay with me for a long, long time.*

## SEPTEMBER 11, 2001 (DAY 58)

*9/11 ... the day that rocked the world. I remember it very clearly. I got up early, and drowsily walked up the stairs. I was still spending my nights in the basement, but spending more time in the kitchen and living room. I'd come far the last couple of weeks, but I still wasn't ready to work. Teaching would still have to wait. Because of this, most of my time was spent around the house.*

*At 8:55, I walked into the kitchen. Mom was having her morning coffee. I sat on one of the kitchen chairs and grabbed the TV remote. I turned it on and started to flick the stations. Nothing new, same crap. But, as I made my way towards CNN, something struck me, hitting me hard, as it did the whole western world. I had to rub my eyes a few times because what my mom and I saw that morning was horrific!*

"We are live here in Manhattan and this is truly unbelievable! This is not a movie, folks, we are live! Our cameras are trained on the Twin Towers of the World Trade Center where, at 8:46 am, an airplane suddenly crashed into the North Tower! What you are seeing is truly beyond explanation, and how this happened is just as earth-shattering. We can see smoke and flames coming from the top of the tower. There are actually people waving white towels from the windows above! Need I say it again? This is truly unbelievable! It is just mayhem up there, and people are dying!"

*And it was. It really was. My mom called my dad down and I called my friend. He wasn't an early riser but he had to see this! I was the first to tell him what was going on only hours away from us.*

*"Shut up! What? Are you serious?"*

*He was blown away when he turned on CNN. He was seeing this for the first time, so it caught him by surprise. We both sat there on the phone in amazement at what we were witnessing. How could this be happening? Was this for real? It felt like a movie! The two of us continued to watch and I kept talking to my parents. We were stunned. And then, as we watched in horror, the unthinkable happened. None of us were ready for this.*

"What's that? God, what's that? Oh my God, something just flew into the South Tower! It's another airplane! Did you see that?"

*My family went silent. My friend went silent. We were speechless.*

"This is truly horrific folks! We have seen two planes go flying directly into each of the towers! The last one just flew in seconds ago! God help us all! I have never seen anything like it!"

*It was truly one of the worst things that any of us had ever seen. Thousands would perish that morning. None of us thought this could ever happen, or that it could get any worse than this. But it did that morning! It got worse, and we all know what happened next. The "truly" unthinkable happened. The two towers collapsed under their own weight and fell to rubble, taking with them thousands above and below. Hope was lost, and fear presided among us all. We knew that life would never be the same again.*

*That day substantially changed me. For the first time since becoming depressed, I had awakened to something outside of my own personal struggle. I was finally seeing outward, beyond my illnesses. Personally, I could relate with those who had suffered from this horrendous tragedy. The western world had gone from exhilaration to despondency and mourning, in less than two hours! It closely resembled my fall into sickness. Could I recover? Could we (the west) recover?*

## A POSTSCRIPT

I did make it out of the basement. By mid-September, I had flown the coop, and was making my way outside: of my own will. I was seeing friends, and taking care of some responsibilities regarding my novel. I would subsequently, with extreme hard work and strength, emerge to work, write and live. I would become ME again, but different. I could only do so thanks to perseverance, faith, support, dedication to taking my meds and therapy. In September of 2010, I visited Ground Zero in New York City. My dad and I were there to attend a *NFL* doubleheader and to tour Manhattan. I was determined that we visit Ground Zero and we did. While there, we observed the rebuilding of a site where I could almost hear the voices of the victims rejoicing the recovery. The survivors have demonstrated the same dedication as I have to get back on their feet.

Today, billions of people will pack the subway tunnels and trains, load the bus terminals, fill the airports and crowd the streets all over the big world we live in. Tomorrow it will repeat again. Some will head north or west, east or south. We are caught in the busiest era of our generation, a generation that will likely bury itself under stacks of computer paper, hard wires and Starbucks coffee cups. So many people in a world that, at times, is too busy for a quick hello or friendly smile.

In a world of so many, is it possible that someone could feel truly alone? I used to think the answer to this question was a resounding no. How could anyone ever feel alone in a world filled with so many people? Well, I don't believe that way anymore. As large as the world is, and as many caring individuals as there were around me, I can honestly say that through much of my suffering, I was alone. This void from everything and everyone was what scared me the most. Alone can mean many things, but for me, I'd have to say that being alone wasn't so much an absence of what was around me, but rather an absence of what was inside of me. There was nothing there. My life was stolen away from me and for the first time in this busy world, I felt completely alone.

***"God has given you one face, and you make yourself another."***

***William Shakespeare, Hamlet***

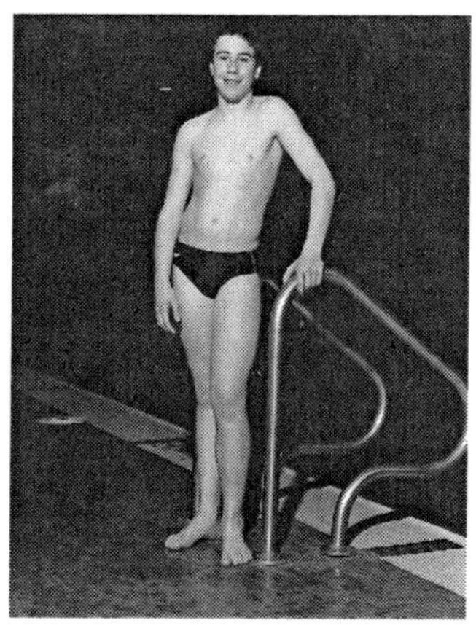

My competitive swimming days – age 13 – Hercules!

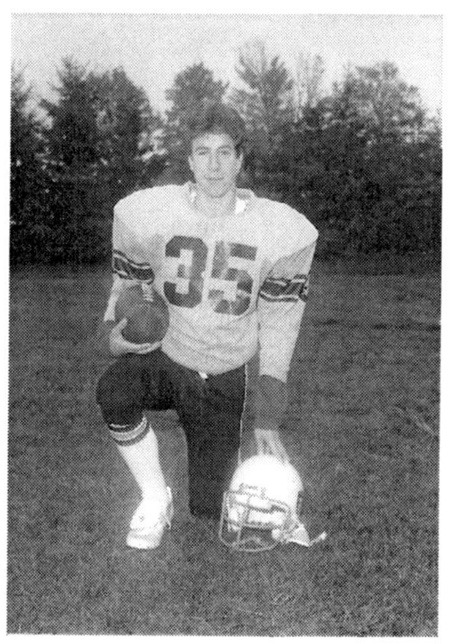


Football with the South Gloucester Raiders – age 15 – Grrrr ...

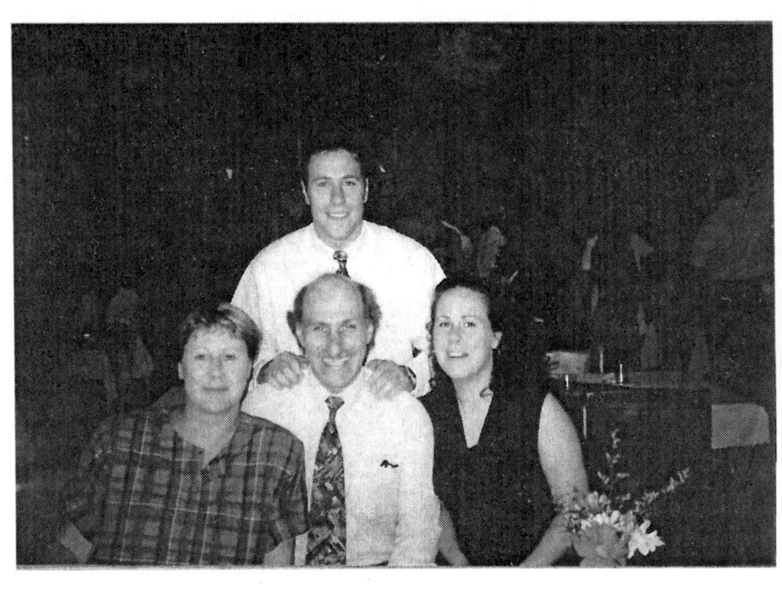

My family at my 1997 university graduation – calm before "my" storm

Recommendation from Dean of Kinesiology,
University of Western Ontario

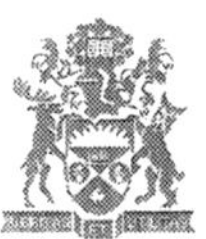

*The* UNIVERSITY *of* WESTERN ONTARIO

*School of Kinesiology • Faculty of Health Sciences • Thames Hall /3M Centre*

January 5, 1998

Dear Sir/Madam:

I am pleased to write a letter of recommendation for Chris Nihmey who has applied to your board for a teaching position effective September 1, 1998. I have known Chris for the past five years in my capacity as Dean of the Faculty of Kinesiology at the University of Western Ontario and as the liaison representative of the Faculty to the Student Council. Chris was president of Council which necessitated our meeting on a regular basis. At the graduation banquet, I stated that the Student's Council under the direction of Chris Nihmey was the finest, most progressive, and best organized of the councils in my 15 years as Dean, and that the success of the Council was a reflection of the leadership of Chris Nihmey. These words were not spoken lightly but were most sincere.

Chris Nihmey has been an exceptional student throughout his tenure in Kinesiology. His grades are representative of his abilities in one of the most demanding programs at Western. Less than 5% of our students graduate with an A average although 100% enter the program with those grades. Chris was able to carry out his academic duties as well as serve as Council President, be a volunteer coach in the London school system, set aside adequate time for a social life and attain the A average. Chris also spent a great deal of time working on special projects such as the Special Winter Games for the Mentally Challenged Children of South Western Ontario. He served as coordinator for this event including fund raising, correspondence, dealing with the several associations which govern these children (including school board representatives), negotiating with businesses and corporations for in-kind donations. Chris was also responsible for the distribution of several thousands of dollars which were raised by the Council for charitable donations.

Chris Nihmey is an excellent academic student, one willing to give of his time and energy tirelessly, and a most enjoyable graduate of our program. Perhaps of equal significance is his happy and positive personality. Chris seems to bring out the best in people, looks for the good qualities in people and loves to communicate. He will be an excellent teacher, an exceptional coach, and a most worthy addition to your teaching staff.

These comments have been made without prejudice and I will be most pleased to comment further upon your request and can be reached at 519-661-4144 (phone), 519-661-2008 (fax) or by e-mail at ataylor2@julian.uwo.ca.

Sincerely,

A.W. Taylor, Ph.D., Dsc.
Professor

London, Ontario • Canada • N6A 3K7 • Telephone: (519) 661-3092 • Fax: (519) 661-2008

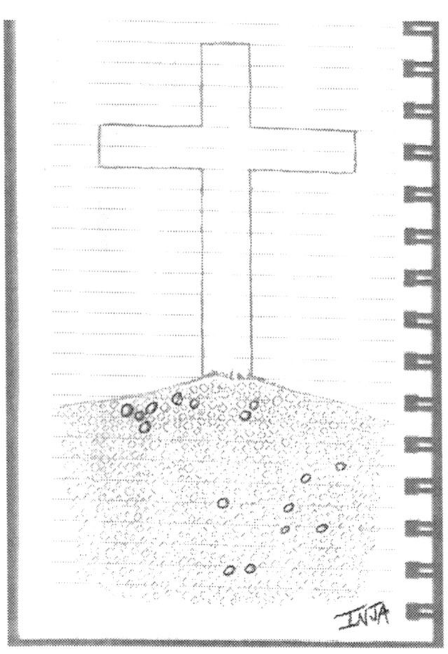

2001 Journal drawing leading to my 9-day fast and escape to Toronto

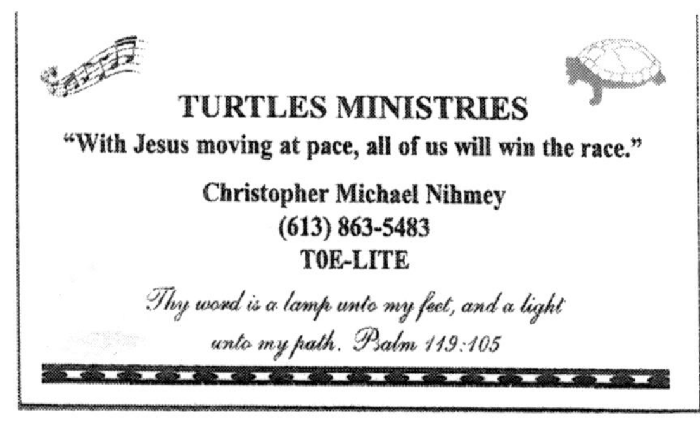


2001 *Turtles Ministries* business card – don't try the number!

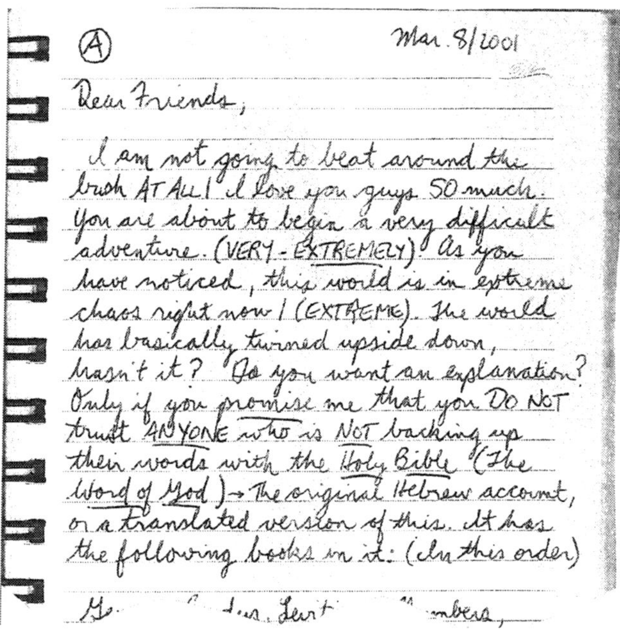

(A) Mar. 8/2001

Dear Friends,

I am not going to beat around the bush AT ALL! I love you guys SO much. You are about to begin a very difficult adventure. (VERY - EXTREMELY)! As you have noticed, this world is in extreme chaos right now! (EXTREME). The world has basically turned upside down, hasn't it? Do you want an explanation? Only if you promise me that you DO NOT trust ANYONE who is NOT backing up their words with the Holy Bible (The Word of God) → The original Hebrew account, or a translated version of this. It has the following books in it: (In this order)

[illegible]

2001 *Revelation* letter, time of "Rapture"

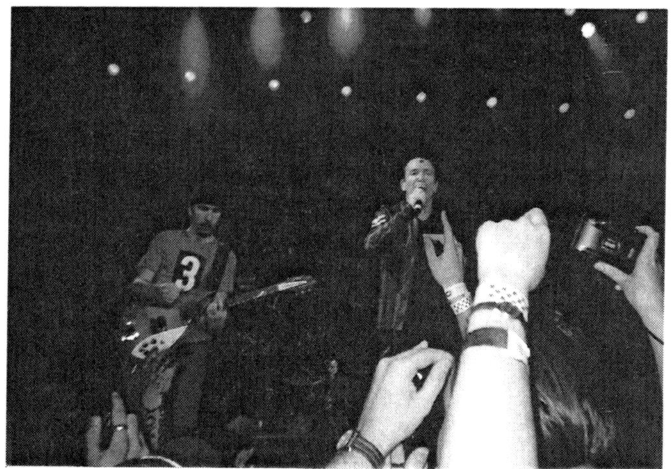


May 2001 – U2 concert, Montreal –
Bono with "my" sticker on "his" forehead!

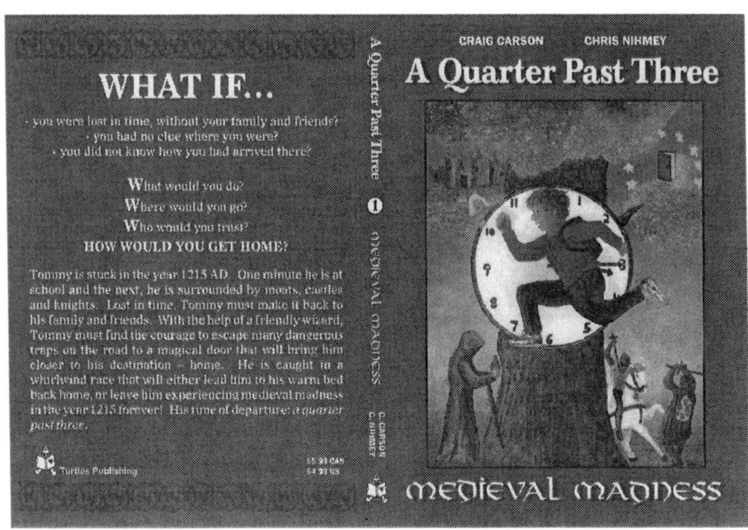


June 2001 *A Quarter Past Three* – my first published novel

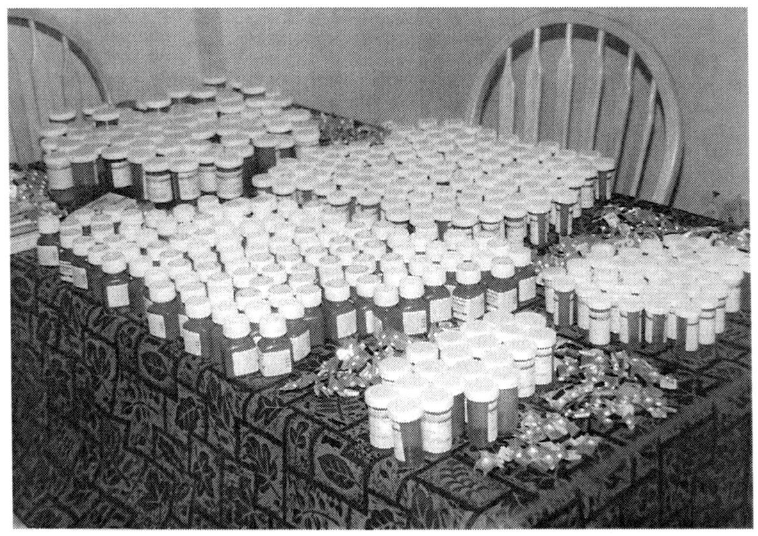

2011 A decade of my meds ...

# PART VI

# THE OCD YEARS

# CHAPTER 1
# WHAT IS OBSESSIVE-COMPULSIVE DISORDER?

I equate the battle against ***Obsessive-Compulsive Disorder*** (OCD) with fighting a war. It's a mental war, one that you cannot see, but one that affects the mind and body of its victim with negative, ongoing repetitive thoughts: **obsessions**. These, in turn, lead to negative, ongoing repetitive actions: **compulsions**. Obsessions came on in full force during my late twenties, although I had traces of this thinking as far back as my teens.

Picture a battle line, where you sit in a trench and are constantly bombarded by thoughts that hamper and ultimately destroy you. Sometimes they attack one by one: most often ... in teams. If you're not equipped, they will destroy you, to the point of suicide. Mental anxiety also affects one's physical condition. Obsessions knocked me down for years. Initially, when I first experienced them, I had no "battle weapons" drawn. With this fight happening all around me, I was constantly knocked over, many times to the point of tears. This led to thoughts of ending my life. How could I live with these obsessions? I just couldn't, and I'd do whatever I could to get rid of the anxiety they caused, even if it meant continuing to repeat the same destructive and irrational actions (compulsions). At the time, it seemed impossible to stop.

As in war, when you are on the battle line, you can never sit back and let up. Even when you think you've conquered the enemy (obsessions), it will make its way back into your thought process again. You must always be on guard no matter what. You can knock'em down and think you've destroyed them, but they keep renewing themselves. I've beaten obsessions for months (so proud I was), only to find that the obsessions had revived themselves, by way of a new experience. I'd say to myself, "Self, good work, put that one up on the shelf as a victory." Then, all of a sudden out of nowhere, months down the road, an obsession would resurface, rearing its evil head again. It may not come in full force as it had initially, but it will try to get back into your thought process again. There, it will fester and build again like embers turning into flames in a fire. The key for me was finding the strategies to ensure this didn't happen.

Obsessing is an incredible process. It takes on a life of its own. Obsessions attack and their goal is to conquer. One needs to learn to be THEIR conqueror, and not their victim, which I was for so many years.

"INCOMING!!! Watch out! It's coming in hard and fast! Do we have enough troops on the line? Oh my God, this is an ambush, a bigger battle than we expected! I don't know if we have enough manpower! Holy shit, this one could blow us over ... ahh! NOOO!!!"

Like a canoe that rocks to one side and starts to fill with water, the boat starts to rock the other way, until the entire canoe is deluged, and then sinks. Overboard! Overboard ... that's right. You saw the Titanic go down ... welcome to the world of obsessional domination.

Obsessions affected my life most drastically in my late twenties and early thirties. Obsessions didn't just affect my life, they dominated and determined its direction. Obsessions became second nature to me. It got to a point where things didn't feel right or normal(?) unless I was obsessing! I didn't feel myself unless I had an obsession I was dealing with. They BECAME "me". They took over my life in every way. Obsessions drove everything; they drove me crazy. At their peak, I would obsess 40 to 50 times each day, a barrage of thoughts that attacked me and kept me from progressing. I would obsess about anything and everything.

People have obsessions about cleanliness or leaving an iron or a light switch on. My obsessions revolved around everything! They were so intrusive. Anything one can think of, I would obsess over. When I had an obsession, my stomach ached and I felt anxious and my head felt light. It caused so much grief and anguish. I just wanted to explode until I could satisfy the obsession by compulsing. These led to ridiculous actions and many a social event was spoiled or sabotaged. Then, when I compulsed, rather than being satisfied, the obsession again appeared in a more powerful form. I found later that, in recovery, and through therapy, not satisfying it actually made the obsession less destructive.

By compulsing, I thought I was relieving stress. But this was false. It would relieve the stress temporarily, but a related obsession would come back again in greater force. Here's an example:

**Obsession:** I shouldn't have hung up the phone so quickly. They must be sad or hurt by how I let them go when I said goodbye.

**The buildup:** Questions like these: Oh my God, I feel awful, what are they going to think? Are they going to hate me? Are they going to think less of me? How will I feel about myself?

**Compulsion:** I pick up the phone and call back immediately to better things. Gives temporarily relief ... aaah ... but unfortunately, leads to repeating the action again.

You may have had similar thoughts, but it's not necessarily the thought that is dangerous. It is the reflex or reaction to perform a ritual in order to relieve anxiety caused by the thought. That is what is abnormal or warped. Also, it is the duration, degree of irrationality and paralytic effect of the obsession and compulsion that determines if one is suffering from OCD. This, therefore, entirely disrupts the individual's **quality of life**. Imagine:

You wake up in the morning, the thought is there. You feel downright awful;

You go to work or school; it is still there. You feel incompetent and worthless;

You come home after; it is still there. You feel exhausted and lethargic;

At bedtime, you hope to rest your mind; it is still there. Anxiety and sleeplessness pervade;

The next morning, it is STILL there. You can barely function. You feel like you are dying.

*For additional information:* ***American Psychiatric Association*** *at* www.healthyminds.org

## CHAPTER 2
## OBSESSIONS GROWING UP

Early on in life, I was hit by the same worries and thoughts that we all experience, but they seemed to affect me more than other kids my age. I had an unusual level of anxiety over things. Maybe I was worried about a test, or a missing toy or a movie I couldn't see or even a girl I liked. I remember ripping the smallest corner of a comic once, at the age of 12 or 13, and I had so much anxiety over that tear that I couldn't get it out of my mind. I thought about it for days and obsessed over the fact that my comic wasn't perfect. The only thing my father could do to alleviate my anxiety, was to take me to the store to buy another one. A compulsion for sure; at the time, we had no clue.

I was obsessed with having things perfect in my little world, and the anxiety over this obsession affected me greatly, especially as I moved through high school. Little did I know, things would get much worse. Even at a young age, you would often hear me saying my two most used words. They were, "I'm worried." Just ask my friends. I worried about everything, and as I got to university, these only became worse. My university roommate, with whom I lived for two years, can testify to that. He became so fed up with my worries and questions, he actually created a question jar, where I would have to pay him a quarter for every "worry" question I asked! Seriously! We joked one day when I walked into his room and threw a loonie on the table, and said, "I got four!" My obsessions never did subside because the "I'm worried" questions (compulsions) persisted, under the mistaken belief that I would find relief by asking. Not so!

Sure, there were "more than usual" numbers of worries as a child, but these usually subsided as I carried on and went through my day. At that stage of the game, I was not yet hit by the storm that was brewing and would eventually devastate me.

Some classic examples of obsessions that I experienced as a child were: needing certain toys long before I was due to get them, and repeating that need ad nauseum, meticulousness about the condition of my possessions and having "whole collections" of toys, comics, sports cards and memorabilia. Where kids grow out of these impulsions, I grew into more ingrained and pernicious ones.

One cannot rationalize one's obsessions. You cannot make sense of them. It doesn't work. Why? Obsessions make NO SENSE! They are NOT reasonable. I tried innumerable times to battle obsessions by trying to rationalize them. You just can't win this game. Their irrationality overcomes any reasonability that one might apply to a situation. I learned the hard way.

***"I know God will not give me anything I can't handle. I just wish that He didn't trust me so much."***

***Mother Teresa***

# PART VII

# LET'S "THINK" ABOUT IT
# OCD STORIES

## CHAPTER 1
## THE SENS STORE

The *Ottawa Senators* are our pro hockey team. We love them, we wear their colours with pride and the city is just not the same the morning after a loss. I have to admit that my attention to the team declined during those difficult years (2002–2008), as I found myself in bed most nights before the game even started, staring at the ceiling in the dark. I would, however, tune into the radio the next morning to hear the result of the game, unless I was too depressed.

There were highlights to being a Senators' fan. Every month or so, my father and I would take the long drive to watch our team play. We loved going but, for me, it depended on what was going on upstairs. Obsessions, anxiety and depression ruined many games for me and my dad, as he had to sit there listening to me spout my worries over and over again. And I had to be coaxed at times to go with him when I was feeling terrible. I was like a runner who had to pump themselves up to go to a race.

Around Christmas time, 2005, my dad and I were going to a *Senators-Philadelphia Flyers* game. I had finished teaching a week earlier, and I was taking six weeks off due to illness to attend the *Day Hospital* program at the Civic. I wasn't keen on missing work like that, but I knew it was for the better and, besides, my days were getting more and more difficult because of how I was feeling: depressed, anxious and obsessed.

We walked through the tunnel and up to the front entrance of the arena. It wasn't extremely cold, but we had our coats zipped right up. There were people everywhere! A sure sell-out. Before going up the stairs, we took our usual detour. We went into the Senators gift shop. There were souvenirs galore. We made our way around one end of the store and slowly browsed the different souvenirs. This is when things got interesting.

We were walking in the back area of the store, my dad leading the way. Then, for some reason, I noticed something on the floor. It was a short crack, and a slight elevation; the surface was a bit uneven. The bump was SO small, no one in their right mind would have ever looked twice, let alone once.

It was really nothing … nothing at all! But guess what happened next …

Like all my obsessions, this was irrational and exaggerated in every way. So, in complete disarray, I stopped suddenly in my tracks and bent down to feel the small bump. Obsession began to flush into my head like a raging stream and I started to go a little crazy.

"Dad, Dad, wait. Come here!"

I signalled for my dad to come back to see the small bump in the concrete. I rubbed the bottom of my foot along the bump as he came over. I could feel a slight difference in the floor's surface. For me, it seemed mountainous! My mind magnified the bump tenfold.

"Yes, son?"

"Dad, look, look at the floor."

My dad looked down and stood for a moment, looking to the left and the right of the bump, but not even noticing the bump itself.

"Here, Dad, here! Do you see it?" I said in frustration, as I bent down and pointed to the uneven surface.

"What? This small bump?" he asked, running his foot over it.

"Yes, this bump right here!" I ran my foot over it again. "Someone could trip on this! Don't you think?"

"Chris, you're being ridiculous. No one could trip on that. An ant wouldn't even trip on that. Let's go get our seats!" he said to me, as he started to turn around. I stood up. I couldn't believe he was brushing this off the way he was.

My mind raced as we walked past the bump and through the store. Before leaving the store, I turned around and asked my dad to wait a moment and made my way back to the bump. I ran my foot over it again. I had developed a fear of someone hurting themselves seriously. This is what was going on in my mind:

1. There was a bump, a big one.
2. I had seen it, and I was now responsible for it.
3. Someone who might not see it could trip and fall and hurt themselves … because of my negligence.
4. Someone could actually DIE if they tripped and landed on their head and it would be MY fault. I would have caused their death!

5. God knows that I now know about the bump, so if someone gets hurt or dies, I go straight to hell!

You can appreciate how carried away I would become. This was the case for ALL my obsessions. It was a cycle that made it from my initial thought to the most magnified and exaggerated thought and subsequent action that one could ever take. And this was just the start of a storm of obsessions that would follow the same patterns over the next number of years. This was complementary to, and with, extreme anxiety and depression.

Dad could tell that I was obsessing over something, but he wasn't sure what. I had so many obsessions all the time, no matter where I was. What is he getting into this time? he must have thought.

I looked around for someone who was working in the store. I walked up to one gentleman and asked, "Can I show you something?"

The man stared at me with an odd look on his face.

"Sure," he said, "but why me?"

I laughed and scratched my head, "Because ... you work here? You do work here, right?" I laughed nervously.

He pointed to another man at the other side of the store. "You'd be wanting him, I believe. I can't help you, and neither can my son," he smiled, as a young boy came up to hug his father.

I laughed again nervously and quickly darted to the other corner of the store, which was conveniently right near the bump. Perfect! I would just talk to the man, tell him the problem and I'd be on my way. I took a quick glance to the entrance of the store where my dad was waiting. This kind of behaviour was not unusual at the time, so he was used to being VERY patient.

"Hello, sir? Can I talk to you for a minute? Only a minute. Come over here," I continued, as I brought the man over to see the bump in the floor. "See this?" I asked. "Do you see this bump on the floor? See how it goes up, how it's uneven?"

He ran his foot over the bump. "Yes, sir, I see it. What did you need?"

I shook my shoulders and shrugged my neck and rubbed the back of my head. I became a little bit frustrated by his reaction, which was that it wasn't much, not much at all. I couldn't believe this and was completely surprised that he wasn't jumping at the opportunity to tell me that I, Chris Nihmey, had done something monumental and profound. That was, in telling him about this bump, I would save countless lives put at risk by this dangerous uneven floor.

"The floor has a bump in it! Can't you see it?" I said in alarm, pointing with both hands. "Someone could trip on that! Can't you see? Someone could get hurt in your store!" I continued, wondering how it was at all possible for someone to be so negligent and so ignorant when something so severe was in play, something that could risk the lives of every person who walked into the store!

"Sir, I will tell my manager about this and he will fix up the problem, maybe put a sign over it or a pylon or something."

I breathed a huge sigh of relief, as I shook his hand. "Thank you. Thank you. You have done the right thing. Just know that." I wiped my brow to show him how relieved I was. We had a little laugh about it, but my laughter was fake because I didn't think the situation was funny ... at all.

I left him and, as I did, I pointed to it again. He waved at me and gave me a thumbs up, assuring me that the problem was taken care of. I must have looked back ten times before exiting the store, hoping, wanting and praying that this guy would go find his manager. But, when I was just about out of sight, I still saw him standing in the damn corner, hanging up some stupid sweater. UGH! I thought, as I joined my dad.

"What did you have to do, Chris? Did you see something you liked?"

"Uh yah, Dad. I did, maybe a Christmas gift for someone ... maybe."

That seemed to keep him at bay and we proceeded to our seats. He would later find out the truth. He always did.

We took our seats way up in section 308. We were in the top row as usual. We had had fun, but for a long time now, I wasn't having fun. I was just obsessing. I was obsessing about the waiter, or my teeth getting stained, or my friends and why I felt they were ignoring me and not calling me back, or the kid at school, or a colleague who didn't like me for some reason because she stared at me strangely. It didn't matter what it was, I was obsessing. But, in this case, it was something different. It was THE BUMP. The stupid fucking bump! As we sat there, all I could think about was the freakin' bump in the store, the bump that I believed could literally kill someone. What if someone fell back landing on their head? This thought cycled through my brain over and over as I sat there trying to watch the pre-game practice. I pictured ten, maybe eleven, victims to the bump that night.

I had to do something more! I thought. This was ridiculous! Finally, I gave in and told my dad what was on my mind.

"Dad, you know that bump that I showed you in the store?"

"Yah, Chris, the bump. What about the bump?" He was only half listening as he watched the pre-game highlights on the giant scoreboard.

"Dad, listen to me!" I said, frustrated, as I nudged him with my shoulder. "The bump. The bump on the floor! Don't you remember?"

"Um ... ah ... yah, you showed me it. Why? What's wrong?"

"Dad, I got to do something about that bump."

"What, Chris, what?"

"The bump!"

"Wh ... what about the bump, son?" he said, flipping through his program. Stupid program, I'm thinking.

"I really think people are going to get hurt, Dad! I examined the area and I looked closely at that bump and I have to say ... Dad ... I HAVE to go back to the store. Someone's gonna fall down and seriously hurt themselves!"

"Chris, don't be ridiculous. I saw the bump. It wouldn't do a thing to anyone! Get it out of your mind, son. You're just obsessing over something that's not worth thinking about. Let's enjoy this game and not ruin another one," he said, hoping that I could finally release these terrible thoughts and focus on happier things.

I tried to put the thoughts aside, sitting through the team introductions and the anthem, but, honest to God, all I really could think was bump ... bump ... bump! I did everything I could to forget it, but I couldn't get the damned thing out of my mind. It was eating me up! All I could picture was someone falling and then me falling into hell for keeping it under wraps. My dad then grabbed my arm and asked me, "Chris, is this why you went back into the store earlier? Was it that stupid bump you were checking?"

"Yah, Dad, and if I don't ensure that the store does something about it, I'm going to lose it. God will punish me! I don't think the guy I told took me seriously enough. He said he'd put a sign there, but I don't think he did. I could just tell. I don't trust him!"

"Chris, it's not your responsibility. If it is a bump as big as you think it is, it's definitely the store's responsibility and, again, not yours! I've seen the bump and it's nothing to worry about at all. No one could ever get hurt from something that small and insignificant."

"But, Dad, I told the guy down there to do something about it and I just have to make sure he did. I got to go back down."

"If you really need to, which I'm telling you, you don't, wait until intermission," he offered, hoping that I might somehow forget about it in time.

"It can't wait!" I said, and I stood up and barged my way down the row bumping into every knee I passed ... excuse me, excuse me, sorry, excuse me. My dad shook his head, and rather than be upset with my decision, he felt awful for me. I felt like I was such a hedonistic rude bastard but it had to be done. Lives were at risk and so was my life thereafter!

I raced down the stairs as the puck was dropped. I took the steps two at a time, hanging onto the railing for dear life because I was moving so fast. I hustled down the hallway in and around the latecomers, who were moving just as fast! Seeing the store gave me such a sigh of relief, as did all obsessions when they were being fed. Like so many obsessions, acting upon them with a compulsion gave me that temporary relief. But it didn't last.

It only made things worse ... far worse. Only thing was, I was blinded to that fact at the time, despite many attempts by my doctor, my psychologist and my family trying to make me see reality. But as much as reality was out there somewhere in the dark, I didn't see it. Not for a long time. All I hung onto was the temporary relief of submitting to an obsession, much like a needle to the arm of a druggie or a tilt of the full glass to an alcoholic. That initial feeling for all OCDs is calm and soothing, however, the storm is sure to follow.

I walked into the store and started to backtrack to the corner where the enemy, the bump, lay. I now hated it with all my heart; yet I couldn't let it go. Hoping, praying that I'd see a yellow caution sign at the back of the store, I zoned in and attacked, and guess what? No fucking sign! ARG! People were walking, prancing, even dancing (not really) over the spot, as I stood there dumbfounded. I started to fret and sweat, and thought about warning people, but I avoided that and knew that, this time, I wouldn't just tell some "kid" to put up a sign. I had to tell the manager: maybe even the owner. Yah, the owner!

A senior gentleman stood at one of the entrances, greeting newcomers and handing out flyers.

"Hello, sir, how are you tonight? Here you go," he said, with a smile. I couldn't smile. I had business to deal with, NOT a smile!

"Can I talk to you, sir, for a moment? Only a moment," I said, but I knew I needed more than a moment for this one.

"Yes, one minute ... Bobby! Can you come here?" he signalled to a kid over by the jersey wall. And guess who? The kid I had asked only moments before! Great!

"Bobby, can you help this gentleman. I have to keep greeting people. This flow of customers just keeps coming."

I felt stressed beyond stress. I was agitated about his pawning me off to a kid who'd done nothing to help me and the other "at risk" customers, only a half hour ago. I nervously rubbed my neck as the man, who it turned out was the owner, turned to face his customers again.

That's when I took things to a new height. I actually reached out and grabbed him by the arm and turned him around.

"Sir," I uttered nervously, "It is YOU I need to talk to, not him," I said. "No offence, Bobby," I said to the kid who hadn't heeded my concerns.

"None taken, sir," he replied.

I took the owner to the area at the back and showed him the floor. Every time I looked at the bump it seemed to get bigger, as my obsession over it grew, and became more exaggerated. I pleaded with him to do something, either stationing a store clerk warning people of the bump or a bright yellow sign, or something! God, something! He told me that he would take care of it for me, but I could tell he wasn't taking me as seriously as I had hoped. He, like the kid, felt that it wasn't a big problem, and that pissed me off dearly! But, to keep the customer happy, because "the customer is always right", he told me he would take care of it.

I thanked him profusely. I felt such a relief that the problem would be handled by the right person this time, and that people would once again be safe. I headed back up to my seat to finally watch the game. This one had come to a satisfactory end. Didn't it?

NO, it didn't! The moment I sat down, with 5:45 left in the first period, I again started to question things. Did he really mean what he said? What if he was just trying to get rid of me? Like Superman in the original *Superman* movies, starring Christopher Reeve, all my mind was saying over and over was, "NOOO ... the people!" Thoughts flooded in again. While my dad was trying to enjoy the game, I was continuing to obsess about "the bump" in the floor. My dad tried to offer relief, but he was unsuccessful. I was stuck with the thoughts, and not only would I obsess about the bump that night (another trip during the 2nd period), and days to follow, and games to follow, I would continue to obsess for months, to the end of the hockey season AND into the next season. This included several phone calls to the store as well.

This story, however, culminates in a victory. I've been in that store dozens of times since, and I have yet to see a sign on that bump! And you know what? That bump is still there! That bump, which was for me, the biggest of mountains, is now merely an ant hill. Perception is everything, and I perceived things in a distorted way then, a sick way. Now that I've come this far in my therapy, I appreciate reality. Sure, the thoughts still pop up, but now I'm able to put them at bay.

That night, like so many nights, I would fall into what I called "the zone". It was a trance-like state that happened whenever I was obsessing. My friends and family knew when I was in "the zone", because I would wear a glassy look on my face, with the brain hamster upstairs running his ass off in hyper-drive, obsessions firing at a high level ... running wild!

But it was my mom, dad and sister who knew "the zone" only TOO well. I remember having many conversations with them where I'd completely zone out and lose all focus on what was being said. This had also happened during my university years. All I would hear was BLAH, BLAH, BLAH, kind of like the sound the teachers make in the Charlie Brown *Peanuts* cartoons. I would lose the ability to take in information and would become a wall at which information would simply bounce off. When I was in "the zone", it was embarrassing, because I would have to either ask the person to repeat what they said, or pretend I heard it and hope to God it wouldn't pop up again. It was embarrassing for sure and a bit scary. Imagine all of the things throughout all the years that people have said to me that I've missed.

As far back as high school, I remember being in "the zone". In hindsight, I realize now that, in class, I would be obsessing, and not focused on what the teacher was saying. Not just thoughts, but worries, worries that were killing my brain. I would go home and have to teach myself. This happened much more in university. I spent many large classes in "the zone". That's why, in my last year, I had to get up for a nine o'clock exam at three in the morning, to read eight chapters I had not yet read! Obsessions forced me into this pattern.

Being in "the zone" was far different from being merely distracted. Distractions are simply distractions. Obsessions are worse, much worse. Obsessions are repetitive, prolonging thoughts invading the mind and working to destroy it, one thought at a time.

Distractions could be forgotten. Obsessions are repetitive, progressively becoming more severe. They shoot to kill, and, in many cases, they do!

## CHAPTER 2
## THE "PERFECT" BODY

"24 ... 25 ... 26 ... phew, wipe forehead, phew ... 27 ... 28 ... 29 ... 30 ...."

That was me working out in late high school into early university. Looking at me today, you probably wouldn't ever think that I was obsessed with my physique. I really was. When it came to my body, I obsessed over it day and night for years. Let me tell you about my late high school years, when it became the most important thing in my world.

I was completely obsessed with working out and, because of this, I became transfixed on my body and how I looked in the mirror or in others' eyes. I would spend hours in the gym, and I would spend just as much time at home doing countless push-ups and sit-ups. I would work to sculpt every body part, transforming each into the strongest and most healthy-looking I could imagine. I became fanatical. Not only would I work out each day, sometimes twice, I would not even eat a tiny cookie or a spoonful of ice cream, or even have a soft drink. My excuse to my friends was, "health kick".

I remember clearly in my last year of high school, my exercise regimen transformed overnight into obsession. And this is how it happened. A typical night at home would transpire in this way.

First, I ensured that everyone had gone to bed. I would then sneak downstairs to the foyer, where I would begin ritually flexing my body in a full-length mirror. Systematically, I would flex all my muscle groups and watch scrupulously, making sure that my muscles looked toned and defined. In my mind, I had to feel really sure and confident about what I was seeing in the mirror. If not, which was often the case, I'd have to flex even harder and longer. I would stare at my "bulging" muscles and then look away, and stare ... and look away again and again. I had to have the "perfect body", thinking of all those who would see me without a shirt. So, I continued ... I flexed harder and harder, more and more. I did this hundreds of times; an episode might last over thirty minutes! Multiply this many times. I would not leave that damn mirror until I felt ready or heard my parents from upstairs.

"What the hell are you doing down there? Go back to bed!"

"Nothing! Gheesh! I'm coming up!" But when they were asleep some nights, I would head back downstairs to sneak yet another peak!

The thought pattern was simple. The "perfection" obsession would enter, causing an uncomfortable feeling in my stomach, and so I would have to relieve the obsession by flexing in the mirror. This happened countless times throughout those awful years. They were repetitive and intrusive ... and ultimately, destructive. This would go on past high school and into my university years where I would continue to obsess over my body and, eventually, in other ways that you can't imagine.

## CHAPTER 3
## BRUSH AWAY!

I obsessed over my teeth for years. I know, we all think about our teeth some of the time, but this became ridiculous. It was more than just your average minor worries about one's teeth. These endless worries controlled my thinking and ultimately my life.

This recurring obsession drove me crazy during my early years of teaching. I was preoccupied with the thought that my teeth were becoming stained.

"Are my teeth white enough?"

I would say this to myself over and over, sometimes 40 to 50 times a day! It got so bad that I still have flashbacks of the repeated rituals (compulsions) I would carry out to try and relieve my anxiety.

Again, the mirror! I used to take whatever measures I could to hunt one down and make any excuse to look at my teeth. I had to make sure that they weren't getting darker. This disabled me, keeping me from living a normal life. These thoughts, the obsessions, were on my mind day in and day out, especially after eating and drinking.

I spent countless hours checking my teeth over and over again to see that they were still clear and white. Each time I looked, even though they NEVER did change, I was convinced that they HAD!

My mind would play terrible tricks on me, under the control of this obsession. I truly believed that my teeth were stained. With that, the obsession took on a life of its own. I would spend days, countless hours, looking in the mirror. After each glance, I would ask myself, "Could I be wrong? Did I miss something? Maybe they are stained!" This would lead me to recheck, which would drive me insane! This vicious cycle took me for a ride, a shitty one. "Oh God, they look stained, don't they?" It was an unending battle with my mind, one I could not win. My mind would not allow me to see reality: a set of clean white teeth. It only showed me what I feared.

One of the places I repeatedly checked my teeth was in the rear view mirror of my car. I hated having that friggin' mirror and, although I would try everything to avoid looking in it, the uncontrollable urge would cause me to take a quick glance. This would lead me to a pattern of peaking repeatedly while driving. Not safe, I know, but I just couldn't stop myself. It became a compulsion that I used to relieve my anxiety. I would look and look and drive and drive and stress and stress and brood and brood. This behaviour continued for a long time.

Besides the never-ending saga with the mirror, a second compulsion developed. It consisted of ordering an extra glass or bottle of water so I could splash my teeth to avoid staining from foods or drink. I would seek out the closest water source to ensure that my obsession would be satiated. When the anxiety would hit, I would swish that water around my mouth, hoping to "wash" the obsession away. Sipping at my coffee or coke and then splashing my teeth, sipping and splashing, sipping and ... you get the point.

A third compulsion: I would never be caught without my sidekick, Mr. Gum! Everywhere I went, I'd rub gum over the front of my teeth! This was a poor substitute for the other two, but "desperate times called for desperate measures".

All of this was obviously very difficult for me. It took its toll. I remember constantly lying in bed thinking about my teeth, wondering if they were okay. I would then race to the washroom to carefully check them. I was so exact in my search and very meticulous. Slightly relieved, "Ahhh." And the moment I left the mirror, guess what? I'd arrive at the same conclusion. Maybe they ARE darker! Back to the mirror ....

I had to be sure each time; and, yep, I'd look again. I never believed my eyes. When the obsession re-emerged, I'd react on it, and the best way for me to relieve my anxiety was, you guessed it, a mirror. This lasted briefly until the thought resurfaced again, only minutes later. This pattern stayed with me for years. Sadly, even a natural act, such as brushing my teeth, became a compulsion.

A visit to my dentist in 2009 confirmed just the opposite (of my obsession) when my dentist, without my prompting, commented on how healthy my teeth looked. This observation was repeated by her subsequently the next two visits, six months and a year later. However, I have to admit, I still obsess occasionally over this issue. But it doesn't control me anymore. I now control it ... better.

## CHAPTER 4
## YOU OBSESSED ABOUT WHAT???

Now for a big one ... or a SMALL ONE, depending on how you look at it!

I actually obsessed for the longest time, BIG TIME, over the size of my penis. Let me explain. This one really screwed me up in a huge way at the time.

It was actually this obsession, and the ensuing anxiety, that kept me from pursuing my dreams of playing professional football. My biggest goal, growing up, was to be able to play in the *NFL* or *CFL*. I know, kids have these dreams and they usually subside as they get into high school. For me, however, the dream stayed alive ... until ...

I was invited to play football with both the University of Western Ontario and Queen's University. However, what stopped me from fulfilling this ambition to play was my obsession with the size of my penis. I lived in fear of my teammates laughing at and making fun of my penis size. This transformed into a huge obsession.

Therefore, I made up a lie. I told everyone I was not going to play university football because, being in Engineering, I needed to have an academically successful first year. To avoid too many questions, I used the excuse that I planned to play the following year. The coach at Western even gave me a year's gym pass to the varsity athletes' gym, hoping to entice me to try out the following season.

The real reason was my fear of what was "below the belt"! I spent hours, and even months after my last year of high school, obsessing over what players would say during football initiation or in the locker room. Have you ever heard of the "elephant walk"? Look it up! And I knew that, unlike high school where no one showered after practice, in university, all the guys did! I thought of all the possibilities. I wouldn't measure up with other guys, even though girlfriends I had been with before had never brought up the issue. It was in my head!

But that didn't matter because, in my mind, I still felt inadequate. Pornography and locker rooms fuelled this terrible obsession. My mind became the match that would ignite this flame. Because of this, in 1992, I made my own decision to give up contact football forever. No one, including my parents, knew the real reason.

But that was only the start of this obsession. I took it to a whole new level in the years to come. We all go through thoughts such as these, I'm sure, but most of us don't act upon them. We just pass them by, until other thoughts take over and help us forget. However, suffering from OCD, I acted upon these thoughts for years later. Here is what happened in the summer of 2000.

When I first started teaching full-time, far away from the football locker room, I was re-introduced to this terrible obsession. These can resurface anytime. I started to obsess over the thought that my penis was also small, not only when flaccid, but even when it was erect. This was prompted by a visit to Chapters, where I happened to come upon a book referring to the human body. There were boobies and asses, and, of course, penises! Everything you'd expect in these types of books! But what came to my attention was a statistic about the average erect length of the male penis. AHA ... it made me think. I NOW had to explore this. I just had to! I remember how discrete my search was, as I continued to look over my shoulders to make sure no one was looking at what I was reading. Then I had an idea. A very bad idea!

I raced home and headed to my parents' basement, where I was living. And I did it! Literally, I began to pull … and pull. I would go into the washroom, put a sexual thought in my mind, or use an image from TV, until I was fully erect. Then, I would pull out my dad's tape measure (sorry, Dad!), and check to make sure that I was of average length according to the book. And guess what? I was … thankfully … but did that matter?

NOOO!

I actually ended up spending one whole summer, hundreds of times, measuring over and over every time this obsession surfaced.

"Chris, are you in the washroom again?"

I would sweat it out lying on the bathroom floor, trying to give myself an erection so I could measure the length of my penis and reassure myself that I was "normal"(?). And it wasn't even for pleasure! Just measure! I remember being so exasperated, doing this same action over and over ... always the same result. I was the same size, of course. BUT, these compulsive actions continued again and again. This would include further visits to Chapters, time and time again, to make sure that I had read the book correctly, and checking other books to make sure the original book was accurate. I would spend a good hour going through these books and finding out the same thing every time. Then I would return to the basement and go at it again. Now that's OCD!

The thought would come (too small?) and I'd act with an awful compulsion (measuring). Returning to Chapters, over and over again, became a related compulsion. Stress and anxiety felt by the obsession would always bring me back to the horror. I'd like to forget it all happened. Not that easy. I can say, however, that this obsession no longer controls me.

## CHAPTER 5
## PAPER OR PLASTIC?

I had an obsession with cleaning up our city. Garbage, garbage and more garbage! I became madly obsessed with cleaning and, more dramatically, recycling! Actually, when I think about it, I didn't just HAVE an obsession, I LIVED it, which is true of all obsessions. In 2001, I was so obsessed with cleaning my environment, I used to drive all over Ottawa, filling up the trunk of my car with ANY garbage I would see along the way: paper cups, straws, cans, boxes, even cigarette butts! Thankfully, my obsession did not include doggy poop! Phew! You name it, it ended up in my trunk. And yes, of course, it smelled badly! I clearly remember pulling over time after time, to collect any garbage in my path. Obviously, it got tedious at times, but I kept on going and going, because of my fear of a place we all want to avoid. I'll get into that shortly.

I would stop the car, annoyed and fed up, with a stabbing thought that pounded in my head, "YOU BETTER, OR ELSE!" At times, I tried to avoid picking things up, but looking at them in my rear view mirror, I had to go back. The guilt that motivated this obsession caused me to turn around and go back, every time! Slowly but surely, my trunk would fill to the top. Then, I would pull into my roommate's garage, and separate the garbage into recyclables and non-recyclables. I would pester my roommate/landlord into obtaining larger bins appropriate for each type of trash. I became the "King of Recycling"! Touring the city, though, became a real pain in the ass because I would take so damn long to get anywhere I was going! That would have been a good reason to fight this obsession. Ironically, instead, this obsession was spent due to the emergence of new and more intense obsessions.

Paper or plastic anyone?

In 2004, I transferred this obsession to my new digs, my apartment on Riverside Drive. Garbage and recycling continued to preoccupy my mind. My kitchen became a repository for cardboard. Piled to the ceiling, in one third of my kitchen, I became motivated to save the world, one box at a time! The pile remained in my kitchen for months: my "collection".

I can recall, many times over, having to return to the lobby from my 11th floor apartment, because I feared that I had mistakenly put a recycled item into the garbage can. I looked pretty foolish dumping the trash can and recycling box onto the lobby floor to ensure that I had placed these materials in the appropriate receptacles.

I still recycle today, but not in such an "off the wall" manner. My kitchen, thankfully, is no longer a dumping ground!

## CHAPTER 6
## SHOULD I PULL OVER ... AGAIN?

In 2006, I began to form an obsession about pulling the car over to ask somebody, who appeared to be stranded, if they were "okay". As this obsession evolved, I found myself pulling over anywhere, anytime, ALL the time! I made it my new "mission" to help those who I assumed needed help.

I remember how agonizing this became, much like the garbage obsession. This, too, prolonged my various trips and, at the same time, was not at all safe. I would pull over, to either talk to complete strangers, or to "rescue" them and drop them off at a safe haven. I met a lot of new faces that winter, but I hated it when I pulled into my home two to three hours later than planned.

In one case, I took this "pulling over" obsession to a whole new level. In this particular instance, I was on my way home from Toronto, on the 401, after visiting a close friend over the weekend. Driving along, I noticed an orange SUV parked at the side of the road with its blinkers on. An alarm went off in my head and it had O-B-S-E-S-S-I-O-N written all over it.

I fought it, for seconds, and then I just had to pull over. I said to myself, "They could be stuck, they could be in danger, they could be dying, and of course, if I don't pull over, someone's going to be really mad!" Long beard, white robe, you know Who! My obsessions with hell were that extreme. So I immediately slowed and pulled up behind them. There were two people sitting in the front. Oh, and I forgot to mention, it was raining ... actually, pouring! I stepped outside. Rain was pelting my head. I didn't even have a coat! But did that stop me? OH NO! I quickly hurried to the driver side window and waved at two young ladies who had surprise written all over their faces. They hadn't expected anyone to pull over in such terrible weather.

"Hi," I said to them. We exchanged introductions and they proceeded to tell me what was wrong.

"Look carefully at the windshield wiper," the driver said, as she turned it on. "When I'm driving, my driver side wiper lifts off the windshield and it doesn't clear any water at all. I can barely see!" she exclaimed, as she continued to fiddle with the wiper lever.

And so, I thought for a moment and said, “You know what? This happened to a friend of mine. Do you have anything that you can tie the wiper down with?”

“We've tried that already,” she said dejectedly.

Meanwhile, I was getting soaked! The rain was continuing to pound the road as I stood their strategizing. To find a possible fix, she handed me a small piece of cord. “Here, you try.” I took the cord and attempted to tie down the wiper, but it just wouldn't work. Then the girl said to me, “We should be okay. We'll just take our time, because it seems to work when we're moving slowly, like a turtle.” Hah, a turtle! I thought. Sound familiar? Ah-ha, a sign!

“Are you sure you'll be okay?” I asked, as obsession continued to brew. Stranded, starving, abducted? Maybe even murdered!

“Sure ... you go ahead. We'll try driving slowly.”

We said our goodbyes and I headed back to my car. I got inside and sat for a minute, waiting for them to head off, but they seemed to be waiting for me to leave. I finally decided to pull out and head away after waiting five minutes. As I passed them, I waved and honked, and entered the busy highway. After a minute or so, IT hit me again ... O-B-S-E-S-S-I-O-N!

Huge thoughts ran through me, causing much panic and alarm. How could I have left them like that? I should have let them go ahead of me! What if their wiper stopped working completely and they got stranded again ... or crashed, and died? Holy shit! I said to myself.

By now, I'd come up with ten, maybe twenty, reasons why I HAD to go back and “save” them from this imagined demise. It was my duty to go back! It was my obligation and, besides, if I didn't go back, I knew where I'd be going. I'd be cast into hell for eternity for this one!

With that, I decided, at the next exit, I would whip back around and go to their rescue. Little did I know, when making this decision to return, that the next exit would not come for the next 20 minutes! I couldn't believe there was no freakin' exit anywhere, as I stared out my rain-soaked windshield. I was frustrated with my decision to go back, but you know! I had to ... my eternal salvation depended on it!

I drove for the next 15 minutes and finally reached the exit. I got off the highway, crossed a bridge and headed back towards Toronto. I continued along the highway, searching for the girls on the opposite side. It was difficult to see in the heavy rain, but I was determined to find them. "Where the heck are they?" After about 25 minutes, not seeing them, I pulled off the highway, again, turned around and started back to Ottawa. I continued to look for them.

Looking out my window, I surveyed the side of the road, searching closely for the girls, who needed my help desperately. I'll tell you who needed the help, dammit!!!

I drove for about 10 minutes and then I said to myself again, "Where the hell are they? Man, where ARE they? Maybe I didn't go back far enough towards Toronto? Maybe they were further back than I thought?" I shook my head in dismay. I couldn't believe it! How could I have missed them?

"I fucking missed them!" I said, wiping my brow. Cursing, under these conditions, seemed no longer a problem. I was sweating now, as I mentally prepared myself for the inevitable: acting out a compulsion. Like all compulsions, I just had to do it! I HAD to! So, I decided that, at the next exit, I would head back again towards Toronto, even further this time. I had to find them! This was the right thing to do. I just knew it!

I drove another 15 minutes and ended up exiting at the same place I had before. I crossed the same highway bridge and started to head back to Toronto ... again. The rain continued to pour. I drove for 30 minutes more this time, and was sure that I'd gone back far enough.

I again exited the highway and hopped back onto the road to Ottawa. At least I was going in the right direction, I reassured myself. I drove for another 20 minutes without seeing them, and slammed the steering wheel furiously. "FUCK!" I exclaimed, as I continued to look along the side of the highway. Maybe I missed them? I thought to myself. Maybe I wasn't looking closely enough? Was it possible? So you know what I did!

OH YAH! The whole damn thing again! Off the highway, over the bridge, back towards Toronto, 40 minutes this time, off the highway, back towards Ottawa. The only reason I didn't do it again (I came very close) was that I called my friend in Toronto and told him what I had been doing. He told me how ridiculous I was, and that I should go right home, immediately. I had already added almost four hours to my trip! I heeded his advice and thankfully headed home. It was the longest trip from Toronto that I had ever taken. Added to that were a few other stops for other perceived victims in need! Total time for the trip … 9 hours! But, come on, it WAS raining!

I continued this practice for years, wherever I drove. It was not pleasant. It was downright dangerous and life-threatening.

## CHAPTER 7
## LET ME JOT THAT DOWN!

In late high school, and throughout university, I became obsessed with writing notes. It didn't matter what time of day it was, or what I was doing, I wrote notes everywhere about everything! In my last year of high school, one could find little sticky notes all over the house: in my bedroom, in the kitchen, in the living room, and even on the washroom mirrors! My mom loved that one! Went great with the decor!

What did I write on these notes? It ranged from things I had to do, to thoughts I was having, to where I was going, to what incredible ideas I might have had. I would even write notes to pump me up before a football game or a test. My mom used to walk around the house finding notes in the plants, or in cupboards, saying things like, "You can do it!" or "Keep going!" or "Yay, Chris!"

You had to see my rooms in those years. There were notes everywhere! Any thought or obsession I had (an uncomfortable feeling that was killing me that I had to resolve) would be attacked with a compulsion (an action of writing the note to relieve the anxiety I was feeling).

I was caught in a real mental prison. I felt the need to write down any thought I was having. Any thought! You couldn't avoid the notes in my residence dorm at UWO. Little yellow "stickies" plastered all over my room: on the desk, floor, bed and walls. My university roommates would mock me for my tendency to write these notes all the time. At the time, we just thought I was a "worry wart". We never saw the severity of these actions. Walking through my room was like walking through a minefield. You'd often hear visitors saying, "Holy shit, Nihmey! What's up with all the notes?" With a shrug and a nervous reply, I would answer, "I don't know."

Get this. I even wrote notes based on my dreams! What the hell am I trying to say? Well, I actually had a piece of paper up on the wall beside my bed, with a pencil hanging on a string. This was for writing any notes I needed to write if I woke up from a dream and had a thought or idea. Notes ruled and controlled my life. I was held hostage by this obsession. I eventually escaped, with a lot of hard work. I try now to apply logic to any note-taking that I do. I don't have it under complete control yet. I am progressively improving, but there's still a lot of work to do.

A few times throughout the years, I did something that helped me to battle the "notes" obsession. I had to do it. I'm convinced that my life depended on it at the time. Three separate occasions, with as much strength and courage as I could muster, I actually rounded up every single note that lay on my floor, my bed, my cupboard and my closet, into the biggest of piles. I then sat, cross-legged in the middle of my room and, one by one, ripped each and every note up. Without even looking at them, I threw them into the garbage. The feeling was excruciating and it burned inside me. I felt incredibly awful, but I still moved forward. The second and third time I did this, I avoided the ripping and just dumped them!

I recall how hard it was to do at the time, but I also remember the satisfaction and relief of letting go of so much. For days following these toss-outs, I would worry and stress that bad things would happen because of the notes I threw out. But you know what? There were never any negative repercussions. Throwing those notes out became pivotal events in my healing, in overcoming and controlling my OCD as a whole.

## CHAPTER 8
## THE CALL BACK

This is still one of the obsessions I struggle with. A bit funny when I think about it now, because I have a better handle on it. But, at the time, it wasn't funny at all. It completely affected my well-being and anyone with whom I was involved. Let me give you a simple, but familiar, scenario.

I would be talking with a friend, hanging on every word to make sure that all was "perfect". Our conversation would be wrapping up and ...

"So, good talking to you, Chris. Thanks for listening. I'll take your advice."

"Glad I could help you," I would respond.

"Take care, Chris."

"Okay, bye."

I'd hang up the phone and, all of a sudden, my body would cringe. Immediately, anxious thoughts would set in. A feeling of dread would take hold and shake me silly like a ragdoll. I would go through a series of rote questions every time this obsession occurred. It sounded much like this:

"Aw... man. Maybe I should have said that, too. Maybe he thinks I don't care. Maybe he thinks I hung up too early. UGH!"

This would lead to worse feelings, as sweat would form on my brow, and I would feel deep down that there was definitely more that I had to say or should have said. "This could completely RUIN my friendship with them! They'll hate me!"

This happened with friends, and family. I thought I would lose them all. I thought the world would cave in on me if I didn't call them back at that exact moment. I even felt deep down that they would be relieved to hear from me again. I assumed that THEY wanted to talk with me and hear more from me. So I was even thinking for them! This also became a common behaviour that I adopted. More later.

My mind would conjure up a reason, any reason, to call them back. I felt there was something so important that I just HAD to tell them that, for some reason, I had forgotten. I would actually convince myself that making a call was a MUST and that they were expecting it. I had to remedy things that may have gone awry and, I felt that, without calling, I would struggle with this for the "rest of my life". This was the case with all my obsessions.

"Call backs" had obsession written all over them. It got so bad at times, that all my family and friends knew that, when we hung up, it meant a call back (compulsion) was coming. They had come to expect the phone to ring only seconds after hanging up with me. This became the ritual for years, day after day. I still catch myself doing it at times, today, but I have a much better handle on this obsession. The feelings still come up in my stomach when I feel I haven't said all I need to say, or if I felt a conversation didn't end on a positive note. That's when I pick up the phone and dial. God bless my family and friends who received the calls graciously, when I'm sure what they wanted to say to me was, LEAVE ME ALONE!

## CHAPTER 9
## UP OR DOWN?

This is an obsession that I have battled most of my life, and probably will for the rest, even though it has decreased in intensity, thanks to therapy and hard work. I touched on it earlier, but I feel the need to elaborate further. At one time, not so long ago, in a very powerful way, this obsession pulled at every fibre of my well-being and affected every aspect of my quality of life. This became lethal during months of both mania and depression. It has been the cause of more compulsions and anxieties than I could ever have imagined experiencing. After countless hours of therapy and many drastic life changes, I have managed to better control my thoughts and subsequent actions.

My doctor and I zoned in on this very obsession over many sessions of psychotherapy. We felt that this one concept was the definitive cause of hundreds, perhaps thousands, of obsessions through the years. This, in turn, led to a myriad of compulsions, in the hope of relieving anxieties and fears I was feeling. I then learned, early on, that the obsessions, although relieved momentarily, returned in a much more intense way the next time. Yes, it sucked, and I fell victim to it time and time again.

So, here it is. Here is the thought or the question I have asked myself, over and over for years. A simple five-word question, but it became deeply rooted and profound in my mind and my physical being. Am I going to hell?

Does it scare you? Maybe not, maybe so. It certainly scared me. Can anything be more extreme or more frightening than this? Hey, I'm a horror buff, and I've seen all the horror movies on the shelf, but this one thought makes all of these movies pale in comparison. Shit, my eternal salvation is wrapped up in those five profound words:

**AM – I – GOING – TO – HELL?**

I have lived with this fear for as long as I can remember, right from my first introduction to it as a kid. But it only started to affect me adversely in my late teens, with the onset of my disorders. I used to wonder why I feared hell so much more as a teenager than others. Why did I have this overabundance of fear that eventually controlled all my thoughts and actions, when others were able to live without it? Hadn't we all learned the same things in our Roman Catholic environment?

However, after extensive therapy, research and contemplation, I started to understand things better and found some answers to my questions. Let me explain what my doctors and I discovered.

When I started to write this book, I didn't quite know where this consuming fear of hell came from. I just thought it was fuelled by things like school and church and the media (horror movies ... our two friends, Jason and Freddy ... you know them, right?). But therapy and research taught me that this fear had nothing to do with the information that I was TAKING IN. We all learn about hell in so many ways growing up and how terrible it apparently is (shit, we celebrate Halloween with our stupid red devil horns!).

Rather, it had everything to do with HOW my OCD processed the information and was input into my life experiences. For some reason, once the information was being processed, something different was happening in my head, compared to what was happening in the minds of healthy individuals. While so many others were able to see these things as fun, exciting or entertaining, my mind processed this information differently.

This five letter sentence burned inside me for years when sickness hit and took over my world. These years eventually became years of a "sick mind" trying to bob for air above the turbulent waters without a life preserver.

Even up to a couple of years ago, I wanted to lay the blame for my infatuation with hell on others, namely school, church and media. At least this is what I thought. Shit, *Looney Tunes* painted the picture of the devil and his workers walking around poking us in the ass with pitchforks, working those same asses off, in the excruciating heat: tired, exhausted and restless forever. Hell, as they described it, as even Freddy described it, was your worst nightmare!

And SO, what happened to me? What did Chris Nihmey's sick mind do? While 99 out of 100 people brushed hell off as merely a passing thought, nothing to worry about, and continued to live their lives peacefully on earth, I bought it all.

Because my mind was so unbalanced, I ended up fearing hell more than anything I have ever feared! I was unable to comprehend it rationally. The fear then grew from there as I began visiting the confessional far more than what was normal.

I tried always to be a good person from a young age but, as I grew, I remember changing many things in my life to ensure I stayed in "God's Little White Book". And so, for more than ten years, I took being a "good" person to new heights. An example of this is the fact that I remained a virgin for so long. Have you seen *The 40 Year Old Virgin*? That's me, and Steve Carrel! This is a profound example of the obsession with "goodness" and God. I tried to do everything right; I tried to follow "goodness" and be the best that I could be. And what came of it? It was what my therapist called ***perfectionism*** (a need to be perfect in every way), an obsession I am battling alongside all the other shit. Boy, was I fucked up or what?

At that young age, I thought I knew what hell was ... I knew it was a bad place ... I knew you NEVER wanted to go there and I hoped I knew how to avoid going. So, where did this intense fear come from? Why did it keep taking over my mind? If it wasn't my family, school, church, friends, movies, television or books, what was it? It was more than that.

Through much therapy and research, I've come again to realize that it wasn't WHAT I was learning that affected me so much, but rather the WAY in which my unbalanced mind was registering and interpreting what I was learning. Without any of us knowing, my mind had become conditioned to obsess. When this happened, my mind would catch onto a concept and take it to a ridiculous and ludicrous extreme. My dad often joked, "How come there's a "Chris" in ludi'crous'?" Yah, I know it's misspelled. Oh-oh, my perfectionism just kicked in again!

So, I took the concept of hell and muddled over it, recycled it, regurgitated it, ruminated over it and, in turn, made it the "Be All and End All"! It was OCD, and it almost destroyed me.

How? Following are many compulsions or rituals that I would undergo when I was obsessing over hell. Mania and the resulting anxiety made things even worse. While so many people of faith were secure in their beliefs and their status with God, I would act in perverse and insensible ways to keep myself from going to hell. I had a really misshapen view of everything. Here's what I did. Some may have been mentioned earlier. Here are MY *23 PSALMS*:

1. I would go to church over and over, several times a week, even when it was completely inconvenient and unnecessary.
2. I would go to confession weekly, and bend on knees several times a day to ask forgiveness for something that was really nothing.
3. I would give money to charities over and over, sometimes in the hundreds of dollars, including several churches I frequented during my mania. I remember tossing a fifty dollar bill into a basket one Sunday, like I was throwing a toonie. I felt God would bless me for that one! Give and you shall receive.
4. I would pray repetitively and redundantly for mine and others' salvation and needs, morning and night. Over and over, whether I was lying in bed, taking a shower, driving the car, with friends, wherever and with whomever ... I was praying!
5. I would seek spiritual advice from priests or pastors for guidance and direction in my life. I did this to find the "way" to Heaven. My address book was completely reconfigured with numbers and addresses of people I'd met at all the churches I attended. I found a whole new "Christian" clientele, and barely saw childhood friends at this time.
6. I would read the Bible meticulously, memorizing and studying it verse by verse. I knew that I needed to know His book real well, or else. I became well-versed in *Revelation*, of course, thinking honestly that the end of the world was just around the corner.
7. I would blare Christian music in the car and sing aloud while driving, just to get the negative "hell" thoughts out. I even left my car and danced at intersections. At times, I honestly felt that if I didn't embarrass myself for God, He'd be mad.
8. I called prayer lines over and over many times a day. Up to 20 different ones! I would constantly

call whenever someone was in need of prayer, no matter how big or how small. If I deemed it important, and invariably it was, a prayer was going to happen. I remember the prayer line people snickering or acting astonished when I called for things that didn't quite need a prayer.

9. I started my own prayer group online and took part in help-lines where I provided spiritual guidance and wisdom. Imagine ... like I knew what I was talking about! I hoped, though, this would bring favour with the "Big Guy". Wink, wink, nod, nod.

10. I would watch spiritual programs ALL the time. I subsisted on *Vision TV*. My roommates rolled their eyes and would constantly bug me when they turned the TV on to some preacher preaching! They laughed at me; so I prayed for their salvation!

11. I would preach to kids, while supply teaching, and even leave pamphlets titled, "Get To Know God!" on the teachers' desks upon leaving. It gave the reader the steps to take to find God and bring Jesus into their lives, to be "born again". This, at Catholic schools, where I was convinced that they weren't spiritual enough!

12. I would preach to friends, family and even people I didn't know; often, I was overly forceful. This would lead to arguments and negative vibes for all involved. I had to share my new knowledge, no matter the cost. Everyone was a possible victim for hell, a sinner, and I had to steer them in the right direction. "The end is nigh!"

13. I would attend church functions or meetings, whenever possible, and, during my high, avoid the Catholic ones.

14. I would attend Bible courses in different churches, which taught about certain principles such as forgiveness, prayer and salvation.

15. I would pray repetitively the *Salvation Prayer* to assure myself that I was saved and not going to hell. Obviously, I was worried it wasn't working, because I kept praying it over and over.

16. I would attempt to purify my "evil" thoughts through repetitive prayer (mantras) and Bible readings. It was never enough, so the Bible, in its little velvet case, stayed perpetually opened.

17. I would have direct conversations with God, calling him Dad. I believed that I had a direct line to Him. At least I thought I had. I talked to Him 24/7 like He was "attached to my hip". I believed that. I looked pretty crazy at times, appearing to others that I was talking to myself.

18. I would verbally attack those who did not follow Christ, even strangers. Remember the Jehovah's and my teaching colleague?

19. I would be judgemental, even when inappropriate, especially when I felt I was being confronted. I never fought physically, but came close a few times.

20. I would carry crosses or wear religious paraphernalia, hang stuff in my car, and carry my Bible everywhere I went. You never knew when there'd be a fight or a bad word and reconciliation would be needed!

21. I would never, ever, kill a bug. Big sin, that one ... hell immediately. He who killeth a life, his life be taketh!

22. As previously mentioned, I would register a business called *Turtles Ministries*, a helpline for reaching out to others looking for spiritual reflection and renewal. The number was 863-5483 ... TOE LITE. I saw this as something "happening for a reason". God lights the path for my feet (toes)! Get it? I even had thousands of business cards printed with the motto, "With Jesus at pace, we'll win the race."

23. I would say grace at every meal, often minutes long, even forcing it on friends who didn't say grace at all, even in a restaurant. This became very uncomfortable, but they had to hear God's message, beer or no beer, wine or no wine!

With all this, I still felt I was heading down the long road to hell. How can one win if these things don't save you? I couldn't. I never felt assured of salvation. My obsessions never left me, ever. I was caught in a negative whirlwind bringing me down, more and more, with repetitive, arduous compulsions to relieve(?) the pain, no matter how high or low my brain chemistry took me.

For as long as I can remember, I've dealt with this "hell" obsession. During my sick years, it took a hold of me and changed my whole quality of life into something completely unmanageable. It was an unbalanced and unhealthy mind that took everything to heart and made life unbearable. It was awful but, with a lot of hard work, perseverance and rationality, I've moved beyond these terrible days. Yes, I still have post-traumatic experiences which trigger "ups and downs", and obsessions causing anxiety but, hopefully, these terrible days are behind me.

***"Our greatest glory is not in never falling, but in rising every time we fall."***

***Confucius***

# PART VIII

# STRATEGIES TO COUNTER OBSESSIONS

## CHAPTER 1
## STEPS TO RECOVERY

I was diagnosed with obsessive-compulsive disorder in 2003. By 2004, my obsessions were at an all-time high: in fact, in the hundreds. My psychiatrist, my family and my friends had come to the end of their ropes with me. I had used them so much during that time. By trying to console me, each unknowingly was reinforcing my bad habits. I would constantly foist my obsessions onto them. They became frustrated, fed up and irritated with me while, at the same time, sympathetic. It was difficult for them to be empathetic, since none of them, thankfully, were afflicted by the disorder.

My psychiatrist referred me to a psychologist, Dr. Tate. The first time I met him, he shook my hand, but I sidetracked the introductions and started to fret. I had parked on a wintry side street and was unnecessarily worried about getting a ticket for being illegally parked. Most people think this way for a moment, but rid themselves of these notions. Well, I'm a different cat. When a thought begins for me, I ruminate over it excessively and it forms into an obsession. And with most obsessions, *a* compulsion (checking my car) is sure to follow, as it did in so many different situations. So what did I do the minute I walked into his office? I immediately shared what was on my mind.

"What is parking like out there? I parked on the street in front of your building. I don't know if I'm illegally parked. I can't tell with the snow. What if I get a ticket, what if I get towed? Oh God, can I just go check my car?"

His firm handshake and friendly greeting didn't matter to me at all. He could tell right away why he was going to be working with me. Like Dr. Boyles, Dr. Tate also said that I was really "the perfect patient", but for different reasons.

For the next year, a whole year, I met with Dr. Tate once or twice a month, depending on his schedule. He was a knowledgeable man, and we bonded well, but he knew I had a real problem, a problem that was affecting my life in every way. Although he helped me out tremendously, even in the first few sessions, I remember feeling the opposite. I told my parents numerous times, "It's not working! I hate it, I hate him, $150 a session and he's not doing shit for me!"

I was sure he wasn't helping and, at the time, I felt nothing would. I always felt that way because, although our sessions were intellectual and informative, when I had an outburst of obsessions occurring the next day or days to follow, I couldn't help but feel defeated, depleted and devastated. It wasn't Dr. Tate's fault at all, or mine. It was a problem deeply rooted within me, and now it was at an extreme. The fires were burning and the wood was piled high! Dr. Tate wasn't the firefighter either, he was just the "directions" out of the building, and I had to start putting my trust in him. I had to learn to put the fire out myself.

Dr. Tate and I would use many charts and his whiteboard to help me to understand a number of things. First, what an obsession really was, and second, why obsessions were happening and what I needed to do to overcome or manage them.

He decided to use the *Cognitive-Behavioural Approach* to help me, trying to counteract my thoughts using an array of mental strategies (see below). He knew I was already taking medication to fight obsessions, so he made it his goal to help me to work on the thoughts taking over my mind, and the behaviours required to overcome these thoughts. He told me, and I'll never forget it, that medication is a great blessing and works miracles, but it only takes you so far. The rest is up to the work you put in, (the mental part) that makes all the difference in improving your lifestyle. This, I definitely needed to do. The more you put in, the more you improve.

Each time we met, I was given homework (see chart below). And I hated it! The homework was meant to change my way of thinking, and that bothered me because I was so used to living the way I was. An obese person finds it so hard to eat healthy because they are used to living an unhealthy life. Why eat celery when you can eat a Big Mac? An alcoholic continues to drink because he thinks it makes him feel better.

I needed to experience life in another way, a more positive way. I needed to change my way of thinking because the type of thinking I had become accustomed to was literally killing me. Denzel Washington, in the movie, *Remember The Titans*, states, *"Everything we gonna do is changing, we gotta change. We gonna change the way we run, we gonna change the way we eat, we gonna change the way we block, we gonna change the way we tackle, we gonna change the way we win. It is desire. Desire!"*

Well, I definitely needed to change the way I lived. Like an anorexic, I had to eat. Like an obese person, I had to lose pounds. Like a drug addict, I had to quit "cold turkey". I had to change everything I was doing. Would that help me? Was that it? I hoped so, because I felt like a wall was now in front of my nose. I couldn't even see the bricks above or below. I was too comfortable in the shit that was suffocating me. But I came to know it was time for change.

So, with that, we zoned in on the obsessions that were most dramatically affecting my well-being. The first thing he asked me to do was to make a $20.00 "getting your life back" investment, by purchasing a book called *THE OCD WORKBOOK*, written by Bruce M. Hyman, PH.D. and Cherry Pedrick, RN. And boy, was I blessed to have used it. I took ten steps (of thousands) forward by reading this book and implementing the strategies involved. We incorporated the book into our sessions, and I was given homework using it, and the exercises inside.

We had one-hour sessions every few weeks, where we worked on trying to understand where my obsessions were coming from and figuring out when and how to leave them behind. From him, and the book, I learned many things:

- **Types of Obsessions** that I was having (which helped me to realize I wasn't alone); mine were hoarding, collecting, ordering, religious obsessions, scrupulosity, somatic obsessions, sexual obsessions, physical checking/mental checking, pure obsessions (thought on thought), and the compulsions that followed;
- **What is Obsessive-Compulsive Disorder?** I learned what OCD was all about, and we worked to define thoughts and better understand them;
- **OCD and Shame (stigma impeding the sufferer)**;
- **Genetics (inheriting the condition)**;
- **Solutions and Strategies**;
- **Cognitive-Behaviour Therapy (the lifesaver)**;
- **Response Prevention / Response Delay**;
- **Dealing with Compulsions**;
- **Facing fears and anxieties**;

- **Scrupulosity** (realized that religious and moral views were warped, and affecting everything I did);
- **Subjective Units of Distress Scale (SUDS)** – measures the amount of anxiety the person feels when they are obsessing (Higher SUDS level = Higher Anxiety).

For SUDS, we formulated a chart for the things that I was struggling with the most and looked at the level of distress I was feeling for each at a given time (see chart below). When an obsession popped up, I would give it an initial rating, a level of distress (*SUDS)*. For example, 80 or 90 was a high level of distress. Most of my obsessions were at that SUDS level or higher. 100 was the highest it went. The stronger or higher the SUDS level, the more it affected me and the more likely a compulsion would follow. I then had to learn to do everything possible to avoid a compulsion from happening (eg., avoiding grace before a snack). A compulsion would only nourish the obsession.

If I managed to avoid the compulsion, I would then rate the anxiety or SUDS level. At first, it didn't decrease significantly. I had a high level of anxiety and distress all the time and fell subject to many compulsions. What I found in time, however, with Dr. Tate's guidance and direction, was the level of SUDS actually did start to decrease, which lowered my need to compulse! It was amazing. It actually worked! The chart denoted what I had to fight:

- no grace after or before snacks;
- swimming trunks off in the change room;
- self-pleasuring when feeling the urge (I had avoided this at all costs because of religious guilt – once for a whole year);
- no water on teeth after drinking dark liquids (coffee, soft drinks);
- no "I love you" before hanging the phone up with family;
- no repeat calls home;
- no unnecessary "sorry";
- no checking and rechecking repeatedly (ex., emails);
- no calling people back after hanging up;
- no long prayer sessions before bed;

- no prayer requests to friends through my online prayer group;
- avoid attending church (for 3 years, I've had to avoid going due to extreme obsessions);
- try to make attempts to displease God (counteract the obsession);
- no weight or food obsessions;
- no looking for hair thinning;
- if upset, no calling home or friends. Take a walk instead;
- STOP thinking what you "think" others are thinking.

My chart looked something like this:

The first number (90) in the first column represents the anxiety level out of 100 when the obsession first appears. The second number (80) in the first column is the anxiety level AFTER the obsession is ignored. Each successive column represents the recurrence of the same obsession. Only this time, the anxiety level has decreased. If the compulsion is not acted upon, the next time the obsession appears, one can see that the anxiety level will continue to decrease. Hopefully, the obsession will eventually weaken and disappear.

The chart is illustrated as follows:

| **ACTION** | **SUDS** | | |
|---|---|---|---|
| No call backs | 90 S 80 | 80 S 70 | 65 S 60 |
| No grace after snacks | 95 S 85 | 85 S 75 | |
| No weight or food obsessions | 100 S 90 | 95 S 85 | |

I was with Dr. Tate for almost a year. Needless to say, he played a critical role in helping me to come out of the cave I was in, but I wouldn't say that I left Dr. Tate with everything figured out. I didn't. I couldn't. There was so much more to know and learn. But I do say that he played a vital role in getting me to where I am today, which is not completely healed, but making the illness liveable and manageable, as long as I continue to work at it daily. I will always have to work at it, but I am now able to live a quality of life that I've never lived. If you suffer from obsessions, even minor ones, I can't encourage you enough to seek help for your problem. You can't do it alone and hopefully with the help of someone you can put your trust in, you will find exactly what you need. I also encourage you to purchase the *OCD Workbook*. It was a godsend for me.

Medication and therapy could only take me so far. Defeating obsessions would begin with a decision that I needed to make. I had to accept that I HAD to change, and take the next step on my own. Applying his strategies was essential for my healing. I also had to employ some of my own strategies to further my healing. I had to apply rationality to all my behaviours.

***"Our greatest weakness lies in giving up. The most certain way to succeed is always to try just one more time."***

***Thomas Edison***

## CHAPTER 2
## MY STRATEGIES

Here are some of the strategies I adopted in those dreadful days. Success wasn't immediate and didn't come easily. These were some of the worst years of my life. I accepted the journey I had to take from the hell generated by my sickness.

### I THE CLICKER

In October of 2004, when my obsessions and compulsions were at an all-time high, depressed and beaten down, I walked into a Canadian Tire Superstore. I hated going into stores like that, with their hundreds of aisles and tens of thousands of store items. I knew what I was looking for, but I had no idea where I would find it, let alone whether it would be in this particular store. And guess what?

Yep, you guessed it. This stressed me out. I was stressed, as I had been hundreds of times before. It had built up all morning and, because I was suffering so much at the time, even doing simple things like going to the store were a challenge for me.

So with all my strength, I started to walk up and down the aisles searching feverishly and anxiously for something that I felt I needed more than anything. I had read a book that gave different tips or ideas concerning strategies that one could use to conquer obsessions. This strategy would be used to defeat the urge to perform compulsions. Many strategies had failed for me, as did most ideas, and being near my wits' end, I decided to try out one more. I hoped so much that this one might work for me, but doubt was in my head as I raced up and down those aisles, dodging around people to find the "Holy Grail", the gift of eternal life! Yes, I know, I'm exaggerating, but I really felt that this would extend my life in some magical way and help me to finally enjoy some things because, right now, I was hating my life entirely.

I looked around more and more, doing everything to avoid the store clerks. I didn't want to talk to anyone. I felt shitty enough that I didn't need to converse with anybody. I just wanted to get what I needed and get the hell out! Finally, after about twenty frustrating and pain-staking minutes, I found what I was looking for. It was a miracle! I remember feeling as though a beam of sunlight had shone on me, with the word "Alleluia!" being sung aloud.

I grabbed the first one I saw and looked at it. This is it? I thought. This is what I spent all this time looking for?

"Shit, I could have made one of these," I said to myself.

I stared at it for a few minutes before walking to the front cash. I bought it.

Alright, time to tell you what I bought, but remember, don't laugh. There was a reason, a good reason. I purchased what turned out to be a wonderful tool. It was something that, according to my reading, would help me counteract the urge to perform a compulsion when an obsession arrived.

In my hand was an object called "The Clicker". It was the perfect title, because that's what it was … that's all it was … a small handheld clicker. It was tiny enough to cup in the palm of my hand. With my hand closed over it, I was able to hide the entire thing easily, which was good, because I didn't want people to see me using it. So far, I'd managed to keep my OCD under wrap. Others just would not understand.

It had a metal lever, and a small screen that displayed 4 zeros in a row (0 0 0 0). It also had a dial on the side for resetting. Maybe I've spent too much time describing the damn thing. If you are confused, all you need to know was that it was a clicker. Okay, a clicker! It clicked!

I had purchased the almighty clicker, an object that was able to count things. It would count up to 9999. Could I ever get that high with the task and the goal I was setting? NEVER! I thought. But at least it gave me hope. I was to "click" each time I was successful attacking an obsession. Whenever an obsession would appear, and I had an intense urge to act upon it, I was to fight/avoid the compulsion at any cost. If I succeeded, I would click the counter once. This, in turn, would cause the number to move from (0 0 0 0) to (0 0 0 1) and so on for subsequent successes. Then, I was told, if I fell to an obsession, I was supposed to reset the counter back to zero. It was all pretty simple, but my job was not. Not at all. Although the "clicker" was supposed to be the motivator for me to fight against obsessions, I found at first, that it actually did the opposite. Why?

This was what really happened. In the months of using the "clicker", I don't think I ever brought that stupid counter above the number (0 0 1 0). 10 dammit! That was the highest I made, and resetting the damned thing was so frustrating: seeing the numbers flip to zero again and again. I remember, time and again, watching the counter flip back to zero, almost like it was in slow motion. It was failure for me and it hit hard. However, this failure started to drive me to get higher than 10, so I kept it up. Maybe this was a stepping stone to success ...?

The "clicker" lasted about four months ... four long months. Out of frustration, I threw the damn thing in the garbage, but somehow it ended up back in my drawer. I still have it to this day. I definitely made some progress with it, but I became frustrated resetting it over and over. At the time I felt as if it weakened me rather than pumped me up. Although it worked some, I'd hoped for more. In retrospect, however, it was definitely a good first step. I would recommend giving this strategy a try. It did take me forward because I was ready for change. But after these months, rather than just a step, I needed to take a leap. The "clicker" was a good initial step, but it was time for a new strategy.

## II THE DELAY

"The Delay" was a technique re-introduced to me by my on-call doctor during a six week stay at *Day Hospital* in 2005. I was taught to implement this clever technique which proved invaluable to my healing. Typically, I saw Day Hospital as a waste of time. In retrospect, I was wrong. My days there were building blocks towards my healing and have contributed to where I am today. The techniques and strategies I was taught were entirely worthwhile but, at the time, there were several I wasn't yet ready for.

Here's how this strategy worked. First, Dr. McBride chose one of my obsessions, one of many I was having. He assured me that if I could make an effort to keep myself from acting on the obsession, I could succeed. "Try delaying the compulsion for one minute, then try five, ten, thirty, and then one hour. With each delay you will head towards the goal of defeating the obsession for good."

It sounded simple, but I learned quickly it wasn't. It would take a lot of work on my part. He said, however, that I had to be committed to it; if so, I would find it highly effective. Delay, and the mind will relax more. The first delay would be the most difficult to apply, but subsequent ones would be easier to endure. They would last longer and have a much greater impact, thus decreasing the desire to act on the obsession. Although the delay technique was not yet effective for me at the time, it was actually one of the beginning strategies that helped me to counteract obsessions like the following, and to live a better quality of life.

I often obsessed about friends and family. When I spoke with them on the phone, I always felt the need to do "the call back". You know this one already ... real pain in the ass. Dr. McBride and I decided to use this particular obsession to put the technique into play. This is what he told me.

"So Chris, you're talking on the phone and you're having a conversation and your friend has to go. You can't talk forever, you know that, although you'd like to, but conversations naturally must come to an end. So your friend says to you that they have to go.

You feel uneasy, wondering what you did wrong to cause them to say that, but you shrug that off. You know that conversations need to end sometime. You say bye and you hang up. Thoughts flood in and you suddenly feel the urge to pick up the phone and call back, and also to make up an excuse as to why you needed to call. Here's what I propose. Next time you talk on the phone, use "the delay". You are going to delay the act of calling back. You're going to prevent yourself from picking up that phone again."

I naturally questioned this. I asked him how this was possible? I just couldn't imagine doing this. How could I possibly succeed? He told me to give it a try. He said that every time I delayed, the stronger I would get, and the weaker the obsession would get. I needed to delay the compulsion. The compulsion was the danger. If it happened, the obsession would strengthen. If the compulsion was blocked, the obsession would eventually weaken and disappear.

I decided to try. I went home and called a few friends and attempted to apply the technique. I didn't succeed right away, or on several occasions that followed, but I noticed this. Over the next few months, as I delayed the compulsion even a little bit, progressively the obsession lessened. With consistent delays, the obsession got weaker and weaker and the need to perform the compulsion was far less.

At first it was tough. I would walk away from the phone, or try to read or watch TV. I wanted so badly to satisfy the urge. I might have waited thirty seconds or so before I picked up. The doctor told me that this was a success on its own. The commitment I made was decisive ... an important first step. The thirty-second delay eventually became a minute delay: a difficult minute where I would think of every possible reason as to why I should call back. What are they thinking? Are they mad? I hung up so quickly! They hate me!

But I persisted. Over the next few months, seconds became minutes and minute delays became victories as I avoided picking up the phone again. Today, it is something I rarely do, but it is still a battle I fight. I continue to use this technique successfully to fight other obsessions.

## III DO THE OPPOSITE

I was not able to use this technique at first. I thought it was impossible because of the difficulties I'd have to put myself through to succeed. Dr. Tate and I had explored this concept, but I was unable to put it into play for several years. I tried but failed ... miserably.

Basically, it worked like this. I was supposed to do the opposite of how I naturally would react (compulsion) to the obsession. Here is an example. All of these examples are true life situations that I experienced battling my OCD.

The phone rings. It is a good friend. They tell me that they "burned" a movie. Right away, the hair on the back of my neck stands up. I know that burning a movie is illegal, and I feel the immediate need to "right the wrong" by telling them, "It is illegal and you should not do that." I did this often with many other obsessions, and with anyone, anywhere. However, I had been working on this new technique. It told me to do the complete "opposite" of what I was thinking, even though it would burn in my gut and be very difficult to do. This is what I would try to do. I would hold my tongue and let the conversation roll on. In other words, the opposite of what I had been conditioned to do … making a value-laden comment, which contributed to making me sick and was often "over the top".

Alternatively, I might turn the conversation to another topic to fight the urge to say something. Where I would earlier have reacted immediately, I would now refrain. Instead of compulsing, I would redirect my thoughts to another topic, countering the original.

It is a very simple strategy, but very difficult to put into practice. After years of struggling, I can now apply it and make it work.

## IV WORST CASE SCENARIO

This strategy also took me a while to put into play, but once I was able to use it, it worked very well. Here's an example.

After a great time, I'm saying goodbye to a friend and his family after watching my godson's soccer game. They are inside their van and I am standing beside it saying goodbye. They roll away and I hear my godson say, from inside the van, "Dad, I need to tell you a secret." That's all I hear and they start to pull away.

I stop in my tracks, and the following questions start to pile up. "Why did he say that? Was he going to say something about me? Does he like me? Was he going to tell his dad that he didn't like his Uncle Chris?" All of these thoughts start firing and, in my gut, I feel like shit. After taking two steps towards the van, I instead turn and walk to my car. I'm now thinking about these things and getting sick to my stomach, however …

I suddenly think of a strategy that I'd been using and that had been helping me get through some obsessions. I apply the "Worst Case Scenario" strategy, which is a technique I read about in Dale Carnegie's *How to Stop Worrying and Start Living*. I purchased this book in 1998, my first year of teaching, when I was looking for answers to deal with the way I was feeling. Although I hoped to derive help from it, I was unable to, because of my condition at the time ... depressed.

After years of healing, thanks to therapy, medication and hard work, I eventually found the book helpful. Here's how the strategy works.

Okay, so he said that to his dad. He told his dad that he didn't like me.

So then, maybe he doesn't like me. I'll just have to accept that.

Another thought enters. What if the parents don't like me because their son doesn't?

Okay, so he doesn't like me, and neither do his parents or any of his family. So what? What does that mean? I'll accept this as a possibility.

Applying the "worst case scenario", I will never see them again in my entire life. That is officially the end of my friendship with them and I am no longer "the godfather". C'est fini!

I've taken a stressful situation and shone a new light on it, actually making it less important. I've imagined the worst possible scenario. Nothing worse could happen. Nothing. That is the most that would affect me. I'd never have to see them again. Oh well! Shit happens!

This is how the strategy works, and it does work, but not immediately. It takes time and practice, as do all the strategies. But they work and they work well. Ultimately, the worst case doesn't occur. I've applied this technique repeatedly with success.

## V THE FLOOD

"The Flood" was a technique I devised a few years into my battle with obsessions and it worked well for me.

You're obsessing about having left the front door unlocked. You've driven away, you are heading downtown and, all of a sudden, you think, "Did I lock the damn door?" This has happened numerous times, but you can't EVER remember going back and finding it open. You think about it over and over. You even picture yourself standing at the entrance turning the key, but you just can't convince yourself that you did lock it. You know that there is a 99.99% chance that the door is locked, but it's that .01% you fear. What if it isn't locked? What if someone gets in? What about all your things, your computer, your TV, your documents? Oh God!

Should you go back? I did, for years, until ...

A strategy that worked for me in this situation and those like it was the following:

Try everything you can to take your mind off the obsession by invading your mind, or "flooding" your mind with random positive thoughts that will distract you from thinking about the initial obsession. I'm not saying that you should bring on other obsessions: not at all! Bring trivial, menial, unimportant things into your mind to help you take your thoughts off that door. What will you eat for dinner? Who are you meeting and what will you say? What happened in that movie you watched ... what was it about? What will you do tomorrow? Take thoughts like these, simple thoughts, and flood them into your head like a waterfall. I have found that this is an excellent tool to put off or forget the obsession. Once you "flood" your mind, you will find that the obsession will gradually lessen and hopefully disappear. Flooding works well if done properly, and the more you do it, the better you get at it. It does take hard work and practice.

## VI ONE YEAR FROM NOW

I stumbled upon this strategy around the one-year mark of my long and arduous battle with obsessions. It became very effective in time. It took awhile for it to have an impact, but when it finally did ... it did!

I was on the phone late one night with a friend. This night made a big difference for me. My friend was about to go on a date with someone she had just met. We had a good talk about him and she was excited. It was her second date and she felt that things were going in the right direction. She told me she was to go out with him the next night. She would then be visiting a friend in Toronto the rest of the week.

"So I meet him tomorrow night and I head off Wednesday morning until Sunday. An exciting week!" she shared.

"That should be great!" I told her.

I was really happy for her, because she had experienced a lot of turmoil with dates in the past and she was really excited about meeting him again. She was just as excited for her trip to Toronto where she would see a good friend from university.

"I better head off to bed. I have a busy week," she said.

I smiled and said to her, "Well, have a wonderful and safe trip and we'll talk when you get back."

"Okay, bye!"

"Yep, bye!"

I sat back and, as I did all the time, I replayed the entire conversation in my head. I always did this and it was a bad habit, often leading me to obsess and be anxious about things I may or may not have said, or what I should have said, or, even worse, things I shouldn't have said. Suddenly, my stomach started to feel uneasy. I put my palm on my forehead and I started to feel some anxious sweats coming on. I stood up.

"No, No, NO! I wished her a good trip, but NOT a good date! Oh my God! I've got to call her back ... NOW!" I frantically grabbed the phone.

The normal mind would have grasped the reality of the situation, and would have said, "Of course, within that half hour conversation you must have said that once, or twice or even more, especially you!" But NO, that didn't matter here. I was convinced that she was now devastated at the other end of the line. She would have thought that I just didn't care. I had to do something. I just had to!

Then, a thought occurred to me, one that only a year ago would never have popped into my head, because I was so deep into my obsessions over everything. I started to think about this obsession, which I never did, because I was too busy compulsing spontaneously. I pictured my life a year from now, and said to myself, wiping my brow, Chris, if you can avoid this one "little compulsion" NOW, it will make ALL the difference in the world "One Year From Now". You will be that much further ahead because you will have shot down this one little, simple obsession.

I literally threw the phone down on the couch and marched into my bedroom. I lay down and the obsession began to fester. At that moment, a dozen reasons why I should call her came flying into my head. It was like an onslaught of thoughts that overwhelmed me and actually made me dizzy. I took my pillow and covered my face to shut everything out. With any thought that entered, I repeated over and over to myself that, in one year, the fact that I didn't act on this obsession will make ALL the difference in my life.

I'd like to say that I succeeded that night, but I didn't. And I wouldn't for awhile. But, I worked hard at making this strategy an important part of the armour for my battle against obsessions. Several months later, I would succeed, and the ball would begin to roll. Now, in 2012, I can say that this strategy has been one of the strongest in my battle against obsessions. Again, simply say to yourself that, one year from now, the fact that I haven't acted on this one little obsession will make all the difference in my life. And it will. And it did.

## VII WORD PUZZLES AND CHARTS

I devised this next strategy, one that I put into play in 2006. It helped me to prevent compulsions which, in turn, made a big difference to my healing. Things happen for a reason, and this is a good example. Here's what transpired.

One night at home, I was searching the web for something, I can't remember what, but I came across a site that had some "dot-to-dot" pictures. I love dot-to-dots, I thought at the time. So, for fun, I printed one out to try. I grabbed the picture made up of numbers and remembering when I was a kid, tried to figure out what the image was. I couldn't figure it out by just looking at it and I felt like such an idiot! I was a full-grown man for godsakes! Anyway, I took a pen and joined number 1 to number 2. Yah, that's how it works. As if you didn't know!

In joining 1 and 2, something suddenly clicked. I thought to myself, there's something neat going on here. How about this? Every time you fight an obsession, why not join one dot to the next dot? Even for the simplest of obsessions! If you don't act on it, join a dot. And so, that week, I kept track of the obsessions I was having at school, at the gym, with friends and at home. For every compulsion I avoided, I put a tick on a piece of paper. Every night, I would come home and count the ticks and join the number of dots. And so, slowly but surely, the picture started to take shape until, eventually, I would find myself staring at a rabbit or maybe even a turtle! I remember feeling so good when I completed the first one. But, more importantly, I could count all the obsessions I had attacked, day after day, over a couple of weeks. It was a very positive feeling and it led me to want to do more. I would then start another puzzle and, after a few, I started to award myself incentives for completing a picture: a dinner at the Keg, a movie I wanted to buy, or even a junk food night. Small rewards, but they did work as incentives. I felt my confidence building.

Eventually, I started doing the same thing with "word searches", highlighting a word every time I avoided a compulsion. I did this also with daily charts and graphs. I got really creative. In the end, when I stopped using this technique, I actually had a pile of papers almost ten centimetres (4 inches) thick! I made "charts", and used "word searches" and "dot-to-dots" for all kinds of obsessions. These included hell and God, perfectionism, food, my body, old habits inhibiting my progress, anxieties and phobias, unnecessary telephone calling and dealing with frustrations and anger. The list was endless.

I even kept track of things that weren't obsessions but would better my life, such as being patient, asking people about themselves, physical exercise, being assertive, trusting God, driving the speed limit, and so on.

I used this chart for many years. Here's an example:

**CHALLENGE AND CHANGE**

| | Jun 28 | Jun 29 | Jun 30 | Jul 1 | Jul 2 |
|---|---|---|---|---|---|
| No call home | | | | | |
| No call friends | | | | | |
| No comparing | | | | | |
| Watch a movie | | | | | |
| No approval | | | | | |
| Listen/Inquire | | | | | |
| No perfection | | | | | |
| Read a book | | | | | |
| TSTTS writing | | | | | |
| Walk if I feel rage | | | | | |
| Positive re: God and faith | | | | | |
| Edit email once | | | | | |
| No Rigidity | | | | | |
| Solve Your Own Problems | | | | | |
| Live with your Action/Decision | | | | | |

| | | | | | |
|---|---|---|---|---|---|
| Obsession delay and drop | | | | | |
| Facing fears | | | | | |
| No emailing friends | | | | | |
| Self-Acknowledge | | | | | |
| No punching walls | | | | | |
| No call backs | | | | | |
| NEVER miss taking MEDS | | | | | |

This technique worked wonders for me but, without the earlier strategies, it would not have succeeded. For me, these techniques built on each other. This technique gave me a concrete hands-on approach and made me feel stronger with each stroke of the pen or highlighter. I strongly encourage sufferers to try it.

## VIII THE MONEY JAR

In 2009, I took my battle with obsessions to a new level. I was lying in bed one night, staring at the ceiling, obsessing over something that would definitely roll itself into tomorrow and beyond. This was always the case. It pissed me off every time it happened, many days ruined even before the new day began.

As I was lying there, an idea popped into my head. Chris, you've come a hell of a long way, but you've reached a plateau. There's much more to climb. You're defeating obsessions, which is great; but, at the same time, you're acting upon just as many. You're at a standstill; this war can't be won in this way. It's time to step up to the plate and bat these obsessions out of the park, once and for all!

I ran to the computer to devise a plan that would hopefully give me the "balls" to win this "tied" game. And so, I adopted "The Money Jar", a strategy to counterattack my negative, unwanted thoughts and to climb the next part of the mountain that was ultimately ... my sanity.

"The money jar" was a simple, yet effective strategy, with a powerful punch to it. It built on earlier strategies of rewarding yourself for successfully saying "NO!" to acting out a compulsion. But with this strategy, I would actually be earning money! There was a catch, of course. The money would not be deposited INTO my account, but rather withdrawn FROM my account and put into the jar! Rewarding, eh?

You may be thinking, what? Are you crazy? How could you afford to do that? Well, let me explain, and yes, it was worth it ... it saved my life.

Here's how it worked. Before starting, I settled upon an appropriate amount of money (one dollar) for each victory. This one dollar would be placed into the jar every time I avoided a compulsion. To say the least, it wasn't an amount of money that would cause me bankruptcy, but enough to help free myself from the heavy burdens of OCD.

For every obsession I fought during that time, I flipped a dollar into the jar. I then made a promise. I decided that each dollar earned would be a dollar that I would give back to mental illness, considering the success I had been experiencing each year. The earnings would go to fight against the stigma of those suffering and to support the battle against mental illness.

One by one, the jar filled up, dollar by dollar for the cause, inspired by a yearning to reach out to others who may not have any support. I also saw this strategy as a call to others who live free of mental illness, to give to those who suffer. To reach out to organizations and businesses to donate, and who could, in turn, reach the darkest corners of the world of mental illness—a world I've been part of for so long. Thankfully, I have had support. Many others don't.

The rewards of doing this were endless, even though I received nothing financially. The intrinsic feeling of watching the jar rise until I couldn't put the lid on was priceless. I kept this idea hush for a long time. I feared that my loved ones, and my doctor, would try to cut me off for financial reasons, since I was struggling. I understood my limits. After a couple of filled jars, I transformed the dollar into a quarter, a little more affordable. This strategy finished with five full jars of change, close to $600! It was a good amount of money, but more importantly, a lot of progress in my healing.

What if you can't afford to give money? It doesn't have to be a dollar. Use a quarter, a nickel, even a penny. It all helps to inspire and heal, while at the same time being able to give to others. Help others, help yourself. Simple. Complex. If you can't afford money, try buttons, or bread clips. The strategy can still help you improve and defeat obsessions. Never feel that money is essential for this strategy. Remember, YOU are the key. If it helps you to improve, that's what matters, because just you being healthy will help others through your love, your story and your triumph.

Change YOUR world, change THE world.

***"I've gotten used to ignoring them and I think, as a result, they've kind of given up on me. I think that's what it's like with all our dreams and our nightmares ... we've got to keep feeding them for them to stay alive."***

***A Beautiful Mind, 2001***
***Sylvia Nasar, Akiva Goldsman***

## CONCLUSION

There were several other strategies, alongside the aforementioned, which I employed through the years to attack obsessions. Some, I used simultaneously. Goal setting became a key to survival, to success. I also adopted countless motivational lists and necessary changes I wanted to achieve. You won't always succeed. I haven't been able to say that I beat OCD. Dealing with OCD is a lifelong process, as is dealing with any mental disorder. You trip and you fall hard, repeatedly, and we all have the bumps and bruises to show. Strategies will not always succeed, but don't give up trying no matter how many times you stumble. I do promise, though, with ***hard work from you***, the ***support*** from loved ones, an ***effective and trustworthy doctor(s)*** and the ***proper medications***, you will cope. With coping comes strength and with strength comes success and, in turn, happiness.

I've learned that life takes you on a ride; there's no doubt about that. We go through experiences that definitely blindside us and knock us silly, and it hurts more than we can ever imagine. We'll never solve it all, but I hope that you, even in your times of suffering, can find a smile now and then. Isn't that what becoming healthy is all about?

***"It's been a long road,***
***Getting from there to here.***
***It's been a long time,***
***But my time is finally near.***

***And I can feel the change in the wind right now.***
***Nothing's in my way.***
***And they're not gonna hold me down no more.***
***No, they're not gonna hold me back."***

***FAITH OF THE HEART – Rod Stewart***

# PART IX

# THE DARK AGES

## CHAPTER 1
## EDUCATIONAL SHAKEUP!!!

June, 2005, I got the call, sometime around 3:30 on a Thursday. I'd just finished a satisfying supply teaching day and was ready for some R & R. I was in my living room watching *Seinfeld*, which I absolutely loved. You might remember the episode. Jerry was planning a comedy gig in a new city, while George fretted about having no job and no money. Elaine was complaining about a new guy she was dating. And then there was Kramer, you know, just being Kramer!

As I watched, my mind started to wander and I began to obsess over a few things that had happened that day. I always did this after work, and today was no different. I could never seem to follow the old motto of "leaving work at work". *Seinfeld* helped me put things in perspective and relaxed my mind. The phone rang. It was from someone entirely unexpected ... a school principal.

"Hello?"

"How are you, Chris?" she asked.

"I'm fine and you?"

"Doing well, thank you," she said, introducing herself.

"And how are you?" I asked again ... stupid! Why was she calling me? I thought. Had I done something wrong? I always felt that way about everything at that time, like everyone was out to get me or something: paranoia.

"I'll cut right to the chase," she said bluntly. "Chris, listen." I could see that she was a woman who spoke her mind. I liked her right from the start, but I didn't know how best to approach someone like her.

"Chris, I understand you've been supply teaching with our board for several years now."

We talked briefly about my experiences working full-time and then supply teaching and why I supply taught instead of teaching full-time. She was curious, as were most people. People continually wondered why I wasn't working full-time; few knew the real reason. This was my fear of being labelled "insane" and being subtly excluded from the profession. I had made a living doing this in spite of being sick, and feared that my phone would stop ringing.

We chatted; she never pried. I was always nervous about that. I had managed to keep everything a secret up to then. There was such a stigma surrounding mental illness, and I felt it was better to keep my mouth shut at this stage in my life. I dared not put my teaching career in jeopardy.

We talked about my writing. Principals and teachers were always excited to talk to me about my two children's novels. After some small chit-chat, she got down to the reason she had called in the first place.

"Chris, I'll just cut to the chase. I want you teaching here this fall, and I never take no for an answer!"

I sat back, running my hand through my hair. "Okay, uh ... I don't know what to say."

"Say nothing, except yes. I want you here and I always get what I want, Chris. Besides, I've got a handful of teachers over here who know you or know about you. I want you to work with them."

"Really?"

"Really!"

"Okay, well can I ... think about it?" I asked, practically pleading, realizing that she intended to hire me. This was nuts, but I felt honoured that she'd ask.

"Yes, you can have a few minutes," she laughed.

"Umm, can I ... call you back?"

"I'll be waiting, Chris. Here's the number."

I hung up and sat back. I looked at the time and kept the TV on mute. I could still see Kramer acting the fool, but his lying flat on the floor wasn't so funny now. All I could think about was the contract this principal was offering. God, I hadn't worked full-time since Christmas 2000! It had been four and a half long years! I had been offered contracts repeatedly, and declined them all. Jesus, what was that all about? I thought to myself. Was she for real? I knew that she was. Did I feel comfortable being with a principal that was so straightforward and blunt, so "in your face"?

A lot of things ran through my mind in the next few minutes, as obsessions started to fester. This would continue for the next few days before I actually called her back. Here were some things I pondered, and obsessed over:

- Was I ready for this? Again, I hadn't worked as a full-time teacher since 2000. I hadn't been well enough.

I'd been offered almost fifty contracts through those years and many had been for permanent positions.

- Was I the right guy for the job or was I fooling myself? Could I really take this on?
- Was my head ready for this? I had been through a lot of ups and downs through sickness the last number of years: three life-debilitating disorders were taking their toll. Was I really ready to take on something this important?

These questions circulated over and over and, of course, my thoughts became obsessions as I pondered all these things way too much. It ruined my weekend, as I couldn't get them out of my head.

AHH! UGH!

I obsessed over every possible thing I could think of, the most intense being my inability to stay healthy in order to meet the demands of the job. My folks continued to remind me of my teaching talent, but that didn't matter here. I really felt that I wasn't capable, but I know now that it was sickness talking. I'd always been capable; that had never been the problem. The problem was my fucking head, and it was killing me, and NOT softly!

A couple of days later, early Monday morning, I gulped and sat upright and dialled the school's number.

"Hi, can I speak to the principal, please?"

"One moment," the office administrator told me. In no time, the principal was on the line.

"Yes, hello?"

"I say YES!" I told her.

"I knew you would," she smiled; at least that's how I pictured her. So it was fixed; it would begin in September. I was officially a classroom teacher once again! She assured me that this would eventually become a full-time permanent position.

I was set to go. I was really nervous, of course, but I was excited. Really excited! I'd been through so much shit the last eight years and it looked like things were finally taking a turn for the better. I was used to the opposite, but this time, I was healthier than I had been only months before. No, I was not close to being healed from my crap, but healthier for sure. I had a long way to go but, with this assignment, it seemed like things were looking up. I was so happy that I wouldn't have to rely solely on a supply teacher's salary anymore! Yay! I would finally have stable work, more money and my own classroom!

I sat back and closed my eyes. I started to think about my past. God, I was so sick and tired of supply teaching. I had done this for over four years because of my mental state. I wanted to work full-time, but it just wasn't in the cards. Supply teaching had its perks, definitely, but it also had many downsides. It was stressful. Waiting for calls drove me silly; missing days here and there drove me crazy. No benefits, no job security, no steady paychecks. Not to mention, dealing with different classes each day. I was so far behind my friends when I compared myself to them. I shouldn't have, but I did. At least five of my high school friends were already easily clearing 100 K a year. I could only dream of that!

I was slated to teach a grade six class. I would be working with another teacher.

**I really felt I could handle the job, finally.**

I was thrilled. I have so much to do and prove, I thought. I'd left teaching twice before and I would not let it happen again. I was sure. But as I look back, what I was really doing was setting myself up for failure. Why?

Right from the get-go, I started to think way TOO much and I began to make the job bigger than it was, bigger than me, actually. I hadn't done anything as yet, but my head was already in September! Perfectionism began to kick in immediately. I had plans to be great, which brought on so many pressures of their own. I was to begin my stint in two short months. Man, I had so much to do!

Just days after the call, I looked around my living room and started talking to myself. My talking started out promising good tidings, but it quickly took a turn for the worst. It took but a few minutes for the anxiety to set in.

"Okay, I need those books."

"I can plan in the evenings. I can mark at school, but not at home. Yah ... no ... well, maybe, I'll have to mark some at home. Maybe."

"My partner can be useful. What if she's awful? That would not be good. Man, I already said yes!"

"What if I fail? What if the kids don't like me? What if I do a shitty job? God!"

"That could mean the end of me, dammit, and I would be known across the board as a failure, a dud in the classroom. Can I take this? Oh my God! What have I done?"

By the end of this, I was no longer sitting on my couch. I was lying on it!

I was nervous and anxious about the whole thing, but I managed to bring myself to think more positively using strategies I was given by Dr. Boyles. I thought maybe this anxiety was a "good" anxious; at least I hoped so. This time, I felt ready to take something on. I was healing more and more every month, I was stronger, my chemicals were better balanced and I was visiting my doctor regularly. My family too, I knew, would be there for me.

I actually started to feel better. I had worked on my thoughts and I finally felt I could handle the job. Who knew what I'd be thinking in September, but it was June and I was finally grasping things and taking control of my life. I had a lot to prove to myself. For now, I had to try my hardest to put my feet up, put things on the back burner and enjoy the two months ahead of me. This did not last, however. During the summer, I really didn't give my mind much of a rest. I was always looking ahead and preparing. Not a good thing.

Thoughts were firing off in my head. Thoughts turned into obsessions which, in turn, led to actions that were very dangerous and detrimental. Negativity then took over.

Although my mood was relatively stable at the time, situations like this caused stress that would also cause shifts in my chemicals. This could cause me to go into a high, or into a low: depression.

That summer, I felt like a beleaguered medieval knight trying to protect myself from a dragon, a three-headed one. I was being hit and almost destroyed by something so menacing, so conniving and so powerful that I almost lost my life. I discovered that I wasn't a knight, not courageous, not valiant. I was just a normal guy trying to live a normal life, but very sick.

By mid-August, the dragon showed its menacing heads! Number one was the most vicious, the leader of the three. This was *Bipolar Disorder*, a terrible beast whose job was to destroy everything in its path. It breathed fire and bared the sharpest of teeth. Undaunted, this head could completely annihilate its victim.

Number two was the manipulative and conniving head, full of lies and deceit. It was *Obsessive-Compulsive Disorder*. When it grasped its victim in its teeth, it not only destroyed the body but also the mind.

Number three was *Generalized Anxiety Disorder*. It too, was an awful head to deal with because it created doubt, and took away reason. It worked at an alarming rate to create fear in every way. The victim would be timid, anxious and lack confidence.

The dragon emerged from the cave. I was immediately hit hard with an influx of negative spiralling thoughts. Amidst my planning and preparation, I worried obsessively about the job and wondered seriously if I was ready to do this.

Finally, September came. It was time to get the classroom ready. I walked in one week before school would begin. I purposely waited until a week before, because I told myself that I wasn't going to overwork ... this time! In and out: in at a normal time, out at a normal time. That was my new philosophy, one I had not applied previously. I discovered subsequently that it was sickness that caused these ill actions.

My new philosophy lasted ... a day! By the second day, I was back to my old antics: overworking. I had so much to do, and so little time to do it! I needed to be there; and besides, the job required it—even if it was only three days a week, sometimes two!

I had all my resources ready. I met my teaching partner and we hit it off right away. She was fantastic, and enthusiastic about the year, as was I. From the moment we began, I knew we'd be a great match. Watch out kids, here we come!

"This should be a great year!" I told her, oblivious to what would eventually unfold. Although I really felt overwhelmed talking to her, I pretended that everything was grand. I was good at this. I had practised countless times before, especially in my previous jobs.

So the week passed by and our classroom was finally ready. I had spent way too many hours that week, but it didn't matter. It looked amazing! Our class was ready ... but was I? The year began, and it began with a bang.

**I just knew that this was going to be a good year.**

Surprisingly, I actually survived the first day of school. I was nervous and really anxious, and I worried obsessively. I did have a pretty good day with the class. I liked their energy. It was going to be a good year.

However, I never expected what would happen day two, the next week. It caught everybody by surprise, especially me. I will now give you the play by play of the first morning of my second week of school, like a sportscaster describing a main sporting event.

*At 6:15 am, the alarm clock goes off. He's up!*

*6:20 am, look at him gulp down his usual bowl of cereal, a banana and some juice (same every day).*

*6:30 am, he jumps in the shower, careful landing, no slippage. Whoa!*

*6:40 am, ALL HELL BREAKS LOOSE!!!!! AHHH!*

I dried off and, at first, began pacing my living room from one end to the other. I was wearing only boxer shorts. I started to recycle my thoughts over and over, and repeated them under my breath. These were thoughts I had been having for many days before. These were definitely obsessions.

"I'm awful, I suck, I can't do this, I'm weak, I'm going to fucking fail!"

Thoughts like these continued to roll through. I felt anxious, nauseous, and thought I was going to faint. I felt horrible. I walked back and forth, muddling through these thoughts. It was so intense, more intense than I'd ever imagined. I started punching my fist into the palm of my hand, as I walked around. And then ... it happened. I completely LOST IT!

SMASH! I took my clock radio into the living room and slammed it onto the floor, breaking it into small pieces.

"Fuck!" I yelled loudly. I then punched a wall repeatedly. Yes, it hurt, but I just didn't care. Bruises or no bruises, blood or no blood, I let that wall have it like it was a punching bag. My knuckles were left bloody.

I stomped into my bedroom and picked up the cordless phone and lay back on the bed. I dialled my parents. My father answered the phone at 6:45. He was supposed to supply teach at his old school that day.

In complete desperation, I bellowed, "Oh my God, oh my God, I'm losing it, Dad, I'm losing it!"

"Chris, what's wrong? Chris, relax," my dad appealed. "Tell me what's happening?"

"I'm losing it, Dad, I'm really fucking LOSING IT!" There was heavy breathing and more whining: then loud moaning and groans.

"Just relax, son. Chris, just relax."

"Dad ... Dad ... I smashed my radio, Dad, how can I fucking relax??? I've punched the wall over and over and my hand is bleeding."

"Just sit down, Chris, and take a breath."

"I am fucking sitting down! I can't take this! I can't take this shit! Ahhh! FUCK!"

With that, I took the portable phone and hurled it across the bedroom, smashing it into pieces against the closet wall. I got off the bed and punched more walls in my room leaving blood marks.

"I fucking hate this, I fucking HATE it!" I screamed out loud.

I raced into the living room. The other phone was ringing but I wasn't answering. I didn't care about anything. I felt so bad, worse than I ever thought I could. It was unreal! I was not just trembling, I was literally shaking. I was breathing quick hard breaths, and I was totally out of control.

I plopped down on the couch breathing as hard as I could. I moaned and groaned more, I yelled and swore more and, with that, I kicked my coffee table across the living room floor. The table went flying into the wall. Then I grabbed the end of my couch and lifted it up over my head and, BANG, drove the couch down onto the floor. The people below must have wondered what in God's name was happening above them at that time of the morning! I then overturned a dining room chair and screamed, "FUUUUCCCCKKKK!!!" as loud as I could.

The phone rang again, and I picked it up this time. I was breathing very heavily.

"I can't believe it, I can't believe it, I broke everything! Dad, I broke everything!"

"Chris, just try and relax. Breathe," my dad said, trying to calm me down, worry in his voice.

"I am fucking breathing! What the fuck do you think I'm doing!"

"It's okay, Chris. Just try to relax. I'm on my way over. Did you call the school?"

"AHHH!" I yelled, and hurled the other phone across the living room.

**I'm losing it, Dad, I'm losing it!**

I remember that morning so clearly, feeling worse than I ever thought I could. It was unbecoming, awkward and crazy all at the same time. It was almost 7:15, and school was to start in an hour. I had to get ready! OOHHH! I felt so terrible. What in God's name was I going to do? I remember that I started to panic right there, picturing the principal and the other teachers looking down on me. What would they think? Good God!

I curled into a ball on the couch, but I remember that I couldn't cry. I was too shaken by everything that had happened. Why was I feeling so bad? Why did this have to happen? I lay there on my couch, staring at the ceiling, my hand on my forehead, breathing heavily.

I stood up and punched more walls, as I walked around the room and then plopped back onto the couch again. I tried to relax and control my breathing and gain my bearings, but I was blown away by what had just happened. I'd been really angry before, but I had never flipped out like this. My family and I had never seen quite this much chaos from me. It was, unfortunately, an introduction to a new way of life for me. Little did I know that much of this same behaviour would continue for a long time after.

I rolled onto my side, bent my body into a ball and started to repeat the same sentence over and over under my breath. "Oh my God, Oh my God, Oh my God, Oh my God, OH MY GOD!" You can add a few fucks in there too. I was never a person to swear, but in these times, I got re-acquainted with the colourful words that I had learned as a teen.

I stared at the blank TV screen and could see myself in the reflection. I looked like shit lying there in my boxers. I kept looking at the TV, without saying or doing anything, and I waited. I waited for help. He would soon be here. But how long would I wait? What was next? Oh God!

My dad arrived at 7:20. He came into my apartment and looked around. The place was a disaster. There were pieces of broken radio on the floor in front of the TV. My cordless telephone lay broken on the bedroom floor. Blood was splattered on the walls. My coffee table was at the other end of the living room and my couch was off to the side. My small one-bedroom apartment looked like a war zone or more like a tornado had hit.

"Son, are you okay? Chris, are you okay?" my dad said, putting a hand on my shoulder.

"NO!" I yelled exasperatedly. "Do I look fucking okay?"

"Here," my dad said, passing me one of my t-shirts. I put it over my head.

"What am I going to do, Dad? What the FUCK am I going to do?" I said in pure agony, with my arms outstretched in front of me.

"Don't worry, we'll figure something out," he reassured me.

**You are not working, not right now.**

And we did. We figured something out, but it wasn't easy.

That morning was an anomaly, a freak, an accident that was waiting to happen after so many sick years and life experiences. It was something that you'd never want to happen but, in my case, it was unpreventable and inevitable. It was bound to happen, if not that morning, then the next or the next. My mind let it happen that morning. What happened in my apartment in September of 2005, just before 7 am, was the accumulation of long years of distress fuelled by spiritual guilt, perfectionism, anger, over-dependence and fear of failure. Add to that, the combination of three highly active and volatile disorders, and you have one incredibly awesome occurrence that I have coined simply, THE PERFECT STORM. When you look at all the factors involved, it really was.

## CHAPTER 2
## DIAGNOSED HYPOMANIC

Obviously, I didn't go to work that day, or the next, or the next. My dad called the principal about the situation (I didn't dare talk to anyone at the time), and a supply teacher came in for me that day. My dad didn't reveal any secrets as to the real reasons I wasn't coming in, but he did tell her that I wasn't feeling well. Both my parents and sister were good at hiding things about me by this time. They knew that this information had to stay under wraps ... for now. Forever? For how long, we weren't sure. Curiously enough, the principal did query my mother as to what were possibly the actual reasons for my absence. We were convinced that my teaching career would be doomed if news of my bipolar leaked out.

My dad then called the hospital to speak to my doctor who told us to come in as soon as we could and he'd fit us in. We got to the hospital around 9 am, and took a seat in the waiting room. I was accustomed to this room by now, as I'd waited numerous times for appointments and for emergencies. I felt like shit. We were hoping that Dr. Boyles would be able to shed some light on my situation. Sitting there, I remember thinking that maybe I'd be okay in a couple of days. But my doctor had other plans.

"WHAT? TWO WEEKS!" I freaked out and yelled at him. I nearly hit the floor, or the roof ... how does the saying go, anyway? Again, I wasn't someone who swore a lot, but I just couldn't contain myself.

"That's a damn lifetime! I finally have a fucking job and you're gonna put it in jeopardy, just like that!"

"Yes, Chris ... two weeks. Now calm down. You are not working ... not right now," he said, in monotone. I hated it when he was so matter-of-fact. But, he was right. I wouldn't work for two weeks. I COULDN'T work for two weeks. He had made his diagnosis. He said that I was hypomanic.

"Hypo what?" I asked. I'd never heard that word before. Hypochondria, I threw at him at first. "No, hypomania, Chris." I had only known highs and lows, but my dad remembered my being labelled hypomanic in 2001 after my coming down from mania. In hypomania, he told us, a person sits uncomfortably between a normal balanced level and full-blown mania. I had experienced this condition leading up to, and following my months of mania. I knew right away that hypomania and work did not mix, and I felt anguished. I'm going nowhere again, I thought to myself, as I stared at the floor and put my hands over my ears. My mind began to play its tricks on me. Thoughts of failure and then devastation crept into my head as he handed me a new prescription. I fretted as we drove from the hospital. I began to whine to my dad about missing work and I swore at Dr. Boyles and his "dia-freeking-nosis"!

"He doesn't like me! He wants me to fail ... fuck him ... fuck all of this!" I declared, as we drove down Riverside. I crossed my arms in disdain.

"Chris, he told you. Basically, you've had a nervous breakdown." At the time, I did not realize that I was being SO adversely affected by GAD.

I was really angry, as I slammed the dash and I took it out on my dad. I had finally gotten my chance to work on a permanent basis, and here I was being robbed of my golden opportunity. It was shitty and so unfair! I leaned my head against the window and bawled uncontrollably. My dad tried to console me, but to no avail. I could only concentrate on the negative, which was common over the last few years. I couldn't help but be pessimistic. Glass half-empty became my motto. Shit, I'd been through it all, so much lost and so little gained over so long. It hurt to think about all of this, and my family was the first to hear about it and to try and offer consolation. We stopped to eat and got to my folks' place around noon. We talked in the kitchen for awhile and I lay downstairs, trying to rest.

Now that I was diagnosed hypomanic, I had to try and accept that I was on a high. Not a major one but, nonetheless, a high, a "bad high", according to my doctor. I had to try to gain my bearings and find out how I could live with this condition. I reflected on it downstairs and we talked more as a family throughout the day.

Hypomania could be very dangerous. In hypomania, as in mania, I felt rebellious, but in a destructive way. It was that "rebel" that tore my apartment apart. In the past, that same rebellious state had destroyed relationships.

The most important question my doctor now had to face was how to be able to bring me back down. That worried him and my family tremendously. Subsequently, I did end up deriving some relief from not having to teach for awhile.

The main fear was my going into full-blown mania, and both my doctor and parents were deeply concerned. My doctor had remembered, clearly, meeting me when I was high in the Civic Emergency in 2001. I had been a walking time-bomb in that waiting room, ready to explode. I was talking to anyone and engaging with everyone, including the security guards! I was handing out business cards, I was talking a mile a minute and even hugging strangers in the room. It was comical to the ignorant eye, but my doctor knew the severity of this condition. He didn't find any of it amusing.

My family struggled with the news of my being hypomanic, as did I at first. This tapered off quickly for me, though. At first, I didn't know what to think, but I did feel much higher than normal, and that felt good. My friends were supportive, but they found it hard to understand what I was going through. My family became my number one support group, as they had for years dealing with my mental illnesses. That day, Dr. Boyles adjusted my medication and we crossed our fingers and hoped for the best. It was always a crapshoot.

In hypomania, the symptoms of mania were present, but not in full force. I was talking at a much higher rate and was unable to sit still for a long time. I was talking to strangers no matter who they were. One might think, hey, that's not so bad. But you haven't read the *other side of the story*, where I would:

- have much higher levels of energy and frustration (as Dr. Boyles said concerning my anger over the next few years), along with self-inflicted hurts;
- stay awake late at nights, not being able to fall asleep easily, waiting for the new day, when I could again talk to somebody;
- not sit still, be constantly on the move;
- use poor judgment;
- be loud, rebellious and aggressive;
- be in an overall good mood, unless irritated, which happened readily;
- have racing, unstoppable thoughts which, for me, became obsessions;

- drive and speed carelessly due to oodles of built-up energy and frustration. This would result in red-light running, racing, dangerous passing and innumerable honking sessions.

To give an example of how different I was acting, I went out with a friend one night that week, and remembered him telling me, "Chris, I love hanging out with you when you are like this because you'll do anything!" And he was right, I would. I did many strange and peculiar things in those erratic days.

He loved it because I was so "way out there" in this state. It was really funny to watch me interact with others. I was acting so strange. I was a lot of fun to be with. I would say or do anything and nothing would embarrass me. Only thing was, everyone else around me was embarrassed for me! I didn't care at all. On my major high, needless to say, I was even crazier! In these states of mind, I couldn't even sit long enough for a coffee or a meal, and going to a movie ... well ... that was impossible!

My parents knew something was definitely wrong that fall. Things had to change quickly, my doctor warned. Going higher up or going down would be drastic and he felt we needed to try and control the "beast" as best we could. After adjusting my meds, Dr. Boyles told my dad that I needed to stay low-key. Easy enough, I thought, but I was wrong. I wanted to do all kinds of things, but I didn't want to go back to teach again. I was now totally afraid of that one thing. I did not realize then that I would not be ready for a good long time.

## CHAPTER 3
## WATCH OUT OR I'LL DRIVE THROUGH YOU!!!

Due to the severity of my illnesses, Dr. Boyles felt that, some nights, I should stay over at my parents. Fears of my going up or down predominated, and I was starting to do things, due to anger, that were very dangerous. This happened several times at my apartment and at my parents' home, but the scariest place it happened was behind the wheel of my car.

"I'm not taking a fucking walk, I'm sick of fucking walking!" I yelled out to no one in particular. Walking reminded me of terrible times, prescribed to help me get out of major depression. At that time, I didn't even want to go outside.

I hated exercising! But exercise was extremely important, Dr. Boyles had stressed. The next morning I was supposed to go for a walk. However, I had other ideas. I didn't want to get up! I just lay there looking at the ceiling.

"Chris, everything okay down there?"

"No!" I yelled. I was pissed off! It had been two weeks since I left the school and I was still in this same fucking place, the basement. I still wasn't able to go back to the job. I was losing it! My dad came downstairs and sat beside the couch.

"What's up? What's wrong?" my dad asked, a bit worried. We were all worried since my breakdown in my apartment. Anger was a scary thing, especially when it was happening on and off all the time.

"I'm sick of this, Dad, I'm sick of it! I just spoke to Matt and he's at work and that just pissed me off! Why can't I just go to work? It's been too long, Dad. I've been dealing with this shit too friggin' long! When am I going to get better?" I slammed my fist on the table.

"Chris, Chris, just relax. You'll get there. Come up for some breakfast. Actually lunch," he snickered. It was already 11:30. I had lain in that basement rolling around for three hours! I threw on some jeans and a sweater, and we walked upstairs to the kitchen. I sat at the table and Mom handed me a glass of juice. I downed it quickly and asked for a coffee. "That might affect your tremor, Chris. Are you sure you want one?"

"Fuck the tremor!" I yelled, again slamming a fist on the table. I was so sick of everything. My mom hurriedly poured me some coffee.

"How 'bout the walk, Chris? Mom or I can go with you if you'd like. It'd be good for you to go outside. It's a nice day."

"NO! I don't want to go for a fucking walk! I hate walking. You can saw these legs off for all I fucking care!"

Mom backed off and dad tried to cool me down. They had seen this behaviour several times since my attack in the apartment. Frustration and anxiety were getting the best of me and so was my OCD. I was obsessing about a lot of things. When OCD and GAD were working hand in hand, shit always seemed to happen.

"I'm just gonna lie on that couch down there in the dark. That's what I want!"

"It would be good to get out there, at least for a short walk. Dr. Boyles ..."

"NO!" I slammed my fist on the table again. "I refuse!" I stood up and shoved my chair in hard, smacking it into the table.

"Chris, just sit down!" my dad warned.

"NO! I can't do this!" I pushed a book off the table and pulled my chair back so it hit the floor. I stomped into the living room and threw myself onto the couch. I was swearing and complaining and arguing profusely with them. After a minute of lying there, my dad said something that made me flip. I stood up and stormed down the hall, grabbed my shoes and raced outside to my car. Flustered, I got in, fumbling with my keys. I could see my parents in the doorway beckoning me to come back, but fuck them! I wasn't coming back! I had to get out of there and fast!

I started the car and raced down the road to the traffic light. I was SO pissed off! The anger was unbearable. I could feel it all through my body, especially in my head. It was so out of character for me. I felt a sudden shift in my head that switched me from normal to God-knows-what. My eyes felt almost robotic, and nothing and no one mattered. At that moment, I didn't care if I died or took anyone with me.

***"I feel complete and utter rage. I feel the mind of a madman, ready to explode on anyone who comes my way. It is the weirdest of feelings in my head and eyes.***

***Like the Hulk, I jump out of my body. I don't care who dies ... well I do, but ... you know."***

"How could God have done this to me, holy fuck!" I yelled aloud. The light was red but I didn't give a shit. There was a car in front of me but I didn't give a shit about that either! I looked both ways to follow the rules like I was taught, and I pulled around the car and drove into the intersection. The car behind me honked two or three times and he raised his finger. I waved back just to piss him off and burned through the intersection heading down the road, one of the busiest in Ottawa. Before I got to the bridge down the hill, I looked at my speedometer. I was already driving 120 km/h! The speed limit was 60, but I just didn't care. I would go as fast as I damn well wanted!

I approached another red, slowed and sped past other cars into the oncoming lane. I quickly cut back into my lane, just as a car approached. He honked, narrowly missing me. I honked right back and continued on.

I turned onto Bank Street and tailgated at least the next five cars. I went right up behind them honking over and over, then zoomed past all of them. Anytime someone looked at me, I just stared back at them with a "fuck you" look on my face. I sped up and passed them and turned into their lane. I was like a mad street racer. I was SO pissed off with how I was feeling. My eyes felt weird and the rebel within me just kept moving faster and faster. I cut onto Riverside and got into a race with some young punk beside me in his sports car. I got up to 130 km/h down Riverside. He would eventually let me pass. I was going too fast, even for him, for anyone! I went faster and faster, not a care in the world. I came to a light and the kid caught up with me. I stared at him and, on the green, he gunned his car in front of me and was gone.

A few minutes later, I started to calm down a bit. I was swearing to myself, and starting to feel guilty for what I had done. I'd put myself at risk, but more importantly, others. I didn't seem to care in this state. All that mattered was that I got where I needed to get. The roads became a platform of danger for me during that time. I tended to speed in situations like this, maybe wanting to break free from the bonds I felt around me. Who knows? I was impatient and reckless behind the wheel. One time, I even remember following some guy right to his house, just to scare the shit out of him. I felt awful looking in my rear view mirror when I saw HER step out of her car and run inside. Sorry.

In response to this, and several other incidents, Dr. Boyles suspended my license for a week. I wasn't allowed to use the car the last week of September. I hated him for it, but he probably saved my life, and others' too.

## CHAPTER 4
## EYES WIDE OPEN

Towards the end of September, my dad and I visited the school that I was supposed to be working at, to speak to the principal. We decided to share the truth with her, because she had earlier indicated to my mom that she suspected an "illness". We sat and told her that I would need more time. She was disappointed because she really wanted me to work for her. I told her that it would not be happening anytime soon. Then, I let her know my story. I somehow felt that I could trust her. She was very compassionate. This became a discussion that opened my eyes to something I just didn't want to hear, but needed to. It became one of the main reasons I decided to write this book.

She was a wonderful lady to talk to, and I admired her honesty, but she was very blunt. First, she told me that she had had over 200 applicants for the position I was hired for. She took me without an interview. This, despite my having left teaching twice before, presumably due to too much pressure. Both former principals had nothing bad to say about me. In fact, my evaluations had been superlative.

She told me that the staff knew I was off. She said specifically that I need only say to people that I have a medical condition. Then she went on to say the following. This opened my eyes to the severity of having this illness, and how people would perceive it.

"Chris, tell NO ONE. Be totally quiet. If any principal knew, or word got around that you're bipolar, I guarantee you, you would not get the job; you would NOT work in the board, period! The board is looking for a person they can count on, who they can always trust to be there for the kids they've entrusted you with, 100% of the time."

She then said, "Chris, I took a big chance with you, a big one. I knew there were problems, but I knew if you stayed healthy, it would have been a great chance, and it still can be. A principal doesn't want to have to worry about the teacher, only the kids. We always put the kids ahead of ourselves or the staff. Really, if you can't do this, supply teaching would be suitable. God knows, you've done a great job there."

Then she said something that absolutely floored me. Talk about being in the right place at the right time.

"Chris, I don't tell many people this, but I want to help you out as much as I can. I have a close friend who is bipolar." WOW! She really DID understand. Was I hearing things? I couldn't believe what she was saying!

"Chris, get your act together; you know what I mean by that, and get healthy. That is the most important thing. Your health, and your dad would agree, is first here. Get healthy, get happy. Then your main worry is, can I be there for the kids 100%? Can you stand up and perform and be a support for the little ones day in and day out?"

I WAS in the right place. She understood the severity of my illness. It was reassuring to have her in my court, but also depressing hearing her admission about the stigma surrounding mental illness. It was refreshing to be able to talk to someone in her position who understood and sympathized.

"Chris, don't talk about your disorder EVER until you've proven yourself as a teacher and you are secure in a job, but more so secure in your life. Once you are established, you can talk to a special person, or teacher or confidant. You need to be healthy. Parents don't want a "sick" teacher. They would NOT be sympathetic."

She told me that she wanted me to work with her and my doctor to develop strategies that would work so that I could return to teaching soon. She still had hopes of me returning to her school. She believed in me, not only as a teacher, but a person.

I had the perfect principal. She said that the kids were always asking about me and wanting me to return, even though I had only been there for one day! Even parents had raved about that day with the class.

It was evident that tons of teachers and principals and administration out there would have no sympathy at all for someone suffering from a mental illness. It was sad to hear that. Stigma was written all over it, and she was right. Mental illness was seen as a flaw, a hindrance. In this day and age, if you weren't completely healthy mentally, you weren't accepted as a whole person.

Following this meeting, she told me that she would ask human resources to wait a little longer. They wanted to terminate the contract. I found out later that she actually kept the job open until February. The board complied. February! I guess she really did want me. After our meeting, I went into the classroom to pick up several of my resources. I was distraught and disappointed at the same time. I again reiterated my love of teaching, as I stopped in the doorway of the class and looked around the room at all that I had created and put together. I had a single tear run down my cheek, but I wiped it as quickly as it fell. I really missed having my own class and I wanted to get back sometime. Who knew when though? For now, I had to heal. I was determined to get there. Meanwhile, I had encountered a great person, now retired.

**In spite of your illness, Chris, I still want you to work for me.**

# CHAPTER 5
# ADMITTED TO THE CRAZY WARD

At the beginning of October, after adjusting my medications a few times and seeing no dramatic changes to my mood, my doctor decided to admit me to the Psychiatric Ward at the Civic Hospital.

"Chris, I want you to spend some time here at the hospital."

"What? No way!" I barked.

"Chris, it's not a choice."

"Oh."

I had to spend some time there because he opined that I was "over-stimulated". He prescribed "boredom", and wanted me to be away from anything that would cause me to be aroused. No, not in a sexual way! No television, no computer, no phone, no car, etc..

He described it as boredom, because I needed to cool down. Hypomania caused many problems. I was awake most nights; I was over-excited. I was still speeding dangerously in the car, I was restless and I became agitated very easily, especially with family. I was basically high! It was like I was on a drug. In mania, I was high, but I felt really good. In hypomania, I felt differently. Anger and distress dominated.

"Welcome to the Civic Ward. You can put your things in this cupboard. They will be safe," I was told.

"Can I keep this with me?" I asked, holding up my Bible and a spiritual book. I was again searching for answers that didn't seem to come. I couldn't understand why He had turned His back on me again.

In the hospital, I had my book to read (*The Ragamuffin Gospel*), I had my discman for spiritual music, I had my pj's, I had my Bible and I had my crazy head. Who could want anything more? Oh, and I also had a pen and pad, because I was obsessively writing note after note of spiritual ideals and random thoughts, and even verses from my Bible. As you see, with these highs came a lot of "spiritual reflection". My Bible was a definite companion for me. I would not have it any other way.

Boredom was my prescribed treatment; however, I instead transferred these same energies to the hospital ward. In my short stay, I met more than 80% of the patients on the ward within a few hours! I knew all by name and I knew something special about each of them. They had been admitted for a variety of reasons: bipolar, schizophrenia, depression, generalized anxiety, obsessive-compulsive. You name it, I encountered it.

**They all had a history of bad times.**

I remember meeting a woman named Liz in the ward. She heard voices all the time, and she, too, thought she was on a secret mission, kind of like me during my major high. She had strategies written out and was planning some kind of adventure. I asked the doctor how long she'd been in the ward. He said that he was not able to share that information, but hinted that it had been a long time. Poor thing. Then I met Tom, who had admitted himself for depression.

"I admitted myself, Chris. I needed to."

Tom was a great guy. He was having a difficult time in his life, having recently split with his wife and was currently in a legal battle with her. Work was a problem, also. We chatted a lot, about deep issues such as religion, faith and finances. I told him why I was here and he understood. He had a cousin who suffered from bipolar disorder.

"Yah, my cousin has been in and out of hospitals frequently. Bipolar can be a lot to handle."

"I know," I said to him, smiling. "Look at me!" I said, spreading my arms in a curtsy. Incidentally, I met Tom a year or so later while swimming at a public pool, doing better.

I met many others on the ward, and learned to appreciate where people were coming from. All came from different walks of life. They all had a history of bad times, and, because of that, they were sent to this ward for help. Did outsiders understand? I'm not sure anyone can fully understand what you're going through, unless they walk in your shoes on the same path. All had different stories and different challenges, but they were people like you and me who had experienced unfortunate events and mental difficulties, most due to genetic inheritance, leading them down this road. Most often, they are without support or proper care. That's how people end up living on the streets. I learned this valuable lesson volunteering at The Mission and The Shepherd's of Good Hope, two shelters for men and women in downtown Ottawa. Many street people, I am positive, are dealing with some form of mental sickness. It is hard to be judgmental when one examines the reality of their circumstance.

***"Don't judge another unless you've walked in their shoes. In other words ... don't judge."***

There, I tried to meet everyone and, yes, I loved to hug them too! I played pool (never lost, chalk it up!), watched movies and even played piano for everyone. The patients loved that and seemed to love me. I was so energetic and positive that I became a leader on the ward in only two days. Despite what my doctor hoped, I wasn't bored and I wasn't going to stay put and lie there in my assigned room. I wanted so much more. My doctor wasn't too happy about it, because I was, after all, "sick". We had to learn to accept that. He knew the inevitable. Depression would likely come and put me in my place, but hopefully, we could lessen its impact. Further, we hoped that we could curtail it entirely.

***"It does not matter how normal your childhood was, or your life is—idealistic means nothing—it can be destroyed in a moment. It does not matter how good things WERE—when it hits, it plants a demonic hand. It can destroy anyone. Mental illness has no favourites."***

# CHAPTER 6
# DISCHARGED FROM HOSPITAL

After a couple of days, I discharged MYSELF from the hospital, against the advice of doctor and parents. They removed the figurative "shackles" and "chains" from my body and I made my way out. I'd had enough! I needed more excitement. I was "bored" out of my mind! Dr. Boyles' prescription for boredom worked, but it drove ME crazy!

I noticed one big difference about myself as I left the hospital that day. After spending time with so many good people who also suffered, I realized two things. The first was how normal they really were, just everyday people suffering from sickness, many without support from loved ones. And the second was that "the crazy ward" wasn't so crazy after all. It was no longer an appropriate label for this place of healing and peace.

I thought to myself, where to next?

I was picked up by my father. What the hell did the doctor know? I felt fine! Besides, I'd done my time, hadn't I? I was ready to go!

"Goodbye, everyone!" I remember saying, on leaving the ward. I had gotten to know some of the patients well, as well as one could after just two days. They gave me well wishes for peace and happiness in my life. Some had been there a long time. Mental illness had really beaten us up.

My mom and dad were worried about me coming home, knowing that nothing had changed. I didn't care, I just wanted to be free, and finally I was. I just felt I didn't belong there at all. Even though I was still high, I was frustrated with my life. I was lamenting my inability to hold a job or have a relationship. I felt I'd never find anyone. Why would anyone want to be with a "sicko"? That's how I saw it.

**I just wanted to fold up and die.**

Dr. Boyles, also worried, told my dad that I should spend much more time in my parents' home. There I would have no computer, no email and limited use of the phone. Email was dangerous for me, because I would obsess constantly over it. I would also be very obsessive when it came to using the phone. I was very argumentative with my parents and my sister. I would constantly bicker with them, causing a ruckus about wanting to go to my apartment to use my computer. I had made it seem so important.

By the second week of October, things started to take a turn for the worse. I was quickly falling from hypomania into depression and, because of this, I was not doing well ... again. I had many concerns about work. I felt that I'd never teach again. Why would I want to? I was fed up and sick of everything. I just wanted to fold up and die, as my chemicals took me deeper into the dark abyss of the depressive mind. Desiring normality and independence, I yearned to go back to live in my apartment, although it was a very unhealthy place for me to be. I would continue to punch many walls and doors there, and had the holes to prove it (upon moving to my newly purchased home in January of 2010, I had to repair those holes in my favourite "punching door". All seven of them!).

I was constantly calling my parents when I was in this state of mind, which really rattled them. Or, I would go to their house. This was scary for them, needless to say, because of my impetuous behaviour. They never knew what might happen when I came over feeling shitty. It was for all these reasons that Dr. Boyles had told me to stay with them for now. He felt that being on my own at the apartment was detrimental to my state of mind. I needed people around me.

***"I'm bleeding and who cares? No one. Why should they? Who the fuck am I?"***

Mid-October, I had another attack ("episode"), bursts of anger and frustration due to obsessions, anxiety and depression. Mini-breakdowns, you might call them.

[*One of my first anger episodes occurred on Christmas Eve 2002, when I got into a wrestling battle with my parents and sister at the front door, and drove my sister back into the wall with my fists. I tore outside into the cold and into my car, arriving at my girlfriend's empty house, crying for hours in the driveway. I'll never forget my sister's eyes when I pushed her back against the wall that night. Thinking about it still frightens me, and her, to this day. To think that I had actually done that!*]

The following took place at my parents' home in the early part of morning. I had a "storm" of rage. I started to argue with my mom and dad about something. As was always the case, I got obsessive and anxious, and it led me to turn a table centrepiece over, smash my fist on the glass tabletop and leave the house in a huff. I called twice from my car and apologized. I then returned. This was a constant theme, losing it, leaving, calling to apologize and coming back ... leaving and coming back. On returning to their home, I was calmer, but started to complain again. It seemed never-ending.

**I miss teaching and I miss my life!**

I was definitely feeling the effects of depression and, in this state, obsessions and anxiety were getting worse and worse—obsessions over friends and work and money ... over everything. Mom and dad were adamant that I continue to stay over: doctor's orders. I eventually did so without complaining. I didn't want to be alone.

"I miss teaching and I miss my life!" I would cry to them. My anger and frustration led to several more outbursts. My parents and Julie hated these times. They hated the anger. They were scared; I was scared, but I had lost my ability to care. I didn't care about anything when I was like that. It became dangerous for everyone.

That night, I finally accepted that I was depressed. Dr. Boyles confirmed this and adjusted my medication accordingly. But I was falling quickly, kind of like a rock rolling down a steep hill. I felt very uneasy and light-headed, which was common during all my depressions.

I did go back to my place the next day, against my parents' wishes, but it wasn't a positive experience. I ended up calling home repeatedly. That day alone, I called my parents twelve times! Twelve! This was nothing compared to what would eventually come. I would call some days fourteen, eighteen and even twenty plus times! I called due to an array of obsessions, and that worried everyone, mainly because anger followed. Although my parents reluctantly let me go to my apartment for brief visits, I was still spending nights at their home.

Subsequently, Dr. Boyles told me that I must take more time before returning to work. I was livid, but I knew I couldn't handle going back. At the time, I hated him for doing it though. I was going to lose my teaching contract! I had further outbursts because of this. These consisted of punching walls, kicking tables ... the usual.

I was, my dad wrote in a journal that he was using for his own therapeutic purposes, "impatient, childlike, petulant and disturbed". Dr. Boyles equated these behaviours to "having tantrums". Sickness came in many ways. My sister was very worried.

***"At that moment, I felt sure that, if my parents were to pass away, I'd be taking care of my brother for the rest of his life. That's how sick he was, and I had accepted this path."***

## CHAPTER 7
## THE SLIDE

Memories of my major depression couldn't help but pop up in times like this, something we feared returning with all our hearts. I never wanted to walk that road again, ever. No one should ever have to. I was pushy, domineering and insistent that I could solve my own problems, but in the wrong ways. My thoughts were dominated by fear, despair, anxiety and obsession.

**In order to gain a life, lose the old one.**

Dr. Boyles and my parents strongly endorsed exercise. My mother suggested I start walking the eleven flights to my apartment when I made the odd visit. I did, and hated it, every step. This led to doing some good things, but other "not so good" things. I would call my folks in a panic and scream at the top of my lungs, "I want to kill myself! I've had it!" I was scared. I was alone, either here or there. I always felt alone with this damn sickness! No matter what support came, I felt I was alone to face the fire.

Medication or no medication, I was headed for the deep end. My energy was weakening and I was beginning to feel fearful of what would come. I persisted in calling my friends repeatedly from the apartment. It seemed I needed to prove to my friends that I was sick. I guess I wanted them to appreciate why I had no girlfriend, no house, no full-time job and very little money. These also became repetitive obsessions. I was fed up, but I couldn't attack them in this state of mind.

My dad, however, said that in order to gain a life, I had to lose the old life. I would have to fight for it. By fighting every single obsession, only then, could I have a life. Easier said than done!

As I became depressed, I obsessed more. My worries increased. Obsessions over family, friends, faith and perfectionism continued, always ending with an apology, after having done something outlandish.

At this stage, I was predominantly just eating and sleeping. I did the odd walk or swim because I was urged to. I just wanted to sleep all the time. I was not doing well and I was starting to moan. Moans were always a sign that I was depressed. I couldn't make decisions and my memory was weakening. Dr. Boyles and I talked about the possibility of entering the hospital as an option. He said that I could not work full-time until January, which again, really peeved me, but I knew I was in no shape to do so. He knew starting any work at this time would only be detrimental to my health.

"I feel lousy."

"I hate my fucking life!"

"I don't know how I'm going to get through this!"

"It pisses me off! It sucks!"

"It's been tough, Mom and Dad."

Late October, feeling as shitty as I was, I visited a pastor friend whom I'd met on my manic high in 2001. Although I had cut ties with most people I met during my high, he remained a good friend and a man I trusted. I had let him know everything I was dealing with. This day, he and some elders of the church actually laid their hands on my head and prayed over me. I like to think that this had a part in bringing me out of depression and bringing me to where I am now. No miracle happened that day, but I think maybe the miracle is the fact that I was able to persevere, and find the strength to heal.

Mom and Dad were helping me out financially and encouraged me to keep my apartment, my only attachment to independence. My dad and I applied for sick benefits that month to get some government assistance.

"There's something wrong," I would say over and over. I said that a lot when I was depressed. I really thought there was something physically wrong with me, because it felt so bad living in my skin. It was SO bad; it couldn't JUST be a mental problem. "I'm so fucking sick and tired of this!" That afternoon, Mom and Dad laid their hands on me, and we read a number of *Psalms* and *Proverbs*, hoping for some relief. Mom, out of desperation, suggested having a brain scan, wondering if there was another explanation for my sickness. The subsequent test revealed nothing.

I went to see Dr. Boyles. He said that I was being too impatient. "Bipolar can be balanced; it is not a terminal condition but a treatable one. We'll aim for November to start supply work." I'd like to say that that happened. Nope.

At this time, Dr. Boyles suggested that I consult *The OCD Workbook*, which I had purchased earlier, but not fully applied. Obsessions were affecting my chemical levels, causing me to fall into depression and causing extreme anxiety. He recommended that I start working through it thirty minutes to one hour a day. He also said that if there was no discernible improvement, I would have to be hospitalized.

I cannot stress enough how terrible I felt at that moment. Imagine waking up one moment to see that everything you've lived and worked for has gone down the drain. Your ambitions, your successes, they mean nothing. You feel so low that you'd rather die. Although support is there, you don't feel it and, in fact, you can't appreciate it. For me, depression equalled death.

***"It's that empty feeling. It's that feeling of being behind your peers and seeing them move forward further from you. It's the feeling that you will never catch up and only see life from a distance through their lives, as you remain still. It's a harrowing feeling filled with despair and loneliness."***

Mom and Dad wrote me another cheque that day. Without that support, I definitely would have been on the streets or chained to a hospital bed! I can fully appreciate why many men and women become homeless ... they're sick, mentally, and have no one. I was coming to the realization that I had to somehow take control of my obsessions and fight them, but, in this condition, it was next to impossible. As I fell lower and lower, these were happening more and more, and this caused incredible anxiety. I couldn't move forward. Worries dominated my life. "I'm worried", once again, became one of my predominant expressions,

In November, as Dr. Boyles recommended, I did start to supply teach a little, but it was very difficult. I remember anxiously circling the classroom prior to meeting the kids, in order to find some relief from my nerves and my negative thoughts. If that didn't work, I would end up phoning my parents for consoling. Collectively, we thought that work would be better for my recovery and hoped that it would build my confidence. I would get to the classroom, and first look around the room and see all the resources that were on the walls. I would have this overwhelming feeling of sadness because I wasn't healthy enough to have my own class. I was too sick. I would feel so depressed about everything and, with these feelings, I would then sit down to read the day plan. And man, if the plan wasn't as easy as easy could be, I would start to feel immense anxiety. I would get nervous and start to worry and, at the next sign of trouble on that page, I would feel like the world was caving in. It was awful. If things were not perfect, I lost it. Sometimes, I would stand up and swear and walk around the room shaking my head. What the fuck am I doing with my life? Look at me, I'm worthless, I'm no good, I'm nothing! Shutting the door, I would even break down crying, but no one knew the pain I was feeling.

***"How long could I hide this life ... I was a magician, a deceiver, a good liar."***

A number of times, I didn't even make it to the school. I would pull over and call home from the side of the road. This included coming to a stop on a busy highway. One time, I even pulled my car into a snow-filled ditch, just to avoid having to go to work. Cost? A hundred dollars!

At other times, I would pull over to the curb and cry profusely, yelling at my parents as they tried to calm me down. One morning, on the off ramp of the 417, there was a knock on my window. Three men in uniform stood by my car. They had pulled their fire truck over to see what was wrong with me. I was embarrassed and wiped my tears and told them I was fine. They let me go, thankfully. Another time, I pulled over on a side street near the school. I was bawling to my mom when I heard a tap on my window.

"Hello ... are you okay?"

I wiped my eyes. "Mom, I'll call you back."

It was a concerned gentleman, who walked by my car and saw me crying. He let me be when I told him I was talking to my mom, only to return ten minutes later with a coffee in his hand.

"Here you go. Maybe this will help." I then proceeded to work. Thank you, sir.

End of November, I had to contact the school board again to tell them that I still was not ready for the contract position, and that sucked. Is that ever a nice feeling! The place where you hoped to achieve great things, and now you're calling because you can't do it. I did find out, however, that some highly respected people at the board office had nothing but good things to say about me as a teacher. This was nice, but it meant nothing to me at the time. Compliments just flew off into the wind.

Because obsessions were immobilizing me, I ended up cancelling almost every supply teaching job that I received. Things continued to spiral downward. I was often angry, hurt and frustrated with everything. I even contemplated suicide a number of times.

[*Suicide threats were very common throughout the years when I was feeling like this. I never attempted suicide, but I was close to doing so several times. When I worked full-time at my first school in 1998, I was feeling very low. I would drive to work in the morning and, deep inside, I wanted to crash my car and die. I so feared going to work. I would drive 100 km/h down Hunt Club Road every morning and I would quickly jerk the wheel towards the ditch, time and time again, approaching the school. In 2001, in my apartment on Elgin, I held a knife to my wrist. I contemplated cutting myself, but managed to ward off the thought. In my apartment on Riverside, from 2003 to 2005, I had threatened to kill myself several times.*]

In early December, at my apartment, I was not doing well. I was sobbing and crying, yelling, "I hate my life!" over and over. I was swearing and I called up my parents and swore at them. I was practically screaming! I was yelling so loudly and I started to threaten to kill myself. I said it several times. I threw things around the room and lay on the couch continuing to yell at them. My parents tried to calm me down, but I was irate and pissed off with everything. Then, there was a hard knock at my door. It was two police officers and two ambulance attendants. Someone had called 9-1-1!

The police officers came in and saw me sitting there wearing only my boxers. My dad, who heard the ruckus over the phone, told one of the officers that he was on his way over, as the other one handed me a t-shirt. Both officers and paramedics stayed with me, asking a number of questions until my dad arrived. Dad remembered me sitting, head in my hands, leaning over a coffee table. He mentioned to me later how heartbreaking it was to see his son in that state. He spoke with them. We told them about my battle with mental illness. Dad assured them that he'd take care of me and bring me to his home. They were comfortable with this.

Their compassion and respect for my condition made all the difference that night. Had they reacted in an adverse manner, like forcing me out in handcuffs, I would have been destroyed, impeding my progress insurmountably. Add to that, I would have lost my apartment, my job and my self-respect.

I cancelled work the next day. We talked about my actions and my parents told me that I could not act like this, because I WAS going to lose everything. This would be disastrous, now and in my future.

In subsequent sessions following this incident, Dr. Boyles and I talked in-depth about eliminating symptoms of obsession, guilt and worries which continued to fester. At one session, I recounted to my doctor regretting telling my mom to "fuck off". She, in turn, had told me to "fuck off"!

"Good for you, Mom," asserted Dr. Boyles. "She shouldn't have to put up with that!"

On another visit to my doctor that month, my dad was with me (happened many times) and I remember being so frustrated with the two of them that I walked out of the office, slammed the door and actually pulled a "Purell" tab off a soap dispenser in the hallway! I did return and apologize, but Dr. Boyles was not impressed. Another time, he even threatened to let me go as a patient, commenting that I might need to see a new doctor. He was concerned that he was not being effective for me. That shut me up pretty fast! Never would I have wanted this. Looking back, I think he was just using reverse psychology on me ... smart bastard! But it worked in the end. Maybe this day was critical to me moving forward? Maybe?

The next day, I had another episode. I was agitated, found it hard to focus, was angry, violent and profane. My dad and I went off to the hospital emergency for the next six hours. This happened a handful of times throughout the years, which invariably ended with coffee at Tim Hortons, where we rehashed the episode. The resident nurse said that setbacks were to be expected. Because of the care I had, full-time hospitalization would not be suitable.

"What about part-time hospitalization?" she asked.

Was part-time the answer?

I continued to feel awful that month.

***"I feel like shit. I can't do anything, something's wrong, I can't stand it, I can't take this life anymore, I can't do this!"***

A lot of crying and yelling and moaning always followed comments like this. Perfectionism was starting to take over. I felt I had to be the "perfect person" and the "perfect patient". I was not applying my strategies at all.

On the next visit with my doctor, Dad and I brought up the advice from the nurse regarding part-time hospitalization. The *Day Hospital Course*, Dr. Boyles agreed, might be effective, especially to attack the obsessions and anxiety. These were the culprits causing the shifts in my moods, causing the bipolar to be triggered. He would enrol me that day, much to my chagrin. It was necessary, however. We were at our wits' end.

***"One step forward, two steps back was often the case. This had to change. Eventually, it did. It became two steps forward, one step back."***

## CHAPTER 8
## DAY HOSPITAL

In the second week of December, I began to take a path to healing, but it was not going to be easy. I was so negative about the stupid course that I felt I was forced to take. I had:

1. lost a full-time and lifelong career;
2. lost huge amounts of income;
3. lost many amazing women;
4. lost opportunities to own a home;
5. lost my faith direction;
6. lost my health;
7. lost my self-esteem noting that my friends had moved on;

AND

8. NOW, I had to sit in a circle like a kindergarten child, and talk with a doctor and ten other unfortunate souls.

How would you feel? What would you think? How could you live with that?

OH, AND THEN YOU GET THE RULES ... yah, they actually had rules! Day Hospital presented us with things such as, you MUST attend each day, don't be late, no disruptions, no going to the washroom during group sessions, respect confidentiality. You get the point ... can you say primary school again?

Welcome to *DAY HOSPITAL*, a day-to-day, 6-week intensive course, running from 8:30 to 3:30 daily, at the Civic Hospital, one of Ottawa's biggest and most trusted. Like *Alcoholics Anonymous* or *Gamblers Anonymous*, *Day Hospital* would act as a support group for me, for six long weeks. When I first got there, I absolutely hated it, as did the others. You could tell that no one wanted to be there, but we all knew we needed support, even from people we didn't know.

"Hi, I'm Chris. How are you?"

"It's Kev, I could be better."

"Nice to meet you, Dev," I responded, avoiding his eyes. I felt pretty shitty and not in conversational mode.

"Kev, I said. It's Kev."

Whatever, whoever, I don't really care. I'm really bothered by you. You're already getting on my nerves!

Slips like these were happening because my head was dealing with so many negative thoughts. Each day, the course would begin with a group talk. One by one, the ten of us had the floor to discuss how we were feeling at that moment, what was bugging us, why we might be anxious, etc.. I found this to be the most stressful part of the day, when it definitely should not have been. Why?

Well, if you know me, I'm usually outgoing, not shy and love to meet people. But something was stressing me out: having to talk to a group of strangers who carried completely different diagnoses (we were not to share our afflictions), along with feeling absolutely crappy. Not to mention the obsessions I had developed for the lead psychiatrist, the onsite DH doctor, Dr. McBride, and his many mannerisms. Perfectionism led me to constantly think about what I would say ahead of time, and I often felt the need to jump in to give advice to others. I worried so much about what HE thought, even to the point of sweating. I would watch his facial reactions and even his stupid beard—boy, that beard really got to me. It was hard for me, but I got through it. When it was my turn to talk, I was always beyond ready because I had thought about it so much. I'll admit that I wasn't really as focused as I should have been in group. Often I didn't even hear others' stories, but I didn't care. I just crossed my fingers and hoped for the best, my best.

On board was the lead psychiatrist, a registered nurse, a cognitive therapist and a social worker. They were all wonderful supports for the six weeks. What did we learn? I'll spare you too many details, but we focused on the following areas, delving deeply into each:

1. Stress Management
2. Anger Management
3. Expressing our thoughts
4. Affirmations / Negative and Positive thinking
5. Goal Setting
6. Cognitive-Behavioural Change (much emphasis here)
7. Assertiveness

Our afternoons focused on these topics, and we worked with the cognitive therapist who was fantastic. Mornings were with group. Did DH help me? At the time, I would have said no, but looking back, in hindsight, most definitely. It was what I needed at the time: a way to feel a little bit better about myself. One "head-scratching" story I want to mention. As you've read, during my mania, I would constantly see turtles everywhere. Well, midway through the course, a group member, without knowing anything about my past, without knowing we'd published our books with a company called *Turtles Publishing*, gave me a small magnetic turtle that said "You'll get there!". She did so because she had noted how badly I had felt the day before. Can you believe that? What were the chances?

Overall, *Day Hospital* was a refuge for all of us, a safe haven. We all came in with no expectations and different stories, along with a certain attitude about ourselves. We left feeling a little bit better than when we arrived, lives that had more hope and more promise. What mattered most is the support we gave each other when we needed it at a very difficult time of our lives. The match was lit ... it was time to light our own paths.

After Christmas, things still continued to be a struggle. I would still get angry often and yell and swear. Episodes did continue to happen, many walls to be punched and yes, my hand was very sore.

I continued with *Day Hospital* through January. I remember feeling, even at the end of *Day Hospital*, that it did nothing for me. The reality was, though, that once I was convinced, in my mind, to put into practice what I had learned, I could then make progress. It wouldn't happen for awhile. I did discover that the biggest part of recovery requires hard work, by ME! This included:

- Faithfully taking my medication (I've never missed);
- Keeping all doctor's appointments, including psychotherapy;
- Attending focus groups, like *Day Hospital*;
- Regular exercise (gym and walking stairs in my apartment);
- Fighting obsessions and anxieties using strategies;

- Building positive faith (finding the "real" loving God);
- Strength and courage;
- Working as much as possible (self-esteem and confidence);
- NEVER GIVING UP!

By the end of January, I was starting to realize that I had to leave my childhood shit behind. Obsessions of friends and worrying about everyone had to stop. I had to stop catering to my obsessions and start focusing on healing my own head. Of course, when you're hit by illness in your late teens, you have a tendency to want to recreate the good times with old friendships. Not possible. I knew that I MUST confront my many demons. They had been with me for far too long.

I did not work on a consistent basis until late February, almost six months! Since, I have continued to battle a number of issues derived from my illnesses. Despite dealing with these assorted issues due to my three predominant mental disorders, I have, since 2006, maintained consistent employment as an occasional teacher, while writing this book, a book I hoped to use to reach out and help others. I sat and planned with my father on Boxing Day, 2005, but I didn't start writing for at least three years. Mount Everest stood in my way, as I looked up, holding merely an ice pick and winter boots. But, boy, was it ever therapeutic! As I healed more and was able to immerse myself into it, it gave me a purpose and a meaning beyond my torments; a reason for continuing to improve. My doctor has reiterated, time and time again, that he can tell when I'm doing well. "Chris, I can finally see that sparkle in your eyes." Well, it has returned, and hopefully it is here to stay.

In spite of a number of blips, I have carried on. In 2007, a contract I took on led to innumerable anxieties. Consoled on the library phone by my mom, finding myself in tears each morning before the kids would arrive.

Then, in 2009, an attempt to get back on to the Catholic Board's "teaching eligibility list" ended in ....

[Anxious and obsessed, I sat alone in an empty testing room staring aimlessly at a blank bulletin board. After what was, in my warped mind, a terrible interview, I secretly stormed out of the testing room leaving the essay section blank, except for a simple note written in the centre of the page which read, "Sorry, not a good day."]

Somewhat embarrassed over my failure to complete the process, I slammed on the gas of the car and never looked back. However, as I neared my parent's place to commiserate, I felt more of a relief than remorse. I was clearly not ready for this giant leap forward. Supply teaching would remain my staple but, after that day, I couldn't help but feel a bit paranoid. Would they try to steal supply teaching away from me, my only saving grace? Would I be left with nothing?

Despite persistent anxiety, ongoing obsessions and ups and downs of bipolarity, I have made considerable progress.

I have since completed several books (for a year and a half, I could not write), purchased a home and have worked every day for over two years. Through my psychiatrist, I was also given the wonderful opportunity of speaking to numerous Ottawa police officers about my story, my path to healing and the dangerous consequences of stigmatizing the mentally ill. My doctor wanted them to see that there are many mental illness sufferers who live normal lives and have just been tripped up with misfortune and untimely circumstances. In other words, we are not all “crazy”, as society believes!

It is possible. It is attainable. I’ve proven this. Sickness knocked me off my feet in an instant. I now stand strong. The best treatments are out there. You just have to reach out. Several sources have stated that 70 to 90% of people diagnosed have a decrease in symptoms and a higher quality of life when they combine medication, psychosocial, psychotherapy and cognitive-behavioural treatment, along with finding the best supports.

***"Success is to be measured not so much by the position that one has reached in life as by the obstacles which he has overcome while trying to succeed."***

***Booker T. Washington***

# PART X

# GENERALIZED ANXIETY DISORDER
# "I'M WORRIED"

# CHAPTER 1
# BUT EVERYONE WORRIES, DON'T THEY?

Before delving into this section, it is very important that we differentiate everyday "normal" worrying that we all experience, versus someone who suffers from ***Generalized Anxiety Disorder*** (GAD). There is a monumental difference, and one you've read about consistently throughout this book. It is called "quality of life". With the former, one continues to live and can prosper. With the latter, it is almost impossible to live a fulfilling and peaceful life. Like the previous mentioned disorders, anxiety destroys your sense of reality, immobilizes you and leaves you isolated in a world of despair and inner turmoil, leaving its sufferers with very sick minds.

"Normal" Worry Vs. Generalized Anxiety Disorder

**"Normal" Worry:**

- Your worrying doesn't get in the way of your daily activities and responsibilities;
- You're able to control your worrying;
- Your worries, while unpleasant, don't cause significant distress;
- Your worries are limited to a specific, small number of realistic concerns;
- Your bouts of worrying last for only a short time period.

**Generalized Anxiety Disorder:**

- Your worrying significantly disrupts your job, activities, and social life;
- Your worrying is uncontrollable;
- Your worries are extremely upsetting and stressful;
- You worry about all sorts of things, and tend to expect the worst;
- You've been worrying almost every day for at least six months.

***Taken from the files of "HELPGUIDE" at*** www.helpguide.org

## CHAPTER 2
## THE EARLY YEARS

From my teens to the present, I experienced anxiety constantly. This would lead to enormous amounts of energy, if I channelled my anxiety properly, or a lack of energy and resulting apathy. Anxiety took over my thoughts and actions, which often left me hibernating in a proverbial hole, obsessing and worrying. I spent countless hours under the blankets in the place I felt most secure ... my bed.

"Worried" was a word I used constantly with family and friends, growing up. "I'm worried" became integral to my vocabulary in high school, university and beyond. I would have feelings of unease, tension and fear. These kept me from performing to my potential. They would lead to feelings of insecurity and instability. I don't remember ever feeling confident in my life situations because I always wondered what others were thinking or whether I would fail.

On the outside, I always carried myself with confidence and authority; but inside, I was like a little lion cub waiting for its mommy. I would often retreat to my family for comfort, especially in high school. In university, I had to find ways to cope. However, my parents remember the countless phone calls at any time of day, relaying my abundance of worries. They got so used to my expressions of dread, that they would often answer the phone with, "What's wrong?" This was obviously a result of the interplay of GAD with BD and OCD, which also kick-started in late high school.

## CHAPTER 3
## IT'S NOTHING TO WORRY ABOUT

I have my grade 6 piano, and I remember the added amounts of anxiety I would have when I had to do a recital or an exam. It was so difficult to do, but I never complained to my parents about it. I've never been a complainer or a whiner. I've always coped and moved on, until adulthood, when I couldn't do it alone anymore.

Entering my teens, my anxiety levels increased, especially when I started to swim competitively. At twelve, I started with the *Gloucester-Ottawa Kingfish*. We had up to six practices a week. Swimming had such appeal, and it began to take over my life. Everything was about swimming: eating, sleeping and training. I was wired mentally to succeed and win. And win I did. In one year with the Kingfish, I put together an array of victories that marked successes that kids would only dream of. My dad would carry the record books with him and we would keep track of my progress versus other swimmers in Canada. At age thirteen, I was swimming in the highest percentile for the 50-metre freestyle. And then ...

BOOM. I hit my first wall of major anxiety. I remember lying in my room, crying and feeling fits of anxiety about swimming. What if I didn't win them all? What if I lost? I would let my parents and myself down. I couldn't let that happen. I started to worry and obsess over the idea of losing and letting people down. I couldn't take the pressure anymore and, early in my fourteenth year, I left competitive swimming for good, on the pretense that I would prefer to play competitive football—you know how that ended—anxiety and OCD prevailed. This became a recurring pattern in my life.

Two years later, I decided to try high school swimming. Maybe there'd be less pressure? I'll never forget the big race. We had a cheering crowd up in the balcony. Many had come from our school to watch the annual swim meet at the Nepean Sportsplex. I was swimming in the 50-metre final and was slotted in the fastest heat, in the fastest lane. I had prepared for this physically and, more importantly, I thought, mentally. As I made my way onto the pool deck, everyone was watching and cheering. Suddenly, IT hit me! I became extremely nervous, my anxiety increasing dramatically as I shed my towel and climbed the starting block.

"TAKE YOUR MARKS!"

My body tensed up, my head felt the fear.

"SET!"

Here I go, here I go, no, no, hold, hold and SPLASH!

I fell right into the water. A false start. At least I had another one, I thought. I looked up to the gallery. Our students were quiet. I hopped out and went back to the starting block, completely embarrassed. The starter readied again.

"TAKE YOUR MARKS!"

My body tensed up again; my head felt more fear. What if I do it again?

"SET!"

Here I go, here I go, no, no and SPLASH!

I fell into the water a second time. A false start again, but this time, I was disqualified! My school was in shock! The place went quiet. We were a medal for sure, if I'd only stayed in the race. I remember sitting off in a corner, tears streaming. Our coach came over to reassure me that things would be okay. These things happen. I started to bawl. I never realized at the time, but that event was pivotal in developing the pattern which would pervade my life.

Anxiety continued throughout the years: on tests, exams, dates. You name it, I worried. Ask my friends about it. "Does Nihmey worry a lot?" "SH-YAH, he does like crazy!" Ask my university friends if I worried a lot ... nothing but the same. You remember the countless quarters I gave my roommate for asking stupid questions. Four for a buck, what a deal ... yah, for him! At least his tuition was going down ... one quarter at a time!

Exams in university were some of the worst for anxiety. I used to get SO nervous for exams. I would prepare, but not for the mental side of things. I would be a wreck before an exam. First off, I would stay up till all hours. I wouldn't eat well at all and I would stress so much about everything. In spite of this, I did succeed, but at great cost. Anxiety would continue to prevail. Forever?

## CHAPTER 4
## FEAR STRIKES BACK

They were the worst words that any baseball player, young or old, wants to hear. STRIKE ONE ... STRIKE TWO ... STRIKE THREE! Remember how awful it felt in grade school when your teacher would say to the class, "Now class, that's two strikes, one more and we are staying in for recess!" We knew at that moment to shut up!

In my mid-teens, I was selected to play on an all-star Little League baseball team. I was so excited! Sure, our team of players weren't really "stars", and none of us ever made it to the "bigs", but we were proud to be a part of that team that summer: a selected group of individuals who would represent Hunt Club where I grew up. I would not only join a group of friends from my school and neighbourhood, but also new teammates who would form their first impressions of me.

I didn't know why it happened but, that summer, something clicked in my mind, affecting me greatly that season, and for years to follow. I was confronted with one of the worst feelings that any kid can experience as they grow up. An eleven-lettered word that begins with an "e" and ends with a "d", and I faced it time and time again that summer. I could barely face my teammates because of it. The word? Embarrassed. And I was!

For some reason, from the beginning of the season, well before being diagnosed with a disorder, I began to form an awful thought about being hit by a pitch when I was up at the plate. I don't know where it came from, or why it persisted, but I remember fearing being hit by a pitched ball. In truth, of the hundreds who would bat that summer, few actually got hit. I would think to myself each and every time, "What if it kills me?"

STRIKE!

It got worse and worse as the summer wore on: so bad in fact, that my teammates actually expected me to strike out every time. I would stand at the plate nervously, knees shaking, and watch the ball coming towards me, swinging aimlessly, missing every single time. Even while I was in the field, I obsessed about my next time at bat. Even while sitting on the bench! My anxiety would build and build as I moved towards the batter's box. I remember it so clearly and it was incredibly awful. And worst, was the embarrassment I felt, as I turned to walk back to the dugout time and time again, facing my teammates, my coach, and the spectators, after striking out.

Slowly but surely, after several games, my coach realized he couldn't depend on me and, instead of giving me a chance to somehow prove my worth, he sat me out one game. And one game led to another, and another. This continued the rest of the summer. I remember sitting in the dugout night after night, watching other players hit and run and catch, while I held my head in my hands and watched. Being out of the line-up not only meant no batting, but also ... no playing. I would cup my eyes and pull my hat tightly over my head, as I watched my teammates play: hiding and wiping small tears that would form in my eyes. This was especially true on nights that my dad came to watch, which were several, hoping for a chance to see his son play ball. Not only was I humiliated, but I was embarrassed for my dad as he sat in the bleachers behind, waiting my turn, which never came. I was devastated. It is still an experience that haunts me when I reminisce. But this was only the beginning of much greater fears and anxieties and obsessions I would face in years that followed. It was a cut that never really healed. I never played ball again after that summer.

In retrospect, at that age, how could I have realized that this type of thinking was more than just a bad feeling, or anxiety? Was it the beginning of an obsessional pattern or was it just a negative thought that fades into the night, the thoughts that everyone experiences? In talking and breaking it down with my therapist years later, we clearly concluded that this was much more than just negative thinking. This had all the elements of an obsession mixed with anxiety that started with a match and ended in a flame.

## CHAPTER 5
## TIED UP IN KNOTS

2006. I stood up from the couch after having had a stressful dream. I started to get ready for the Christening of one of a good friend's son. His little guy was being christened. It was a special day and I was looking forward to being part of it. Why? Because I had to be the "perfect" friend in the "perfect" little world my mind had created. Thinking about this, and I had thought about it the whole preceding weekend, an uncomfortable feeling started to dwell in my stomach.

As I stepped into the shower, I started to get worked up. Why hadn't I had gotten ready at 2:30 instead of now? It's 3:05, dammit! I got out and started to shave. It was already 3:12! Time was ticking away and I was starting to sweat as 4 pm approached. My brow was wet and I tried to cool myself down with a towel. I had hoped so much to arrive at the Christening well in advance of everyone, so I could see my friends ahead of time and have a little bit of chit-chat.

With that in mind, I raced through my shave, put on deodorant and sprayed on my new cologne. I was now sweating profusely. I threw on a dress shirt. It was so uncomfortable ... I was so uncomfortable! Both medication (side affects) and anxiety were contributing. I looked at the time, 3:20. I started to fret and my mind started racing. Gotta go, gotta go, gotta go! I quickly buttoned up the shirt and reached for the top button. Frig ... frig ... fuck! I couldn't believe it! I couldn't fasten the fucking button! 3:26, God help me!

Finally after, yep, you can count'em, about forty-two friggin' attempts, I finally latched the button. Finally! I looked in the mirror. I was standing there with a shirt on, in my boxers, my hair wet and frazzled. Now ... the tie ... where was my tie? I found it and went to the mirror. Practice not needed. Pro tie-guy extraordinaire!

And then ... and I am NOT exaggerating. I tried and tried and tried, over and over and over to tie the goddamn tie! Still sweating, I started swearing and pacing and banging feet on the floor. I called home in a fit, screaming about my tie, and Dad implored me to come over. I slammed the phone down, annoyed at something he said (this happened often), and still attempted to properly knot the tie. I would not fail on this one! With a last effort, I grabbed one end and looped it from behind, trying to tuck it in. Unsuccessful! I took it and threw it into the living room. "ARGGGG!!!"

Exasperated, I stepped into the living room and gave the door a good hard punch. Then I grabbed the top of my really nice dress shirt and ripped it right down the middle, popping off every damn button. I then threw it onto the floor. I felt like the Incredible Hulk, or maybe the Incredible Nihmey. I was raving and raging to the boiling point, breathing heavily. In my head, I felt bubbles on my skin and notches in my neck.

I went over to the door separating my bedroom and living room. I held a tight right fist and BAM! I socked the door one good one, putting a huge hole right in the middle of it. But it didn't stop there. I ran through the living room and threw a wooden chair onto the floor. I grabbed the *Ab Roller* and tossed it on to its side. I looked at my hand, which was starting to hurt, blood dripping down from my knuckles. I ran to the tap to run cold water on it. In my other hand was the phone and I dialled home again.

"Hello?"

"Dad, I did some bad things. I had to!" I was breathing hard.

"Son, slow down, what bad things?"

"My hand! It's bleeding!"

"Why, Chris?"

"Because I fucking punched a hole in the fucking door, that's why! Two fucking holes!"

"Son, just relax. Meet me downstairs. In the lobby. I'm leaving right now."

"Ok. Man, Dad. This sucks ..."

"I know, I'm coming."

I don't know how many times my dad made his way over to my apartment to rescue me in those terrible years. I've lost count. My confidence had abandoned me. This was apparent in doing even the simplest tasks, like throwing a ball, shooting a basket, catching, launching a dart, playing pool (which I mastered in university), and even drawing. Oh yah, and tying a tie, something I still can't do.

Generalized Anxiety Disorder affects even the simplest of life's tasks. The more you think you will fail, the more you do fail. Confidence is shot. Self-esteem is destroyed. Any sense of feeling good about oneself ends. Even my writing, in spite of having two bestsellers, took a place on the back burner. I didn't write again for years! Anxiety led me to do things that were abnormal, things that caused even greater worries and added tension to my life. Before and during intensive therapy, this often led to extreme anger outbursts, frustration and a sense that I would ALWAYS fail at everything I did. Trying to overcome this obstacle was a huge challenge. Adding my two other disorders to this mix made it feel unattainable. It was like a deadly *Bermuda Triangle* that, at one time, I felt I could not survive against.

However, faith, perseverance, courage, therapy, medication, support and many life changes proved otherwise. With success at battling these demons, I finally became convinced that I could take steps forward without falling every time. And so I did.

***"It's awful to think that there are others out there still feeling the way I felt just a few years ago ... others out there feeling the way I had felt."***

# PART XI

# "BUT (S)HE'S ONLY A KID!"
# THE EARLY SIGNS

## CHAPTER 1
## WHOSE BIRTHDAY IS IT ANYWAY?

***"As I look back, and connect the dots, everything that was a mystery then, became crystal clear. That's when reality hit. It had been with me for a long time."***

My sister's birthday, December 1st, 1991: her 16th, the big one. It was a day we would never forget. Not because it was her 16th, but because we experienced something that scared all of us that night. As a family, we were subject to my first ever mood swinging episode. The first of its kind, it was a foreshadowing of things to come, which caught us all by surprise. I had been always one to walk the "straight and narrow". That night, I would fall off the path.

We were all excited for her, but I have to admit, I was a little more excited for my 18th birthday coming up shortly. I would be legal in Quebec! Anyway, that's another story. For birthdays, we had been in the habit of spending our special dinners at Pizza Hut. They treated their customers well, not to mention a cake with candles and a singing choir—at least they tried! Good pizza, though. Our night was filled with smiles, pictures, good chatter and many laughs. We never imagined that this night would be capped off by a life-changing event.

At about 6:30 pm, after an enjoyable dinner, we headed home.

"Happy Birthday again, Jue!" Mom said.

"That was a really nice time. Thanks everyone!"

It was dark and very cold and I remember snow coming down. I cleared off the car for my dad and jumped in. We were freezing. Dad cranked up the heat, we zipped up our coats and we sat on our hands, doing everything we could to fight the cold. A winter we would never forget, because ....

We drove down Merivale and turned on to Hunt Club, and that's when something alarming happened. We were introduced to a taste of what was to come for years after. It is hard to remember what the actual discussion was about and exactly what caused the incident, but it doesn't really matter. What matters is what happened a minute later down Hunt Club.

"Well, I don't care! I don't want to do that!" I said, raising my voice. I was heated, I was upset, I was angry, very out of character for me.

"Chris, your dad is driving. Don't yell," Mom said to stop me. I continued.

"Chris, stop!" Julie said, worriedly; it was slippery and the snow was still falling.

"But I always do it! Always!" I said defiantly, slamming my fist into my hand.

"Chris, it's slippery. Settle down and be quiet. What's going on?" Mom wondered out loud.

"Never mind! God!" I yelled again.

The car pulled up to a stop sign and Dad turned and told me to settle down. Then, all of a sudden, unlike anything we had seen before, I lost it. As he rolled on from the stop sign, I screamed in anger and quickly opened my door. I jumped out of the car and slammed my fist on the roof.

"I'll walk home!" I yelled.

"Chris!" Julie yelled in despair.

Acting the way I was, my family probably would have agreed that a walk might be a good thing, but this WASN'T summer and we were NOT ten minutes from home. Mom rolled down her window and Dad leaned over. He was not happy.

"Chris, get in the car, now! This is ridiculous!"

"NO!" I yelled, and started to walk faster away from the car. Julie yelled again and told me to get in. I pretended not to hear her, or any of them, as I marched away and turned my head. My dad moved the car forward and continued driving slowly beside me, pleading for me to get in. I just wouldn't. In my mind, I was pissed off and I was right ... SO right! They were wrong. They were all wrong! I remember feeling very light-headed, full of energy, but most importantly, determined to prove my point ... whatever that was. It felt so weird and foreign to me, but I didn't care. Who knew at the time that all of this would one day become so familiar to us?

My dad continued to drive beside me and I went on stubbornly. I would not get in the freakin' car! That would only mean I was wrong, and I wasn't. I knew it!

No, I didn't walk home that day. No, I didn't take a cab or hitch a ride. Eventually, after some time, and much pleading from my family, I did get back in the car. Besides, my gloves were in the car, it was beyond cold and I was freezing, and was convinced that this was the reason I got in. Not because I was wrong and they were right. I sat in the back with my arms crossed looking out the window. I didn't say a word and neither did they, but I could tell they were very concerned. I wasn't. I was right, and no one could or ever would prove me wrong. We later reconciled and put the problem behind us ... something that had been so unlike me. But did we really? The real problem still persisted; what the hell happened that day on Hunt Club Road? None of us could really put a finger on an answer that night or that year, but it would become a monumental event. In retrospect, this would make much sense and eventually answer so many questions.

Subsequent to arriving home, I decided that I needed some space and took a walk to my old elementary schoolyard to sit and meditate. This was a standard pattern of behaviour for one who experienced a bipolar episode, mixed with anxiety and obsession. I was to endure this way of life again and again, from here on.

## CHAPTER 2
## THE ZOO

September, 1992. I was dropped off with all my belongings in front of one of the ugliest buildings I had ever seen. With its puke-stained colour and maze of windows, I stood below and scratched my head. What have I done? It didn't look like this in the brochure! I remembered campus being so beautiful and serene when we drove through it, and here I was staring at this eyesore, smack-dab in the centre of campus: an eyesore that I was now stuck with for one whole year! Saugeen-Maitland Hall, the "Zoo", would be my new address.

I stood atop the hill for a moment longer and then marched my belongings down the stairs to the path below that led to the residence's entrance. I looked up again and couldn't believe that this would be my home! The only consolation at the time was the oodles of first-year girls that were also entering this residence. I had a girlfriend back home, so they were off-limits, but I couldn't help but keep my eyes wide open!

Dragging my bags and suitcase into the building, I was greeted by several girls who were decked out in purple paint and brightly-coloured shirts. This was crazy, I thought, but it seemed so cool at the time!

"Welcome, froshy! Welcome to Saugeen!" one of the girls exclaimed, as she threw the grossest of bright fluorescent orange t-shirts at me! I took it off my head and laughed. "Drop your stuff in your room, put that shirt on and get back down here!" she continued, pointing to several first-year students (frosh), who made their way back out in front of the large stone staircase. I laughed and left the three of them, and later realized I didn't even know their names. Shit, they didn't know mine either! Should I go back? Na! I walked through the entrance hallway and headed towards the rooms on A-Lower, the basement of the residence. I asked a few people if I was heading the right way. Many students donning the same ugly bright orange t-shirts were walking all over the building. I noticed them everywhere.

I walked onto my floor and met some first year students. I met Barry and Joe and found out that Joe would be my roommate for the year. He was a really nice guy, but he didn't know what he was getting into. He was about to experience the "full me" that year. Personally, I would experience the "ultra-me"!

"I'm Joe. I guess I'm gonna be your roommate this year!" he said, with a handshake and a smile.

"Great! It's Chris. Chris Nihmey."

"Well, Chris, I put my stuff on this side of the room; I hope that's okay," he continued. I smiled and placed my belongings on the other side.

"Can you believe this shirt?" I said, holding it up. "They want us to wear this? God. It's butt-ugly!"

Joe laughed, "I know what you mean. Barry and I have felt completely weird since we put it on, but supposedly everyone's going to have'em. That's conformity for you!"

What does conformity mean? I wondered.

I put my things down and sat on my bed. This is it, I thought and I put the shirt over my head to officially make me a Sauganite! I walked into our hall and met a few other members of our floor. We laughed and exchanged pleasantries and Joe locked our door. I followed the boys into the main lobby and we headed outside and, again, I noticed how many beautiful girls there were. Holding on to a long distance relationship was going to be tough, I thought, as I glanced innocently, yes innocently, at some long and short haired pretties.

Outside I met a few girls from our floor.

"I'm Chris, and you are ...?"

"I'm Jen. This is Patty. Isn't this exciting?"

It was. It really was. Here we were, all of us, away from our parents, in the heart of the campus of the University of Western Ontario. We were alone and we were free! For the first time in our lives, we were independent, not just me, not just Jen or Patty or Joe or Barry. All of us!

I remember getting to the base of the stairs and feeling an excitement brewing inside my body. I had felt it before, but it seemed to be more intense this time as I stood there. My body seemed to be going into shock, because I felt a surge of energy, mind and soul, much like during the later years of high school. My energy seemed to be very high, and I was restless and wanted to scream! I felt just great as I looked at a gathering of froshies filing on to the steps that led to the road to main campus. You could see everyone donning their fluorescent orange t-shirts, and although they looked corny at first, together, in a group, they actually looked pretty neat. I looked down at my shirt and read the words. "Super Saugeen! Y'all Ready For This!"

Suddenly, Joe grabbed my arm and pulled me towards the stairs. A DJ to the right of the steps was getting ready to play music. There were probably more than a 100 gathered on the stairs already as we approached. My thoughts were racing and I was talking a mile a minute.

"Let's go guys, up to the middle of the pack! Let's go, come on! Let's go guys!" I was now pulling the two of them into the hub of the crowd on the steps. Stickers, pastels and purple paint were being passed around. I grabbed some stickers and plastered them all over mine and the guys' faces. So did those around us. Watch this, I thought to myself, and, to get a kick out of the guys, I lifted up my shirt so a girl froshy could sign her name in purple paint.

"Thanks," I said, as I grabbed the paint and signed her shirt. Man, we were in heaven! We introduced ourselves to those around us, all of us ready to party. Is this what university was all about? I hoped so!

I felt a party in my head many times before this, but this party looked like it was going to last a long time, as I looked around at all the students surrounding us on the stairs. Within minutes, many more joined, and we filled the tall stairway that faced the residence.

A whistle suddenly blew, and a stream of marching students came jogging out of the residence entrance. They were cheering and chanting as they moved towards the stairs. Each was wearing a white t-shirt and blue shorts with Saugeen written right on their asses! We all looked around at each other, wondering what was going on. Everyone was in awe. We actually looked pretty wild, all of us there donning the ugly orange t-shirts. I thought again, maybe it didn't look that bad? A whistle blew again, and the line of runners came to a stop at the base of the stairs. There were approximately 30 students. But why? Then I found out.

"Welcome to Saugeen-Maitland Hall!" one of the guys in the group shouted out through a megaphone. He started clapping against it and all the students donning white started to clap with him. I figured that these were not first-year students. They had to have been here at Western awhile, because they looked so confident standing before us. Joe whispered in my ear that these were the second-year students, sophomores or "sophs", they called them. They would be our leaders for the year at Saugeen. Cool. There were some pretty good-looking sophs down there!

By now, we were well into the hundreds gathered on the stairway. We were all packed in tight on the steps and everyone was ready for a party. I was so excited! I could barely contain myself, looking around at my fellow Saugeeners. I met some more frosh, including Donny, who was also from Ottawa. He would eventually become my roommate in years four and five. I'll get into the reasons for the "five" sometime later.

"Standing before you is a group of guys and gals that will make your stay here at Saugeen one of the most exciting times you've ever experienced!" The crowd of first-year students roared, as megaphone-man continued. "We are your leaders for the year, your sophs! We're here to ensure that you have a fun and ... crazy year! We're here to ensure that you will NOT be a Christmas grad! But we can't guarantee it. We had a few last year!" the sophs giggled and laughed aloud. Christmas grad? Wonder what that means?

Suddenly, the DJ instructed us to follow the sophs' lead. We could hear him loud and clear on the tallest and, I found out, the loudest speakers I had ever heard! His words resonated in the courtyard entrance and the sophs started clapping slowly. Second by second, their claps became faster and louder. There were about 50 of them by now and it sounded really wild. As they clapped, the crowd started to follow and frosh all over the stairway were clapping and cheering and hooting, like a group of landscapers whistling at a pretty girl. I can vouch. I did that for six summers!

I looked at the boys and we were laughing so hard. This was incredible! And then the clapping stopped and the stairs fell silent, until ... the music boomed ... *"Y'ALL READY FOR THIS?"*

Suddenly, all the sophomores below us started to move to the music in rhythm, arms in motion and feet stomping. They were doing what seemed to be a tribal dance, as they tapped their heads and shoulders and knees. They formed a conga line. It looked awesome. Dancing alone? Not so awesome!

We were then encouraged to follow their lead and, guess what? We did. We all bought into the dance, quite easily. The music continued to blare out our theme song and we all partied on the stairs.

"This, froshies, will be your tribal dance for frosh week. You will hear this song over and over, so get used to it! You will see the dance and you will know it and memorize it, all of you! We will be one tight team, and we will show everyone on campus which residence rules Western U! S-A-U-G-E-E-N!"

We cheered and again awaited our next cue to go crazy. I was rip-roaring ready to dance again, as the sophs below directed us.

"Get naked, get purple, GO STANGS GO!!!" The group of sophs started cheering in unison with megaphone-man and then, once again, like little guinea pigs, we followed. And with hundreds of us on the steps now, we weren't just a loud cheer, but rather a giant roar! It sounded so damned cool, and I couldn't help but stop at times just to look around at the neat attraction around us! Not to mention the hot girls!

"Get naked, get purple, GO STANGS GO!!!"

I was having a ball. So was everyone else. We were enjoying ourselves so much, right in the moment. We were frosh … our parents, miles away! Woohoo!

We screamed another cheer about "Pizza" or "Wheels On The Bus", or something like that, and the crowd continued to go bonkers. And then, we heard the heavy bass of the speakers. "*Y'ALL READY FOR THIS?*" Our theme song came blaring again and we did the dance that, at that time, I believed, rocked the world. Not so much now as a thirty-eight-year-old, but then, it was everything! We moved our arms and legs flailing all about and partied like it was "*1999*"! Remember, it was only '92. But Prince's song already existed, and we partied like it, dammit!

While all this was going on, I was beyond the moon. I was having so much fun and enjoying my time tremendously. I mean, everyone was, but I remember feeling something greater, for some reason. Something was going on in my little head that was a bit off-kilter. While most students were enjoying the moment, laughing, cheering, dancing, I was feeling something different and grander, something much more intense, and I knew I had to do something about it. With that, I made my move and, because of it, from that day forward, I was bestowed a new title, a new name.

I was so hyper and so full of energy that, without warning, without even telling my new friends, I began to squeeze and manoeuvre my way down the steps through the thick crowd. I made my way down to the bottom steps, to the front of the gathering. I introduced myself to those around me and kept on cheering and chanting and waving my arms to the cheers, sporting a Western hat over my mullet. We all hooked arms together and laughed and sang. And then ... I did something. I would no longer be seen as just crazy for this one. I would henceforth be labelled ... a "legend"!

Here goes nothing! I leapt off the fifth step and dove right into the crowd of sophs at the base of the steps, much like a body surfer at a concert! A group of sophs caught me and started to lift me up and down while cheering aloud. I was then tipped upside down and then right-side-up as I linked arms with two gorgeous females. I turned to face the crowd of hundreds on the steps and, to my surprise, dozens of frosh started to point at me and in unison proclaimed, "He's one of us! He's one of us!" It was awesome! It sounded like "cheese on a bus"! It didn't take long for that cheer to surface.

This was WOW, I thought, but it wasn't going to end there and I knew it. This was only the beginning. In only minutes, I was titled SUPER FROSH and, crazily, I actually started leading the cheers and getting the party going mad! Those on the steps, from where I was standing, were astounded, and I could see Joe and Barry halfway up the steps having a blast. I waved to them and they shook their heads and gave a thumbs up. They'd have done anything to be in my shoes, I was thinking. At the time, I just thought I was being swallowed up by the moment. Funny thing, later, in speaking to several of the sophs, they couldn't believe that I had not been drinking. They thought I was drunk or stoned! It looked that way on many nights that year.

What was I feeling at the time? I guess you could say I was feeling really weird. I remember an odd feeling in my head, a sort of cloudiness that was so freaky but, at the same time, so exhilarating. It was something I'd felt before, something I was familiar with at different times over the last few years, and something that I'd most certainly feel again and again. It was not like being drunk and it was not like being hyper or over-excited. It was more. Definitely more.

In retrospect, at other times, through high school and into adulthood, I couldn't help but notice that a lot was going on in my mind, kind of like fireworks. First off, my focus was completely all over the place. My mind was running a mile a minute: again, the hamster! I couldn't sit still, I couldn't think straight and I remember loving how I felt. I loved the feeling, as any person who is experiencing mania would agree. My eyes, as they always felt during a high, were shifty and almost robotic. My head felt light and my body was just moving to the motions of my brain. My body really had no say, which was evident in the crazy and many stupid things I did. I remember feeling a need to be liked, rather loved, by those around me. In fact, I was almost obsessed with it, which made so much sense later.

I acted so impulsively, like trying to hug every girl and guy that I met, and doing things that were so unnatural. I did some things that year that were so foreign to me and so unlike me. I shake my head at many of those things, but that's what always happens when you are in a high. When you come down, you have to collect the pieces and start over. That is when things are most difficult because you have fallen into depression.

## CHAPTER 3
## AUTOGRAPH, PLEASE?

Saugeen traditionally honoured its frosh with a visit to what was hailed as, the "pub of all pubs". And it was; it really was. I remember it like yesterday even after all these years. You might ask, why? It was due to my state of mind.

Saugeen was introducing us to its end of frosh week Graffiti Pub. We had heard all the stories that emanated from these legendary nights, back to the first-ever Graffiti Pub. The night was crazy and we'd heard stories: well okay, just rumours, since we'd arrived. Every party paled in comparison to the Saugeen Graffiti Pub nights. We were about to find that out first-hand, but before anything got started that evening, I must say, that none of us, and I mean NONE of us, were ready for what hit us that night. We were unaware of what was coming our way until it came, and it did, in FULL force.

Graffiti Pub nights were nuts. Anything could, and did happen: experiences that could not be fully described once they were over. Many Saugeeners bared the scars that would stay with them for the long haul. What happened at these pubs stayed at these pubs: hard to contain, but a definite cardinal sin to repeat anything that happened on those wild nights. What happened at the pubs, or in the bedrooms after, kept lips sealed forever. It was, however, very common after a night like this, to see a guy or a girl sneak and creep quietly out of someone else's bedroom, in the wee hours of the morning. Maybe they were just sleeping? Hmm?

At 7 pm, pub night, the residence was already booming. The amount of beer and liquor that poured into Saugeen that night was beyond reason. Case after case of beer was delivered by many after-hours campus liquor services. Top the beer off with dozens upon dozens of mickeys and 40 ouncers, and you had one awesome boozefest!

That night, Saugeen would be primed for one amazing night of debauchery and mischief. You were either gonna get drunk, high or laid that night, or all three! Seriously, David Letterman himself, an all-star American hero, had coined Saugeen as "one of the top 10 residences in North America to get knocked up", and I realized that this was most certainly due in part to large consumptions of alcohol! To see the amount of alcohol coming in that day, I had to agree wholeheartedly with his TOP 10 selection!

We didn't really have to dress up for the Graffiti pub, since we all left Saugeen that night wearing our own white t-shirts. Some had regular t-shirts, and others, who were daring like me, donned muscle shirts (no arms attached)! I was in really good shape at the time, so I wanted to show off my pipes anyway!

Every Saugeen night out began with some pre-drinking ... actually a lot of pre-drinking. We gathered in one of the rooms. There were many guys and girls, including some guys that later became my good friends.

Arriving at the bar, I was really happy for the pre-drinking, because things changed quickly when we got there, where I received the most embarrassing welcoming "gift" I could ever receive as a first-year student. The bouncer, a big burly beast of a man, stared me up and down and asked the dreaded question we "under-aged" kids absolutely hated to hear, "Can I see some ID, please?" Since I was still only eighteen, ugh, while others received the "drink 'till you puke" bracelet, I received the "look at me, I'm a pussycat" bracelet. God, I was so embarrassed.

I was pushed to the side, as others receiving the "drink 'till you puke" bracelets brushed by me, including every good-looking girl I arrived with. All that were left were me and some nerdy guy. Great! I grabbed a marker and walked the hall, head-down, into the bar. I'd be scarred for life, I thought, and I couldn't hide the damned thing either! I had no freakin' sleeves on my shirt and, to top that off, it was like a stupid hospital band that you just can't rip off your wrist! Oh, God!

I entered and was instantly mesmerized by the atmosphere around me. Tons of girls and, what seemed like fewer guys, were walking around, ordering drinks and boogying on the dance floor. I met up with my crew and we grabbed a table. I had my stupid bracelet on, that I tried to hide under the table, but it was a little too late. My gang already knew I wasn't nineteen yet.

The whole idea of a Grafitti Pub was foreign to me, but I learned quickly. I found out that we were supposed to tour around and ask people to sign our shirts. Simple enough, I thought. We didn't know at that time how crazy this task would get, but we found out soon enough!

"This place is happening," Ron said, as we scouted the room, holding markers in our hands. The dance floor wasn't crowded enough yet to join in, but it soon would be. We chatted at the table, practically yelling, since the music was so loud. It was similar to the bars back home in Hull, where I could actually drink as an 18-year-old! But I definitely didn't miss home.

Everyone was talking and a couple of girls had joined our little group; but, I remember as I sat there, my mind was in another world. I'd hardly slept all week and I didn't know why. I guess I was just too hyper and excited about everything, and especially tonight. My mind was moving at an alarming rate and my focus on things was a blur. I didn't think anything of it at the time; I just went with it. It was only in retrospect that we now know that it was more than just plain excitement. Something was up. I hoped my mind would change for Monday when classes were to begin. I was just too absorbed in everything that was going on, to realize what was really happening.

As I sat there, I remember feeling something strange. A flame was burning inside of me and I felt the need to get up and walk around. I couldn't sit still. I was so wired; so I got up on my own to tour the bar. I grabbed a coke, planning to tell others that it was filled with vodka! That would do, I thought. Right through university, I often pretended to be intoxicated, in order to be accepted. I definitely didn't want to be labelled a "square" in week one! I was gone for about fifteen minutes and then returned to the table.

"Holy shit, Chris, how long were you gone?" one of the girls exclaimed.

"I don't know, fifteen minutes, why?"

"Look at all the names on your shirt! You got an amazing start!" she laughed, as she popped the top off her marker and looked for a white space to write. She signed "Jenny" and wrote below it "smokin hot". We laughed, but she really was! I had my eye on her the minute I met her earlier in the week, but my girlfriend back home kept me honest. No one said I couldn't flirt though. And believe me, I was good at it!

"Yah guys, it's pretty simple. People are starting to get signatures now," I said to the gang. And I was right. The Graffiti Pub was now most certainly happening. I could see people all over writing names and comments on people's shirts. I signed the other girls' shirts and they signed mine. Even if I couldn't touch, I preferred to have women write on my shirt. It was just better. I remember the feel of the marker on my back and front. It was almost sexy-like. Not when the guys wrote, though ... again, *not that there's anything wrong with that!*

The night went on and the dance floor started to fill up. The music quickly turned from rock to dance, and girls started to flood the dance floor. That was my cue. I was ready to get this party started. I grabbed my marker and again left the group. My head was telling me that I needed to move. I couldn't sit still. I'd been feeling that way all the time. I also remember being super attracted to every girl that I saw that week. But was it wrong to look? It killed me to see girls and guys meeting for the first time on the dance floor and "making-out" right in front of me, but I pushed it aside. God, it would have been nice.

I met up with a group of girls dancing. They all started to sign away and then, I gladly signed their shirts. And while that was happening, I felt really weird inside my head. It was kind of like a switch that went off in my mind telling me that I needed to get crazy. I had to do something to stand out. And it was at that moment, when I felt crazier than ever, that I vowed I would make it my "mission" to meet every single girl in the bar!

So now, while my friends danced in one area, I started to hop from one girl to the next, allowing me to sign them and, even better, getting them to sign me! I was quickly running out of room on my shirt, but the girls got creative. First of all, they would write on my arms, which I liked. Then, others were lifting up my shirt and writing on my abs and back. It felt so cool, and I was enjoying it because I was "ripped" in those days. This wasn't cheating, was it? One really hot girl came up and introduced herself, "Hi there, I'm Cindy. Can I sign your shirt?"

"Be my guest, but I'm getting pretty filled up!"

"You're a cutie," she said, as she wrote her name, and ... yep ... her room number, right on the side of my torso. I wrote the same to her. What a great idea she had! I decided to start doing that. Just flirting, remember?

My whole body was filled with signatures, room numbers, even some phone numbers. It was tough to see which names went with which numbers, because my shirt and my body were just covered in ink. Oh well, I was just having a great time. I looked around while being signed by a Rebecca and a Maria, and I noticed that I had so many more names on my shirt than any others'. I told the girls about my challenge to meet every girl in the bar.

"Well, good luck, Chris," said Maria, smiling. "Don't forget me!"

"How could I?" I said, as I released her hand and moved to the next group of girls on the dance floor. I was having SO much fun as I started to dance in the middle of them. Two of the girls wrapped me up like a sandwich, one behind and one in front, as two others signed my legs. I danced with them for a few minutes and moved along. I told several girls of my goal. They always laughed, and I never got slapped. None of them seemed to care, and some of them even cheered me on my way.

I went to the washroom and I couldn't even pee. I froze thinking about how much fun I was having and I just wanted to get back out there. I went back into the bar and met some other girls I'd met earlier.

"Hey honey," one of the girls said, reaching for my face. One girl signed and, without even asking, lifted up her shirt and asked me to write on her bra! Ha! Gladly. I did it, of course. I'd be an idiot not to! This was getting hot, I thought. Girls were lifting shirts all over the place! Alcohol was definitely a big factor that night. I then met a second-year soph, who actually planted a kiss right on my cheek, but I didn't kiss her back. That was tough. As I moved away, she grabbed my shirt and pulled me into her. We hugged but that was all. She then followed her friends off the dance floor. But before she left, she looked back at me and winked. She ran back up to me and whispered something into my ear. "715." Her room number.

"See you later," she said, running her hand through my hair. I swallowed, "Oh … my … God!" This was completely nuts, I laughed! I vowed not to forget that number … ever, in case things didn't work out back home. I did forget though. Memory loss had been a bit of a problem lately. I graduated high school easily, but my marks went down over the second half of the year. Thank God I had already been accepted to university! A lot had happened that year. We started to see things that were very uncharacteristic of me. My parents had their worries. Not me, I felt fine, but I had done some things that year they had questioned.

The night moved along, and I continued to stick to my outrageous plan. Would I remember their names? Probably not, but faces were the key. I could ask them again, especially the girl in 715. I did forget her name, damn, but her face was burned in my mind. I would not forget that.

I jumped and danced around and, seriously, I was having a grand time, high as hell. My head was really in the clouds. I was, however, accomplishing my goal. I would meet every girl in the bar ... and many guys, too, but who cared about them? It was funny, but every person I met that night was convinced I was drunk, when really all I was drinking was Coke. I had only had one drink before we left the "res"! They just saw me as so hyper and crazy, talking a mile a minute, and assumed I was really drunk—a drunk super-frosh! I did play the drunk-role well. I didn't want anyone to think I was sober. That wasn't cool and I knew it, so I played it up, and I was good. I was, oh so good.

Was it a good night? What do you think? By the end of the night, I had five or more invitations to parties back in "res" after the pub. I was invited to visit at least ten girls' rooms for post-evening drinks and whatever followed. I couldn't read my shirt anymore so I had to go on memory alone. I had accomplished my mission of meeting EVERY girl. In fact, that night, and I'm not exaggerating, I met over 500 Saugeeners, guys included! They estimated close to 600 were there!

There were a lot of memories from that night. The Graffiti Pub was as wild as rumoured. I will always remember it as being "super" crazy, but it was my mood especially that made things so memorable that night. Mania was definitely a big part of my opening week at Western U. It became the reason that, over the next week or so, people refused to walk around residence with me, unless they were ready to stop and talk with every person we met. I knew everyone because of the pub! I was definitely, as they said, a super-frosh that year. Mania has sort of clouded many memories from those years, but there were definitely some "highlight" moments like this night that, to this day, I will never forget. Oh, what a pub!

## CHAPTER 4
## FOLLOW THE "LEADER"

It was aptly named the official Saugeen "party of the year", even before it started! Perfectly named: two simple words, "Float Party". And that's what it was, a party that floated! I had heard about this type of party, even before I came to Western. That was how crazy they were! They were also banned in a lot of places, my residence included. But as high as I was feeling at the time, did that really matter? NO! I didn't care that night, nor any night in those months. I was ready for anything. Any kind of craziness would do, and that night, it definitely did!

Let me take you there.

It was early in the school year, mid-October. The leaves were changing and frosh week was well behind us. However, in my state of mind, frosh week actually became frosh month, which became frosh term. What about frosh year?

Me and some of the buddies on my floor were sitting around in one of our rooms at around 7 pm on a Friday night. The liquor was flowing and music was playing and chatting was happening, but I remember feeling bored. Really bored. We did the same thing every Friday, and being underage sucked. I couldn't contain myself and spoke up.

"Guys, we gotta get out of here. Look at us. We can't just sit here like this until the party upstairs at 10:30, drinking and smoking and listening to music for two hours! Let's get up and do something. What about something wild? We need to get the party started. What do you say?"

The room fell silent as the music was stopped, and the four other guys in the room looked up at me.

"What did you have in mind, Nihmey?"

I knew what I had in mind. It had been in my mind the whole month of September, but it hadn't happened. It was prohibited in all residences, but I dreamt of it in my state of mind that whole month and well into October. That's when I laid it out.

"A float party? What the hell is a float party?" Eric piped up.

"I'll explain, listen ... all of you!"

I went on to tell them exactly what a float party was, how it worked and how risky it was for us to start one. They were literally crazy and got carried away by anyone like me, who decided to get one started.

"I don't want to get written up for this," John said worriedly.

"You only get written up if you get caught! I don't plan on that. Besides, the party moves up, not down towards the lobby, and most of the RAs, I've heard, are away this weekend. It's the perfect time for it. What do you say, guys? You in?"

Three of the five were. The other two stayed put, as we developed our plan for the float party. And then ... it began! We started with the basement: # 1-Lower. Twenty-seven floors later, the party would be at its peak!

I grabbed a ghetto blaster from Eric's room and we entered the main door to 1-Lower. I pressed play on the blaster. The music belted out, and the three of us started walking down the hall banging on room doors, and even washrooms, yelling at the top of our lungs.

"Float party! Float party! Come on everyone!" We made our way down the long hall to the right, around the back and up the left side of the floor hall. Girls and guys started to come out of their rooms to join our little party. It wouldn't be little for long! It was great to arrive at a dorm room where a group of partiers sat drinking. When we got one of these rooms, we ended up with a big jump in numbers and a much bigger entourage. We left 1-Lower with 10 people! Ten! We entered 1-Middle and 1-Upper. By the time we arrived at the 2nd level, our party had turned into 30! The music blared, the people were loud, and we continued to move our way up. "Float Party!"

By the third level, we had a good flow going. I estimated around 60 people by then! "Float Party! Float Party!"

You see, the neat thing about float parties, and I knew it would work this way, was that the more people you got, then the more people you got, then the more people ... you see! It worked that way. God, everyone was looking for a party in Saugeen ... all ... the ... time. We were the craziest "res" in North America, dammit! Remember Letterman?

So we floated, from door to door and floor to floor. By 5-Lower, we figured we had well over 100 people ... just floating! It was amazing! It was really working and so neat to see! Now that we were really moving, each floor went a little like this:

The main floor entrance door would pop open and I would yell down the hall, "FLOAT PARTY!" Then, people would start to file onto the floor, as Eric played the booming music. The crowd would steer to the right, dart down the hall smacking on all doors, come around the back and make their way up the left side to the entrance door once again. By the 6th floor, we had so many floaters, that those who had made it around already had to stop to wait for others who were pouring in! This, before the leaders could proceed to the next level! The party was getting longer and longer and crazier by the minute!

The higher we went, the more people joined in because we had such an awesome party floating by. This was becoming ... one HUGE party! I noticed that about the Zoo. It didn't take much for Saugeeners to find an excuse to party, especially me being so freakin' high at the time! Trust me, it was fun, but coming down in November wasn't.

Both Eric and I, and the other guy, I forget his name, were floored at how well this party was moving. And we were yet to be stopped by anyone! It just kept rolling along.

We finally pulled up onto the 9th levels, the penthouse floors, they called them. The last stop was about to happen. We were hitting the roof, literally and figuratively. Honestly, I'm estimating based on our quick calculations, that when we arrived on 9-Upper, we had well over 250 people! 250! Can you imagine?

At the top, we arrived at a room full of partiers. I told them what was going on before anyone entered the floor.

One of them yelled out, "Wanna beer?"

"Do you have 200?"

"What? What are you talking about?" one of the guys said, as he stood up and looked aghast into the hall. Dozens of partiers were now entering the floor. In only seconds, the place was jammed! The blaster was playing and the floor was jumping.

"Holy shit!" he said, turning to the others. "Check it out! We ARE gonna need a lot more beer!"

The floor was packed. The guy, whose room it was, grabbed the blaster and took out the CD.

"Here," he said, as he put the CD in his HUGE stereo, speakers reaching above his desk! He turned it up, cranked the bass and people started to file into his room by the dozens. People were crowding in, standing on the beds, the dressers, the desk, it was complete madness. I was one of the guys on the desk and I looked at what we had achieved. There were Saugeeners everywhere! There were so many people, the floor seemed to be caving! The crowd, so I heard after, filled the entire floor. Many others waited in line just to get ON the floor! No ID required. We partied for a long time up there. One of the bed boards broke and a chair was cracked, but what a party! My biggest memory was the *Steve Miller Band* being played out and the whole crowd singing to "The Joker". *"Some people call me the space cowboy, yeah ..."* Complete and utter chaos!

I remember the "Float Party" as being talked about as one of the greatest Saugeen had ever seen. There was a risk, but, in my crazy mind, it was a risk worth taking. It was all about timing things properly and taking chances. That's what mania was all about. Doing things without thinking and taking chances, and that night, I did.

What ended the party that night? We got busted. The three of us got "written up" for starting the float party. One more and we'd be kicked out of the "res". But what a memory! I will have it forever. Would I recommend it for my pre-university grade twelve students? No, but man ... what a night! I would repeat it again the following year.

***"It was the best of times, it was the worst of times."***

***Charles Dickens (A Tale of Two Cities)***

And it was nights like these that would eventually be the demise of my first year of university at Western. I ended up leaving at Christmas with the embarrassing title of "Christmas Grad". I guess you can't succeed when you can't focus, your mood going up and down, never resting in the middle for any time. Highs were exhilarating those first couple of months, when I partied hard, studied very little, slept very little, drank my share, and had several relationships after Thanksgiving, when my Ottawa girlfriend and I broke up. Lows were worse, much worse. Unlike the exhilaration of being high, partying endlessly and socializing (I got to know practically everyone in the "res"), I would spend many more hours later that term lying in bed, sheets over my head, or crying on the phone to my parents. I was unable to focus or study in any way, even falling asleep in many classes. My mind was in another world. I could not concentrate. My door would remain locked often in those days and my roommate's trips home that term were a godsend. The last two months were a complete opposite of the first two, and I most certainly preferred the former. Wouldn't anyone? I think I've shared enough information about being in mania to help you understand why this was the case.

At home over Christmas, my family and I evaluated what could have possibly gone wrong that fall. We just couldn't understand it at all. Nothing made sense then. I returned to Ottawa in December, a beaten, battered and broken boy, with feelings of relief that the onslaught was finally over. But this was replaced by feelings of shame and resentment, and most definitely, a loss of dignity and self-respect. We just didn't know what hit me. At the time, we chalked it up to my not having tried hard enough or, as we often told others, not being happy with my choice of study, Engineering. But was all this really the case? God, my first two months, I was as high as hell and did next to no school work: my last two, the opposite, and again, next to no work. Shit, I was told three times that term in classes of five to nine hundred students to be quiet during lectures! "Shut up or get out!" one professor had said. Who gets themselves in trouble in classes that large, at that age? I just had to talk to someone ... anyone, so I did. I honestly felt I would break and lose it if I didn't. This urge to talk was so evident in times of mania, whether a big or small wave was occurring.

That Christmas, we even looked back at high school for answers. I was a strong student in my last couple of years at St. Patrick's, but there was clear evidence, in retrospect, of changes in mood. I had very solid marks, I had been a disciplined worker (and yes, still a talker), I had a strong personality, and was dynamic in every way, socially and mentally. And, we thought emotionally, too. This was all being questioned now. What had happened that term was unlike Chris Nihmey in every way. Superman had his alter-ego, who was opposite him in all ways. It was like my alter-ego, and not me, who had attended Western that fall. But it was me! It really was. We just couldn't understand why. We were left to do that during the break and the many cold, dreary winter months that followed, when I would face the embarrassment of bumping into someone who would ask after Christmas, "Chris, what are you doing home?"

I finish this section with a story, or a "coincidence", you might say, that will explain everything that went on just before Christmas. It is more than just a story. I believe that things happen for a reason. Was God in my court? I believe He was, even in these lowest of times.

[*I remember walking through Saugeen after my final exam, which I had flunked miserably. The residence was pretty much empty, as most students were gone home for the holidays. Engineers always had the last exam. I locked up my room and threw my bag over my shoulder and grabbed my suitcase. I was meeting a friend from Montreal who was going to drive me home. He was waiting in front. I was SO relieved to be done, but that was only because I felt as shitty as hell. I knew I was going to have to face all my friends and family at home and share with them this awful news. Good God. I had avoided most of them over the four months because of my new life, so they didn't know about my academic struggles that term. I was either too high to think about it, or too low to talk to anyone.*

*So, down in the dumps, I walked into the main hallway downstairs and something miraculous happened. I pushed on the handle to go outside and, with one foot in the building and one out, I heard, "Nihmey!" Everyone called me that.*

*I turned. Oh man, it was Donny, my buddy, also from Ottawa. I didn't want to have to talk to anyone else. Couldn't I just get the fuck out? Donny and I had hung out a few times that term, especially during frosh week. He thought I was just crazy, and called me so. He laughed whenever we crossed paths, because I was so hyper and in party-mode all the time. But he could tell I was in the dumps this time, even behind my small crack of a smile.*

*"What's up? You okay?" he asked, concerned.*

*"Hey, Donny. Well, to be honest with you ... I didn't have a good exam, or exams, or term, at that."*

*"Hey, exams aren't returned until January. Maybe you did better than you thought?"*

*"There's NO way. I'm not an idiot, Donny. I know how they went. Shit, I just finished my last exam and was the first person up, not because I flew through it with flying colours, if you know what I mean? I don't think I'm gonna be back after Christmas. Engineering is not for me ... I don't know what is?" I said, shaking my head.*

*It wasn't the first time I had come to terms with this fact. I really felt I'd be leaving after Christmas, back to Ottawa, back to who knows what? And that was exactly when God said his piece.*

*"Chris, come here for a minute. Have you ever thought of Kinesiology?"*

*I closed the door and moved over. "Kinesawhat?" I questioned.*

*"Kinesiology ... I know, it's a long word. You like sports, don't you?"*

*"Yah, I guess, but I'm not going into gym, if that's what you're talking about!"*

*"No, no, Kinesiology ... you're in good shape, I've seen you in the gym lots. Kinesiology is the study of sports. It is NOT gym! It is very different and much more in-depth. I'm trying to get into the program for next year. It studies Athletic Injuries, Coaching, Physiotherapy, Chiropractics, Sports Psychology, Sports History, Sports Wellness. The field is really growing."*

*"That sounds cool, Donny, but I don't know. I'm not really in the mood to think about that right now. After this term, I don't think I'll be accepted back at Western, anyway. I really blew it, man."*

*"That's okay, Chris. So did I last year. I went the full year only to find out I didn't get into Kinesiology, and I worked my ass off! This year I'm trying to get in again. So far, so good."*

*That day, Donny not only told me about Kinesiology, he turned me in the direction of this faculty. "When are you leaving?" he asked.*

*"My ride is waiting in front ..."*

*"Well, it is the 22nd, so they may be gone by now, but you never know. You should take a quick hop over to Thames Hall and see if you can meet with the Academic Counsellor there. She would be worth talking to, even now. After Christmas it may be too late, and they won't be there to call over the holidays. I would see her ... if you can. Just check."*

*Then he said the grabber, "Chris, it could be the smartest thing you ever do."*

*I thanked Donny and decided to follow his advice. On a last whim from a guy I barely knew, my driver and I quickly decided to head over to Thames Hall before heading for Ottawa. I ran in, and as I've said already, things happen for a reason. Strangely, her room light was on, and no one was with her. She was the only one in the office. That afternoon, before heading away from Western, after my terrible term, I sat for fifteen minutes with a wonderful lady. I told her my story; I was pretty down. She praised my courage in coming to see her like this. She couldn't promise anything, but she told me that if I passed at least two half courses, which would keep me eligible as a Western student, I might have a chance. Yikes! We had to wait until January.*]

I was readmitted into the University of Western Ontario in May of 1993, and by September of 1994, I was officially a Kinesiology student. God does work wonders. I had passed my two half courses! Just passed. The rest of my courses that year? I'll keep that to myself.

This "meeting Donny at the door" incident changed the whole course of my life. I look at it as one of the pinnacles in the direction my life took from that day forward.

It is the reason I graduated from Western: Kinesiology with Psychology, Honours.

It is the reason that in my final year at Western, I was voted Kinesiology Faculty President and was, according to the Dean's speech at our grad, "... the best president the faculty has ever had over my (his) term." He'd been Dean for fifteen years!

It is the reason I was voted Student of the Year in 1996–1997, and presented with two scholarship awards.

It is the reason I was admitted to the University of Ottawa for Teacher's College, and why I have taught with the Ottawa Catholic School Board for fifteen years.

Most importantly, it is one of the reasons I was able to write this book for you. God works wonders, and he did in my life throughout the years. On the way, though, I have paid a hefty price due to disorders that have dramatically changed the course of my life. I am only writing and speaking about them now, after all these years.

Despite my multiple disorders, which manifested themselves and continued to build strength and momentum throughout those school years, I proudly accomplished these many things. I had not yet been diagnosed or been under a doctor's care as I battled through school. Little did we know that things would only get worse.

I thanked Donny when we bumped into each other the second week of school, 1993. I remember hugging him that day. I had a whole new direction to my life because he had simply called my name on that blistering winter afternoon in December. He could have let me pass into the night and who knows where I would be today? Precise moments like these can change you forever. It is freaky when it happens, but, when it does, your eyes may be opened to a world that suddenly becomes that much grander and special.

## CHAPTER 5
## SHE WASN'T A HOOKER?

Western's biggest dance club was booming as it always was on a Saturday night in 1997. The crowd would settle in by about 11 pm and would party hard until closing at 2. I had gathered that night with the UWO soccer team, a team that I had spent my final year with as Head Athletic Trainer. Actually, I was the only trainer, but I loved the title and so did the ladies! It was part of a course I was taking that year. My responsibilities as head trainer were really simple ... help hurt people. Really, the job posting should have read "Athletic Taper" because that's mainly what I did that season ... oh, and hand out ice bags, too! Thankfully, there were no major injuries that fall, but I could have made one up and you'd never have known the difference. Like a bad tear or double bone break or a hernia ... yah, yah, a hernia! That would have been so cool!

I arrived at about 11:15 with two players from the team, Sam and Luke, two guys that I had a special bond with that year ... at least I thought so. We were to meet up with the rest of the gang inside. We slipped right past the long line at the entrance. The soccer team, which was on its way to the OUAA playoffs, had instant access to the club, and that included their Head Trainer!

That night, we were to meet up with the girls' rugby team, tough as nails, hot as ever. In particular, I was to meet up with a red-headed bombshell named Nikki, captain of the team and absolutely gorgeous. We'd been on a couple of dates and things were going really well, that was, until ....

"Wow, it's packed tonight!" Sam declared, as we squeezed our way over to the bar alongside the huge dance floor. He was right. The place was jammed and the music was loud, the bass pumping right through our bones!

"Where are the girls?" I asked. "Do you see any of them?"

Sam continued, "Yeah, where are they? Especially, where is Nikki?" he said, sticking his tongue out at Luke. Instantly Sam caught my attention with that one, obviously, as he ordered some drinks for us. Luke was quick to inform me that Sam had been dating Nikki. I was taken aback, but didn't say anything about my dates with her.

Sam handed us some drinks and we scouted the dance floor for the soccer team and, more importantly, the girls' rugby team. For me, though, the night had taken a different turn now that I had heard that Sam was dating Nikki also! I was really upset but I kept it to myself. Not really upset with him ... but with her. How dare she? I thought.

We met up on the dance floor with the guys, who were mixing it up with the girl's team. The guys had formed a circle around the girls. It was, oh so primitive! The girls could handle their own, though. They were a tough group and they were hot: especially Nikki. I would describe what she was wearing but that would have to be censored! She was smokin' and her moves on the dance floor ... well, I can't even go there. I gave her a wave as our eyes met. Then, surprisingly, Sam gave her a "how can I grope you?" look, as he headed over and nestled in behind her. Her eyes lost contact with mine as she closed hers and fell back into Sam. She looked so beautiful on that dance floor and the more she danced with him, the better looking she got. I suddenly had a huge wave of jealousy and it rippled through my body.

"Bitch!" I remember saying, staring at the floor. Did our two romantic evenings not amount to anything? Obviously not, I figured. We hadn't yet kissed but didn't holding hands mean anything to her? I guess not.

I couldn't watch anymore of this display of unfaithfulness, so I looked away, but kept finding my eyes back on the two of them. I hoped to give Nikki a look of disapproval but, honestly, she never opened her darn eyes! She just continued dancing in his arms and, trust me, I've never seen hands work as quick as his did!

I had to get away. I squirmed out of the circle without anyone noticing, and made my way to the crowd along the perimeter of the dance floor. There was a pool table, so I headed that way, continuing to glance at her from many places, but nothing was changing. "Bitch!" I said again, as I put a loonie on the pool table. I was a pretty good player, but that wasn't the reason for playing tonight. I just wanted to kick someone's ass since I couldn't kick hers, though she deserved it. She had barely given me a glance.

After losing at pool, I headed up to the second floor. It was a big club and, from the top, I could still see Sam with his hands all over Nikki's perfect body. And then, something happened and I lost it! I watched, practically in slow motion, Nikki bend her neck back and the two of them started a make-out session right there on the dance floor! That was it! That was the last straw! I was outta there! Great night, thank you very much, everybody, Sam, Nikki, the teams, what the fuck, déjà-vu, I'm gone! I remember this huge feeling of anger, and an even bigger feeling of despair. I felt the need to do something spontaneous; I just didn't know what. I felt shitty, but I also felt "crazy-like". I also felt like I was going to do something I'd regret if I didn't get the fuck out!

I headed back down the stairs and dodged people to the front door. No one had noticed. Everyone was partying, and I just felt like shit. I passed the line outside, keeping my head down. I didn't want to see anyone, but, sure enough, I did. I bumped into one guy from Kin, and another from Saugeen, and then a group from Kin, and then some others I knew. I couldn't avoid seeing them! I was well-liked and a popular guy at my school. Didn't Nikki know that?

I walked over to a fence away from the line and looked through. It was someone's yard. I was so pissed off, and I remember feeling really weird in my head. I'd felt it before, but tonight, it seemed to be more enhanced. I wasn't tired; I felt like I could go on for a long time. I thought angrily about Nikki again and said to myself, "I got to get the hell out of here!" And so I did.

And then ... I walked, and walked, and walked. I headed right down the "main" street, Dundas. Uptown was busy with people gathering at bars and restaurants all over. I didn't care. My head was doing weird things and I was still mad so I kept walking along Dundas. I wasn't sure where it ended, but I'd find out tonight. I was starting to form a sweat because I was moving so quickly. It was then, for some reason, that I determined to keep going for as long as I could possibly go. I don't know why I made that decision, or what went off in my mind, but I felt the need to do this. I seemed to always take things to the extreme.

I stopped at a couple of bars along the way to look in and see if I knew anyone. I didn't, and I noticed that the further I got, the fewer people I recognized. The university pubs and restaurants were now transformed into London pubs and restaurants. Everything was changing and things were looking sketchy, especially the people. I remember approaching a strip joint well down Dundas and, feeling somewhat of a high, I said to myself, "What the heck," and went right in. If I couldn't have Nikki, dammit, I'd have another girl. I looked around at the dirtiest place I'd ever seen and strippers were out to lure me into some lap dances. I didn't have a lot of money, but being just a bit horny, the mere sight of a naked girl turned me on. However, a slow song came on and I looked up at one of the dancers on stage. I noticed that she was as old as my friends' mothers! I stormed out of there quicker than I came in!

I continued my walk further down Dundas. I had been at least an hour and a half on my walk, but I wasn't tired at all. I felt I could go on for days. I was hot, but I was full of a burning energy in my body and in my mind. I started a few conversations with bar dwellers along the street, and lit one woman's smoke with the butt of her last cigarette. I chatted and told them about my predicament that night. Even THEY understood why I was angry.

For the next hour, I went deep into London's outskirts, staying on this main street. If I steered away, I definitely would get lost, I thought. I was pretty far out now and, as I recall clearly, I was so awake and alert: in the moment. I had a flame burning in my head and I embraced it. I was so far down Dundas that I started to wonder how long this stupid street was! Then something really strange happened.

I approached two young girls on the sidewalk. One was walking normally, the other was staggering drunk. Both asked for a light. I didn't have one. They started to strike up a conversation with me. I started to worry about the drunk girl, as she was tripping over and trying to stay upright by holding on to a fence.

"Hey, honey. Why don't you come home with me?" the inebriated girl asked, as she reached for my shirt.

"Please excuse my friend. She isn't normally like this," her friend said, and we both laughed.

We talked for a bit and then I planned to leave them but, before I did, my innate "goodness" took over and I decided to stay with them and walk them home. It wasn't far, they said, but the area was not the safest. I took one of the tipsy girl's arms, and her friend took the other. She was very heavy on my arm as she kept stumbling.

We cut down one street and headed over a bridge. I was now officially lost, I agreed, but for some reason I just didn't care anymore. I would go with the flow and see what would happen!

I walked with them right to their home and got to the front door. The sober one thanked me for being such a gentleman.

"You're welcome. Anytime."

Then her friend slurred some words in my ear and invited me to come in. I told the girls I should leave, but the drunk one seemed to be coming onto me a little. She was tugging on my shirt, and I remember continuing to feel this kind of wildness inside. I sat down on the step outside the house and the sober girl told me she was going to bed.

"Take care," I said. The other girl then sat on my lap, and I couldn't help but get a little excited.

"Won't you come inside?" she said, touching the buttons along my shirt. I could smell the alcohol all over her breath. I looked at my watch. It was 2:30! Oh well!

We walked in. I knew this was wrong and did so with some trepidation. She was drunk and she was nothing like a girl I'd ever be with! We walked into the kitchen and I could see a little girl run by, probably around four years old. Then I saw a black cat follow behind her. I was so confused. It felt like I was in a sci-fi movie or something, a state I never thought really existed. Then I heard an older woman yelling from one of the rooms down the hall.

"You fucking slut! Another one of your fucks, you bitch!"

It was her mother! This was not a well-to-do family, I thought. I should go. She hollered at her mom to shut the fuck up. Slowly we made our way downstairs. I should go. The mess, the dirt, the smell, nothing seemed to register. I should go, but I didn't. It was dark downstairs and she led me to a couch but, before we sat down, we found her brother lying there, passed out! I should go. She tried to wake him but he was "dead to the world", so she shoved him aside and we plopped onto the couch.

"Maybe I should go?" I said to her, but she insisted that I stay. She continued to slur and hiccup but, again, I was turned on and so full of excitement. Deciding to leave her brother lying there, she took me into a room that had beads hanging down at the entrance, and she pushed me onto another couch, a leather one, fake leather, for sure. She then suddenly got on top of me and she started to move her hips slowly on mine. I couldn't believe what was going on, but I liked it. But I was also scared and fearful of the risky situation I'd put myself in. What if her mom or brother had a gun, or a bat? I thought. But that seemed to make things even crazier and more exciting.

She started to gyrate on top of me, forward and backward. God, I barely knew what she looked like, and here we were engaging in the raunchiest of behaviour! Nikki was completely off my mind and I was being turned on by this kid, probably in her late teens. And then ...

As she kept moving on top of my body, something happened. She asked me if I had a condom. I didn't, of course. She reached for my zipper anyway but I moved her hand aside as she continued to move her hips on top of mine, and then, just like that, it happened. Yep, it did! Well, I should say I did. You guessed it!

I was so turned on, and so loving the feelings, and my mind just let go. I was really embarrassed and I quickly slid out from under her. She grabbed my shirt and beckoned me to lie down again. It was then that I said to myself, "What the fuck am I doing here?" I got up and tucked my shirt in. I was suddenly very uncomfortable. Reality set in, and I knew I had to get out. From upstairs, I heard her mom yelling again, calling her a whore, and a slut. I walked to the stairs and she grabbed my arm and tried to pull me back. I yanked my arm away but she pleaded for more. I walked into the kitchen and could hear her mom yelling, "You bitch, bringing home all your fucking men!"

Her mom peered into the hall and started yelling at me, calling me a bastard and a prick. I guess I had been a "prick" tonight, but I had to get out of there. I stepped out of the side door and jogged up the street. I looked back at the shady neighbourhood and headed safely to the lights of the main street. What just happened, I remember thinking? That was the wildest thing I'd ever done! I didn't even know her name! I felt weird, but I still felt the fire inside, a feeling of rebellion. Me, the "rebel". Who was this kid from Ottawa? Was this really me? I hadn't even kissed her, and was thankful for that!

It took me a long time after to put things into perspective from that night, but I remember jogging for close to two hours down a road that, thankfully, led me back to campus and then to my apartment. I was shaking my head the whole way home and laughing out loud. Wow! I had even told her I was from Ottawa! She was convinced we'd see each other again! Sure, I told her.

I ran and ran that night. For some reason I had so much built-up energy, even though it was 4:30 in the morning. I wasn't tired at all, even when I got home. It was an energetic feeling I had experienced many times prior to this, but I never understood any of it until years later when my life changed forever, close to ruination.

***"Early identification and treatment is of vital importance; by getting people the effective treatment, recovery is accelerated and the further harm related to the illness is reduced."***

***Paraphrase from National Alliance on Mental Illness (NAMI)***

# PART XII

# WHERE TO NOW?

## CAN YOU HANDLE THE TRUTH?

The most important thing in my life is sharing my story. So that one day, that kid, who's sitting in the dark, afraid to tell his friends and family that he/she is suffering from an illness, will step forward and be accepted completely by those around them, as they would if they had cancer or diabetes or a heart condition. So that mental illness will be seen for what it is ... a sickness like any other, and that healing is possible. That one day the dreaded stigma surrounding mental illness will forever cease to exist.

Stigma can be defined in one word ... abandonment. Maybe you've never experienced the feeling of being truly detached from the world around you. Many who have are no longer alive to talk about it, but I am alive and I will speak, because I believe it is my responsibility, my reason for having lived through hell. There are no excuses, because I am one of the few fortunate souls who has healed substantially and has survived to share my story. With that, I hope to inspire and help others who suffer to do the same, and those around them to accept them with open arms.

I held off much of the terrible effects of stigma for so long, well over ten years. How did I achieve this monumental task? ***I lived a lie.*** I lived only one side of my life to avoid the terrible anguish, fear, and discrimination from stigma. I've finally lifted the mask, I've removed the disguise and I am ready to live life now, as a whole person; to live ***the other side of the story***. That I've concealed for far too long. Now it is your turn, and it begins with a change in attitude.

Let's be honest. Words hurt. They are powerful. They can kill, and yes, unfortunately, they do ... over and over. Hitler proved this many decades ago through the stigmatization of a culture, of a family, of a people. Today, and even back then, the afflicted had to live with harmful and negative labels that made them inconsequential and seemingly meaningless.

***"I can imagine how the Jews must have felt during the Holocaust, when their lives meant nothing to the Germans. Squashed like bugs."***

We've been fighting stigma since the beginning of time, right back to Adam, Eve and the forbidden apple, changing our world forever, separating us as individuals, making us disparate. Being human, and not perfect, we made excuses to *treat those who were different from us ... differently.* To treat them as unequal. In the playground, it inspires bullying. It exists everywhere today, from the classroom and beyond. Teaching our children, therefore, becomes imperative. If the walls and barriers that have existed in our society aren't knocked down, who suffers? We all do.

Know this. You can still live, but feel dead inside, mentally enslaved by the world around you, surrounded by ignorance and bigotry, prejudice, racism and shame. Stigma has a whole life of its own. It has lived with us since time began, and remains a deadly influential force in a world of suffering and sickness, both body and mind. You will remember what a principal once told me about living with mental illness within the teaching profession. I share her disturbingly blunt, but truly honest words with you once again.

***"Chris, tell NO ONE. Be totally quiet. If any principal knew, or word got around that you're bipolar, I guarantee you, you would not get the job; you would NOT work in the board, period! The board is looking for a person they can count on, who they can always trust to be there for the kids they've entrusted you with, 100% of the time .... Parents don't want a "sick" teacher. They would NOT be sympathetic."***

And what did these insightful, genuine but "difficult to hear" words portend? Silence. Separation. Abandonment. However devastating to hear, at the time, it was a must needed action that ultimately led me to stay hidden. What was I hiding from?

When stigmatized, we choose to hide. We choose to be alone. Wouldn't you? Hitler wasn't the only one to stigmatize a nation. Just look at your reflection in the mirror, or the shadow you carry with you. We've all, including those of us who suffer, used labels such as these: insane, wacko, sicko, crazy, bonkers, dangerous, evil, malicious, cuckoo, delirious, demented, deranged, flaky, lunatic, mad, maniacal, maniac, nuts, psycho, wacky, stupid, loony, idiotic, psychotic, violent."

We are all, as a society, to blame for not only pouring the gas, but lighting the flame.

These are your neighbours, your colleagues, your loved ones. Is this fair? NO! We, who suffer from a mental illness are not monsters! Stigma makes us feel that we are! Being subject to these attitudes, someone who is sick simply gets sicker. They feel inferior, insecure and lack the confidence or desire to heal. They see a wall in front of them. Again, I ask you, is this fair? How can we justify a society being so close-minded? These are our men, our women, our children ... our loved ones.

While millions have been recipient to these destructive labels, thankfully, I found a way to avoid them. It was called lying, and it truly saved me. Sad, but it works, and in this world I had to. I don't have to anymore and neither should you. The stigma from having to reveal an illness prematurely, or having to be hospitalized or institutionalized, knowing the lack of support from society, or its disdain, makes the journey abundantly more difficult. Whether you deal with mental illness or not, we all have things we hide that hold us back, that hurt us, that keep us from moving forward. It doesn't have to be this way, for anyone, for you. You are not cancer. You are not diabetes. I am NOT mentally ill. You have cancer, you have diabetes, I have a mental illness.

People are honoured, people are praised for their battles with ailments such as cancer or heart disease, or even battle wounds, and they should be. My mom was diagnosed with breast cancer in 2010 and survived two mastectomies. She is one of my biggest heroes. She has endured the most difficult of operations, and has found the courage to face the many fears she had endured all her life. People struggling with these sicknesses are seen as heroes, soldiers in their fight. What about those with mental illness? They are rejected, discriminated against, ostracized, misunderstood, ignored, labelled and ultimately stigmatized. Mental illness is only one side of a "double-edged sword" stabbing its victim mercilessly. Alongside having to deal with a terrible illness, the sufferer must also withstand the harsh and cruel stigma carried with it.

Though it is not physical disease, when sufferers "come out", they most definitely have to live a life of wearing their sickness on their sleeve, for all to see and all to judge. They live the "label". It is imperative that the illness be

SEPARATED from the sufferer. The person is NOT the sickness. As long as they are linked, stigma will conquer and destroy, and without any support, it will be deadly.

The Ancient Greeks used the word stigma to refer to body marks or brands on people to be avoided. Millions of North Americans in a given year experience a mental disorder. Very few receive help. The rest stay hidden.

This is not right. This has to change. We HAVE to change and it is critical. No one needs to be labelled "wacko" or "crazy" anymore. Visualize yourself in your neighbour's shoes, no matter what size. At one time, I stared vicious stigma in the eye and asked myself, "How will I ever get out of this?" My answer? It was to stay in the proverbial closet.

## DID YOU KNOW?

According to the *World Health Organization* (WHO), in 2012, *"someone around the globe commits suicide every 40 seconds."* Wow, that is hard to believe, but not when you think about the number of people who suffer worldwide. WHO says that 1 in 4 people will suffer from a mental illness in their lifetime. One in four! We need to open our eyes to a world behind its own closed doors that is afraid to open. And these people are dying.

The *Canadian Mental Health Association* reported, according to the WHO, in 2000, *"815,000 people lost their lives to suicide—more than double the number of people who died as a direct result of armed conflict (306,600)."* As of 2012, this number has increased to almost one million deaths per year! Stigma is one of the leading contributors. People hate to be pointed at, so what do they do? They avoid help, and without help, they die.

On April 29, 2002, at the University of New Mexico, US President George W. Bush announced the creation of the *President's New Freedom Commission on Mental Health*. In his address the President stated:

***"Stigma leads to isolation, and discourages people from seeking the treatment they need. Political leaders, health care professionals, and all Americans must understand and send this message: Mental disability is not a scandal; it is an illness. And like physical illness, it is treatable, especially when treatment comes early."***

Despite this statement from one of the most powerful world leaders, stigma continues to fester and grow worldwide. People who suffer from a mental illness continue to be very fearful of facing their families, their neighbours, colleagues and friends. Stigma continues to prevent millions of people from stepping forward to receive treatment and care, in fear of what society might say or think about them. This is alarming. This is a tragedy. Media (movies, television, newspapers) often portray sufferers as outcasts, as less than, as strange, abnormal, even dangerous, when this is far from the truth.

Why do you think I stayed hidden? Wouldn't you? Many do, and many suffer because of it, and yes, many die.

I had the support which kept me healing within a safe environment, but millions don't. If I can feel as strong and confident as I do today, after all my healing, why can't others? At the same time, I could have healed substantially faster with society's support. We are wasting precious time. Our loved ones are suffering fear, loneliness and death. Everyone deserves to heal. Everyone deserves a life of freedom.

We all know that suicide and mood disorders, and thus mental disorders, are closely related. Those who suffer are at an alarmingly high risk of taking their own lives. Ninety percent of people committing suicide have a diagnosable psychiatric illness. Ninety percent! The most common form of death for those who suffer with schizophrenia is suicide. Fifteen to twenty-five percent of deaths by suicide are committed by those suffering from depression or bipolar disorder. Statistics Canada reports suicide is becoming a grave threat to humanity. According to the *World Health Organization* in 2012:

***"In the last 45 years suicide rates have increased by 60% worldwide. Suicide is among the three leading causes of death among those aged 15–44 years in some countries, and the second leading cause of death in the 10–24 years age group; these figures do not include "suicide attempts" which are up to 20 times more frequent than completed suicide."***

Who? Why? Those left behind go through a spectrum of questions like these, but the biggest decision the sufferer makes in their life is HOW? Gun, rope, car, leap, swallow, slice, "Next Exit" ... DEATH. Suicide should NOT be a choice EVER. That person riding the fence should be able to step back down because someone special was on the right side, pulling them towards healing and living. We have a responsibility as a society to create an environment for our loved ones, where they can feel safe and wanted, not alone and rejected. The *WHO* predicted that from 2011 and forward, depression will be the leading cause of disability worldwide: bigger than cancer, heart disease, diabetes and even AIDS. Doesn't this tell us something?

***"... one out of every four Americans is suffering from some form of mental illness. Think of your three best friends. If they're okay, then it's you."***

***Rita Mae Brown***

Ms. Brown, the great American novelist, tells us that if you live in a family of four, one member of your family may suffer in their lifetime. What about a family of three? Well then, it's your neighbour. To put this into greater perspective, in a football stadium of 80,000 spectators, 20,000 people will suffer from a mental illness in their lifetime. Do we have reason to be concerned? Of course we do. When you add the stigma experienced by this many people, you have one big mess. A cause for alarm? An epidemic. Ask 1 in 5 Canadians. Ask me.

Because of a negligence to learn and change, we end up creating MYTHS that start as rumours and become half-truths. Well ... they're completely false. What if people knew my secret? Would my own students think these things about me? Would I be labelled less of a person? Here are some common myths:

- Psychiatric disorders are not true illnesses like heart disease or cancer; people who have a mental illness are just "crazy";
- People with a mental illness lack intelligence;
- People with a mental illness never get better. They are not treatable;
- You can will it away;
- Being treated for a psychiatric disorder means an individual has in some way "failed" or is weak;
- If I just do enough exercise or yoga, get enough sun or eat the right diet, my psychological problems will disappear;
- Mental illness is caused by bad parenting;
- Kids don't suffer from serious psychological disorders;
- People who have mental illness are dangerous;
- If I tell people I have a psychological disorder, they will treat me differently or even reject me. I will be alone.

Only the last point is not a myth. It is true in every way. We are always alone inside; outside, it doesn't have to be this way anymore.

How can we rid our world of this stigmatization? It is simple. *Think before you speak or find a roll of tape.* Either way, words and discrimination are killing us, don't you see? Yes, regardless of change, there will always be people who will choose to take their lives. We can't prevent this, but we can slow it down dramatically by making a change in ourselves, and how we feel towards others. Can you handle the truth? Can you look within yourself and admit that you have been a part of the problem and that it is time for change? There is no shame in trying. We can make a difference.

Archbishop Desmond Tutu, himself, in an interview I heard on one of the leading websites on mental health, ***healthyminds.org***, stated that the stigma of mental illness in our world today is truly a crisis. He compared it to the stigma of those who years ago were afflicted with the deadly tuberculosis disease, shunned by society because of their illness. He also made a comparison with the agony and despair of exclusion, torment and segregation: deprived, a second class citizen in his own country of South Africa. This was before the democratic election in 1994. Following that day of freedom, he stated, *"... the blue of the sky was a different colour, a glory about it."* I paraphrase a part of his 2011 interview on stigmatization. He went on to say:

*"I think a lot of people want to hide it. Any time you have someone say that they are going to see a psychiatrist, it's almost a swear word ... to say to you that you are "crazy". It's like what people used to think about leprosy. You don't mention it ... mental illness is still seen as you really have something wrong with you ... you should be put in a straightjacket once you mention you have a breakdown. That then affects what gets to be done. Do we really provide sufficiently for that? ... and so it's a crisis. People just don't think of mental illness as an illness."*

Tutu made a parallel between those who stigmatize and talking to someone who is blind. You want to describe to them the magnificent wonders of the world, but the talking language does not make sense. It goes unheard. They can't understand what they don't see. Neither does a large part of this world when it comes to mental illness. They are simply ... blind. Will those who suffer from mental illness one day see this same blue sky that Tutu marvelled about?

In 1963, Martin Luther King Jr. stood on the steps of the Lincoln Memorial, and in front of a multitude of people, spoke the four words leading to his famous life-changing message. He declared, *"I have a dream ...."* If one man took his dream and changed a nation, inspiring them to embrace mankind, despite their many differences, why can't we, as a world, share that same dream. A dream where those suffering from the terrible afflictions of mental illness can finally open their doors, and their lives, to take that first step towards healing. Why can't we find compassion and understanding for those who have been afflicted? It is time for those who hide to feel love and acceptance. To feel the liberty to express who they are and what they've been through, and to ultimately stop ***living a lie***. There are ***two sides to every story***. Isn't it time we read the whole book of a person's life, and not just stare and point at its cover? It is only then that we will accept a person, not only for their great achievements in life, but also for every struggle they've had to endure and overcome.

Change is attainable, but again, it begins with a change in you. And the greatest of it all, is that the *dream* is possible in every single way. We must gain insight and speak out against these things that separate our people, our world. If we join together, we can stop the words of hatred from destroying us. It may be true that words can kill, but it may be our own silence, our own fear of speaking up when it is necessary, that hurts our loved ones the most.

***"In the end, we will remember not the words of our enemies, but the silence of our friends."***

***Martin Luther King Jr.***

## THE BIGGEST DECISION IN LIFE

***"Why dear God, have they begun to miss me?"***

**Do YOU want to live?** Suicide is NEVER the answer … you do have a choice. In the depths of despair, when it seemed like all hope was lost for me, and death was standing right at my doorstep, I had to make a choice, and my choice was YES. YES, I wanted to tie my laces, pack my bag and climb the mountain before me, and you know what? It has made all of the difference in the world. No one needs to die like this. No one ever needs to answer this question with NO. Life is too grand, too precious. The fall into sickness may be an exponential decline, but through my own experiences of getting back on my feet again, I assure you that, fortunately, healing takes the same path in the opposite direction. And once it starts, with proper measures taken, you can eventually soar.

The stands are full, and they are cheering you on. Be proud of who you are, because you are special in every way. Ending your life is never the answer. The answer will lie in the hearts and the lives of every single person you will reach out to, and inspire because you chose to live on and share your story. I am living proof that it can happen. I'm doing it now and it feels unbelievable. You can too, so go ahead and take the first step. It's a tough one, sure, but you are ready, and once you get moving, keep your head up high and don't look back—you're not going that way. The sky's the limit for you. The bleachers are full, and I am also in the crowd. I'm cheering louder than anyone.

***"There's a hero,***
***If you look inside your heart,***
***You don't have to be afraid of what you are.***

***There's an answer,***
***if you reach into your soul,***
***and the sorrow that you know will melt away."***

***Hero – Mariah Carey & Walter Afanasieff***

## THE BIGGEST DECISION IN LIFE

*Why dear God, have they begun to miss me,*
*When I've ended my sorrow and allowed myself free?*
*What makes them cry, the way they do every night?*
*How can I bear to witness, such a terrible sight?*

*Don't they understand that my life was a battle,*
*A never-ending grind, from hassle to hassle?*
*Don't they understand that problems were there,*
*And I felt I was lost, that they didn't care?*

*Why do they weep, now that I'm gone?*
*What have I done, have I done something wrong?*
*I've gone to a place more beautiful than ever.*
*I just won't see them again, I'm gone forever.*

*I watch my mother cry, but I can't lend a shoulder.*
*Her only son is gone, no longer brave nor bolder.*
*Look what I've done, I've left them in tears.*
*Why did I decide to end, my long future years?*

*Now I realize how important things are,*
*How much I was loved, but now so distant, so far,*
*To even say how sorry I am, for the thing that I've done.*
*It's too late to come back, no more rain, no more sun.*

*No more mother, no more father, I can no longer complain,*
*And I no longer feel sorrow, I don't feel any pain.*
*Though I watch my father cry, for the very first time.*
*Maybe he did love me. Why did I commit such a crime?*
*All I can do now is lie here and wait.*
*Will I go to Heaven or hell, only soon God will state.*

*I can no longer see them, it's so dark inside.*
*They can no longer see me, I haven't the choice to hide.*
*I just want one more look, to remember them by.*
*Why God, just why, did I decide to die?*
*I can no longer hear my mother's good cheer,*
*Or wipe off my father's very first tear.*
*I can no longer lend a shoulder, to my sister who cries.*

*To wipe off each and every tear, that enters her eyes.*

*I can only wait and hope that soon I will be free,*
*To run and play, and to find the key,*
*To unlock the memories, I remember from the past.*
*Why did I choose poorly, to end my life so fast?*
*Yes it's hard on so many, when someone special has died,*
*And I ask God's forgiveness, though it was no white lie.*

*Now I am gone, no more life left in me.*
*I can no longer hear, I can no longer see.*
*I have gone to a place, I hope I can soon find,*
*My family, end this darkness and get rid of the blind.*

*I know that when I find them, we can continue to grow.*
*I only hope it's not too late, to come above from below,*
*I feel I've sinned so intensely. Will I be forgiven?*
*I hope I can rejoin them, in one place only, in Heaven.*

**Christopher Nihmey, 1987, age 14**

Was this poem a foreshadow of my future battle with mental illness?

***"Another suicide, another life. Many unanswered questions, but the biggest question of all for those left behind ... WHY?"***

## YOU LOSE SOME, YOU WIN SOME

Mental illness has its ups and downs in so many ways. I learned this the hard way, but I learned it, and that is what matters. Triumphs bring their disappointments, and success does not breed happiness, without the thorn of failure by its side. I was hit so hard, blindsided by the loss of so much in my life so quickly, over a short period, but I can say that it has made me stronger than ever. What was I robbed of? What did I lose throughout all these years of suffering?

I have never married. It was something I always hoped for, but sickness kept me from keeping and pursuing a long-lasting, successful relationship. Obviously, children have been out of the question. I believe I would have been the "perfect" dad. Okay, I need to get out of the habit of using that word! Let's just say, a good father. Since my full-time employment in 2000, I have not worked permanently in a teaching job, a job I am very good at. No promotions, no health benefits, no summer pay. I have also lost money over several long periods of time when I was dealing with too much. As a 15-year permanent teacher in 2012, I would be earning over $90,000 per year. I am currently making less than $40,000. That's if I work every day of the school year (next to impossible in occasional teaching). And yes, this also hurts my pension, but I do earn some ... very little. We've calculated (my father and I) that I've lost close to one million dollars throughout these years. Yes, you are reading correctly. Not to mention thousands of dollars given to me by my parents and the thousand-plus I've had to spend each year, for the deductible on a provincial drug plan. Let alone what I gave away during my manic periods. At that time, I gave away my whole Registered Retirement savings. I have been unable to invest in either RRSPs or homes up to three years ago.

I have unfortunately lost many of my prime years and special moments with friends and family because of sickness. A lack of confidence, self-esteem and stability have kept me away from many important gatherings.

Bigger than anything though, I have lost ten years of my life, years that for many people my age are the most productive, fulfilling, life-building and life-changing. But don't feel sorry for me. I have gained some things too, and I've realized that these gains far outweigh the losses.

Since 2009, I've been working on this book and planning my journey to reach out to others who suffer from mental illness through my story.

For the last three years, I have volunteered at the Royal Ottawa Place, working on writing a book (a collection of residents' literary works). These residents, like me, suffer from mental illness.

I wrote and published two children's novels in the early years of my sickness. Later on, it never would have happened. In 2010, I purchased a 2-bedroom home (with Mom and Dad's help), supported financially by my consistent employment as a supply teacher.

I've kept and made many good and trustworthy friends throughout the years and have finally started dating again.

For the longest time, I couldn't laugh. It took healing for me to see and accept the craziness, the absurdity and the bizarre in the things that I did. Being healthy, I can finally laugh and put on a smile. And when I reflect back to some of these things, I shake my head in wonder and amazement.

I have been embraced by my family's utmost love and care; without this blessing, I'd have never made it. I would likely have been institutionalized, or even locked away. I believe that institutionalization would have inhibited my progress. The stigma alone would have killed me. At home, I was able to heal before facing the world head on. I would bear armour, a shield, a sword, but most of all, strength and courage, to prepare for any future battle. My mom, my dad and my sister were the strongest supports anyone could ever ask for: who stood by my side, day in and day out, regardless the forecast. I am forever thankful. They walked with me all the way, and my life became beautiful once again. We are now closer than ever, as we look forward to sharing more healthy and productive times together.

Most of all, and most important, I have finally found a more realistic, positive and stable faith life, with a loving God. I know now that He never left me.

My three disorders are at bay after a long journey of therapy, use of many medications, hard work on my part, support, exercise, and dozens of life changes. I have found inner strength and a confidence within myself that I believe

I've never had. I was blessed to find an amazing therapist whom I cannot thank enough. I've called him a "blessing in disguise". He truly is. I've felt triumph and success in my healing and plan to give others hope in their difficult journeys. I have discovered courage, perseverance, discipline, inspiration and an abundance of creativity (one of the only benefits of having bipolar disorder) in everything I do.

I still have my many battles; I always will, but I am now confident that with all of these supports by my side, and the triumph of battles I've already won, I can continue to stand tall and succeed—and be damn proud of everything I've accomplished. It only takes one success to get the ball rolling and realize, "Hey, this CAN happen." And with that, it does.

These many gains have made life bearable throughout my years of suffering. Now they make life liveable and fulfilling. You cannot earn or win these latter gains. They don't come with a price or a congratulatory certificate for the wall. They come from deep inside you, and they make continuing life worthwhile in every way. I have now realized that each gain has greatly outweighed my losses. Things happen for a reason, and they were the reasons I kept on breathing. They were the reasons I am alive today to talk about it. One of my mottos is:

***"Trust in the LORD with all thine heart; lean not unto thine own understanding. In all thy ways acknowledge Him, and He shall direct your paths."***

***Proverbs 3:5–6 (KJV)***

## SALLY

I used to complain about being hungry.

I don't anymore.

I used to complain about the cold.

I don't anymore.

I find it hard to complain about anything anymore.

Life has changed forever for me, as I hope it has for her.

Here is my story.

I first came across Sally on a cold day in November. I was walking home from school through town, when an elderly lady approached me from an alleyway.

"A quarter for an old lady?" she asked, as she reached out her frail hand. I remember that her fingers were so thin, her hand red from the cold. I quickly turned a cold shoulder and passed on by. I pretended not to see her ... she was, after all, a stranger. Without thinking much of anything, I hurried home.

That night, I ate dinner, did some homework, watched a bit of television, spoke to a few friends on the phone and headed off to bed. I curled under my sheets. They were warm and cozy. I was safe inside my little world and as I lay there thinking about the day, several thoughts came to mind, but never once did I think about the lady in the alley. She never crossed my mind. I turned another shoulder and fell asleep ... in my comfy bed, under my warm sheets.

6:30 am came quickly, and following breakfast, I headed to school. I entered the downtown area and passed along the same route I had taken home yesterday, but as I passed the alleyway, again, I thought nothing more of the old lady.

The day was busy as I went from class to class. Math, English, History, Religion ... I learned them all, and left school that day thinking I was just a little bit smarter. On my way home, I headed into town, stopping at a few shops along the way. Coming out of a pawn shop, an elderly lady approached me from an alleyway. It was the same lady from yesterday.

"A quarter for an old lady?" she asked again, reaching out her frail hand. With nothing to give her, I just pushed on by, and as I did, I noticed a dime lying on the sidewalk. I bent down and picked it up. I turned around, walked over to her and handed it to the old lady. "Here you go," I said, and then I headed home.

That night, I did similar things ... I ate dinner, I watched a bit of TV, talked to a few friends, but something was different from the night before. For some reason, I couldn't stop thinking of the lady in the alleyway. Why was she living on the streets? Where was her family? Where were her friends? I fell asleep thinking about these many things.

After another busy day at school the following day, I stopped into a corner store to buy a sandwich to eat. Leaving the store, I took a bite and headed through town. Like the last two days, there she was once again, sitting by the alleyway begging for a quarter. I reached in my coat to look for some money, but I'd spent my last bit on the sandwich.

"Here you go," I said to the lady, as I reached down to hand her some of my sandwich. The lady looked up at me and nodded her head. I even thought that I saw a smile. With her frail hands, she ate the sandwich and I headed on home feeling proud of what I'd done.

Days passed, and the weather got colder and colder and each day on my way home, a similar pattern began. Having little money myself, I started to bring a different item each day to the old lady in the alley. One day it was a sandwich, or a pair of gloves for her frail hands. Another day, I brought her a worn blanket and even one of my old sweaters. It fit her perfectly. Not only was I bringing her things, but I was starting to talk to her and was getting to know her more each day. She told me how hardship through extreme depression and stigma had separated her from family and friends, leaving her with nothing but the streets. She eventually felt comfortable enough to share her name. It was Sally.

For the next while, every day following school, I headed straight for the alley to see Sally. She was always excited to see me, wondering what surprise I might bring her next. On this particular day, I had something very special for her, and all day at school, I was excited to see how she would react to it. I arrived at the alley, and as always, she was there.

"Hello Sally," I said, greeting her with a smile.

She, too, smiled back. Then I pulled out my surprise. Reaching into my coat pocket, I retrieved a small harmonica that my grandfather had given me years ago. Sally's eyes lit up. I could see that she loved music, so I started to play. I carried a tune and began to move about the alleyway. Sally clapped and tapped her knee. We enjoyed each other's company for the next hour and then I headed back home.

That night, I thought deeply about Sally. She was really a special lady. It was sad to see her living on the streets like that. It was also sad to see how many people walked by her without even a smile or a hello. But, I guess I had reacted the same way when I first saw Sally. It just didn't seem fair. Why did people have to act that way? What did they fear? She was just like you and me. Why would family and friends turn their shoulders away from such a wonderful lady? How could sickness hurt relationships, friendships? It just wasn't fair. I just couldn't understand it.

Weeks turned into months, and months turned into more months, and I continued to visit Sally in the alley whenever I could. But, as time went on and things got busy with school and with life, I found myself, more and more, drifting away from my visits. I didn't want it that way, but it just happened. Life happened. Although I didn't see her as much, I did stop by when I could to say hello and play a tune.

On one fine day in June, towards the end of the school year, I raced to the alley to see Sally. I had something really special for her. I knew how much she loved to draw, and I had something that I knew she'd love. I arrived at the alley and greeted her with a smile. "Look!" I said, retrieving a pad of paper and some pencils from my bag. "It's a sketch pad, and some pencils you can draw with, Sally!" She was beyond thrilled with the gift, and she thanked me over and over. She even drew me a picture of a cat and mouse. She was very talented. Her drawings were amazing.

Time continued to pass on by and again, days turned into weeks, and weeks turned into months. One day, I had realized that it had been a long time since I visited Sally in the alley. Sitting in class, I wondered what she had been up to. Now that I was taking the bus home from school, I no longer crossed paths with her. I decided to head to the alley to pay her a special visit. I was excited to see her.

Following school, I approached the alley only to find an ambulance with its lights flashing. I stood there in shock, wondering what had happened. Who was hurt? Was it Sally? I wondered immediately. I panicked and ran up to the paramedics. "What happened?" I asked worriedly.

"We found her in the alleyway and she was not doing well."

"Can I see her? I know her."

"Not right now. She can't see anyone," the man said sadly. He told me that she was very sick, and hardly coherent. I stood there for minutes, hoping that I could at least see her face. I was so distressed. Another ambulance attendant then came over to me holding something. "Your name wouldn't happen to be, Tom, would it?" she asked.

"Yes, how did you know?" I responded, surprised.

"We found this in the alleyway. Does this look familiar to you?"

"Yes, I gave that to her."

"She repeated several times that she wanted me to give this to Tom. That would mean you," she said, handing me the notepad. I took it and put it in my school bag. "Thank you."

The attendants closed the door of the ambulance, and it slowly rolled off. I followed along the sidewalk for a few minutes and then they were gone. She was gone.

I never saw Sally again. I visited the alleyway many times over the next year, but she was never there. I like to think that she's alive and well somewhere, but I'm not sure.

The one thing I remember most, was my walk back home on the day that Sally left me. The ambulance had pulled away and I remember retrieving Sally's notebook. I stopped along a fence to take a look at her pad. I was surprised to see that the notebook was filled with many beautiful pictures ... some of fruits, some of trees and animals and people. What a talent she had. But the thing that surprised me most were the pictures in between these ones. They were pictures of me and her, the two of us together. In one, we were eating, in another, the two of us laughing. There was also a picture of me playing my harmonica for Sally. All were pictures of our times together.

I finally got to the last page, and there it was. Sally had drawn a picture of me hugging her. I never knew how much of an impact I had had on her, the strong love and friendship we shared. Now I did, and although we had never really hugged each other in person, she had imagined it within her mind; within her heart. Her picture spoke thousands of words, and each word was representative of love. I only wished at that moment, that I could have truly hugged poor Sally.

From that day forward, I always hoped to bump into Sally from the alley, somewhere, someplace. She stayed in my prayers and every day that goes by, I wish her much health and happiness. She touched my heart forever. She was the greatest act of kindness I ever knew, because she shared her love, even though she had so little to give. I'll never forgot that. Ever.

Life has changed for me. I no longer complain anymore. I just live, like I'm supposed to. Life has also changed for Sally. I hope that she is taken care of, and that she is content wherever she may be. I've written this story for her. Maybe this story will change your life if you let it. It has definitely changed mine. May her legacy and her story live on forever. God bless.

By Chris Nihmey

***"That person on the street is someone's son or daughter … they were in kindergarten just like you."***

I initially wrote *Sally* in 2005, as a picture book for children, because even kids need to be aware of the awful effects of stigma on mental illness in our world. I realized after completing it, that it reaches out to all of us, no matter what age.

It doesn't have to end this way. Ultimately, in our mind, we are alone in sickness, but no one should have to suffer the difficult perils of the illness by themselves, without support and love surrounding them and caring for them.

***"Approximately 20-25% of the single adult homeless population suffers from some form of severe and persistent mental illness."***

***National Resource and Training Center***
***on Homelessness and Mental Illness, 2003***

## IN MEMORIAM
## FLY AWAY

This is a short story of an angel who came into my life. Her name is Nadia.

For the last year and a half, I volunteered helping Nadia, and she has most definitely been my inspiration. Nadia suffered from Huntington's disease, a terrible hereditary disease that took over every muscle of her body, including the ones in her face and tongue, disabling her speech. It caused her whole body to shake uncontrollably, even more than someone suffering from *Parkinson's Disease*. Along with this, year after year, her brain also experienced a mental decline of its functions. The disease began in her early 20's, and by her 30's, Nadia was bedridden, unable to walk or talk, because of the severity of the disease. I first met Nadia when she was 32, a year and a half ago, while volunteering at the residence she lives in, along with many others who suffer from physical and mental illnesses. Early on, I developed a genuine fondness for her, because of the beautiful person she was and the strength that she had, but I have to admit, also because of the reality of the life she lived, a life where she was alone ... she was all alone. At the young age of 32, Nadia had few friends and family, and was surrounded mainly by fellow residents, volunteers and workers who helped her at the home.

Over the many months, I spent much time with Nadia, going for walks, helping her with communication, sharing special times together, watching her favourite cartoons on TV and spending time with her during meals. Although she could never share her words of appreciation with me, I always knew she cherished our times together. We both did.

Just after Christmas, Nadia's health took a turn for the worst. She had to leave the home due to a virus that had entered her body, causing her core temperature to rise dramatically. That, on top of the disease, hurt her deeply. She went into emergency immediately and was admitted into the hospital for treatment. I found this out a week later on my visit to the home. I was very surprised when I entered her room that day and she wasn't there. An empty space grew inside of me. I missed her instantly.

A week or so after she left the residence, I decided I would pop in and visit Nadia in the hospital. I took a stuffed dog from her room and planned to go some time the next week. I was driving home from the grocery store on the Friday night. It was January 7th, around 6:15, and for some reason, and I still can't understand why, I felt the need to turn the car around and go to the hospital that night. I didn't think much of it at the time, but it just felt like the right thing to do.

I took the elevator to the fifth floor and entered her room. There she was, sleeping like a baby on her stomach, head turned to the side. "Nadia," I whispered. "Nadia." She slowly opened her eyes and looked up at me. "Hi Nadia ... it's Chris!" She quickly tried to turn onto her back to look at me. It always took a while for her to do this, but it was good to let her do it by herself, to build her strength. In short time, she was looking at me and answering questions in short small breaths, more like grunts, as her muscles contracted quickly and she actually ended up kicking me in the face! I laughed. She appeared to also. It was so great to see her and we spent a couple of hours together.

Early on, I placed her stuffed doggy on her stomach. She was very happy. Then I took out a little gift I had purchased from the gift shop ... the perfect gift. It was a *Willow Tree* carving of an angel with wings holding a small butterfly, and it was perfectly named "Angel of Freedom". I went on to tell Nadia that she would always be watched by God and His angel of freedom. And that someday soon, she would be free and, like a butterfly, would emerge from the cocoon she'd been imprisoned by for so long. My mother, reflecting on all I had been through, called me her elusive butterfly. Nadia was mine. She would fly to a life free of pain, suffering and hardship. I don't know what she understood from my words that night, it was hard to tell, but I do know she was listening and comforted as I spoke, as was I. I hope she understood. I like to think that she did.

That evening, we cherished our time together and I bade her farewell with a kiss on the cheek and a prayer. My kiss was so rare to her; little did I know that night how important that kiss would be.

Driving home, a lot of things about life came into perspective. What did it all matter? My house? My car? The things I owned? The reality was, none of it did matter. What mattered was the companionship and friendship that Nadia and I had with each other. Wasn't that true of all things in life? It's really not all the things you "think you have", but more so the people "who you have" in your life. Nadia did not have much, but she had me, my friendship, my love and, most importantly, my prayers.

Three days following my visit with Nadia, I received an upsetting phone call from the residence. On January 10, 2011, Nadia had passed away. The pain, the discomfort, the heartache ... it was over. It was a sad call, it was a happy call. She was out of the dark, and she was free. Nadia was finally free! She was now with God, and she had emerged into a life free of the very things she'd been enslaved by. She would spread her wings and fly forever. For once, after a long time, she would feel warmth, happiness and unending love.

I smile when I think about Nadia flying off to her new home. I always thought that she was my angel, my angel of freedom, my inspiration for never giving up. But I guess, too, I was her angel on earth. Like she was an angel for me, I was one for her. I guess that's why our bond was so special, and why my final kiss to her that night was so precious, her last kiss, or maybe her first of many, depending on what side you look at things. I tend to think the latter.

I now dream of Nadia running and jumping and playing like a child. I picture a smile on her face, and words coming out of her mouth, being able to eat on her own, and roll over in an instant. Boy, do I miss her already, but I know that my need to see her means little, because she is now free. Although I'll miss her dearly, I know most certainly that I will join her one day, and we will take a walk arm in arm. This time, however, we'll leave her wheelchair behind. Actually, it won't even be there!

God bless you, Nadia. You're a one of a kind. I can't wait to see you again. Until then, enjoy the life you should have always had. Embrace your new life. You deserve it, kiddo. Miss you ... dearly.

Love Chris (written January 11, 2011)

## I LEAVE YOU WITH ...

That man on the street, that woman isolated in her home, that teenager who feels like dying every time she steps away from her locker. They all began their lives just like you, bright-eyed and optimistic, sitting in a circle with twenty other children who would become friends for several years in school, hopefully longer. But while they sat in their circle, one could never predict that one day, down the road, some might be sitting in an entirely different circle, joining the millions worldwide afflicted and/or affected by mental illness. Their many deprivations would include a loss of reality and ruin, along with feelings of being alone with their thoughts and fears. And that circle would be inundated with much suffering. Prejudice and stigma would surround and separate them from society, day after day. People would fear them, mock them and turn the other way because of misunderstanding, and simply "not wanting to know". It is time to educate ourselves in the things we've been ignoring and bring compassion, sympathy and hope to those who've lost theirs. It is only then that we can truly face each other with dignity and respect, and put our misgivings behind us ... to live in a world where we are equal, and not feel judged because of our differences. We just have to make the choice. From there, change is inevitable. It will happen, but change of attitude is essential. Otherwise as a society, we remain stagnant, and doors stay closed. Is that what we really want? I've thrown the first pebble. I've started the ripple to healing and acceptance. Whether you are sufferer or supporter, it doesn't matter. We are all in this together.

I am Chris Nihmey. I suffer from mental illness. I'll admit, it was the hardest thing I've ever had to endure, but through a balanced faith, support from loved ones, will and determination, hard work and therapy, doctors I could trust, proper medications, daily exercise and numerous life changes, I have survived. I have not given up. And you know what? So can you. And it will mean everything to you and yours.

I leave you with three simple words that will change your life forever. NEVER ... LOSE ... HOPE. I found hope, and healing began.

***"Where I once crawled, I now walk. Where I once walked, I now run. Where I once ran … I now fly."***

## AUTHOR BIOGRAPHY

Chris Nihmey was born in Ottawa, Canada in 1973. He attended Holy Family Catholic Elementary, and continued at St. Patrick's High School, graduating in 1992. He then attended The University of Western Ontario in London, Canada, from 1992 to 1997, and received a Bachelor Degree in Kinesiology and Psychology, graduating with Honours, and on the Dean's List. He followed with a Bachelor of Education at the University of Ottawa.

In 1998, excited to begin his teaching career, he was hired on a permanent basis to teach grade 4 with the Ottawa-Carleton Catholic School Board. He taught for two years before succumbing to his various illnesses. He resigned from permanent teaching and began substitute teaching, which he continues to do full-time to this day. This was a painful decision preventing him from moving forward in his life, which left him in professional and personal limbo.

Alongside occasional teaching, Chris co-authored two children's novels in a series titled *A Quarter Past Three*, the story of a boy and girl who are lost in time. Their adventures take them to many different time periods, where the reader learns what it was like to live in that historical period. To make it home, they must find magical doors which appear at exactly "a quarter past three"; missing a door on any trip, would leave them lost in time forever. These books were written in a particularly difficult and trying time, when Chris was battling three terrible disorders that nearly ended his life. At the same time, they proved to be a blessing, because they served as a convenient alibi for having to leave permanent teaching. This also allowed Chris to avoid the negative effects of stigma, while battling his debilitating mental illnesses. He would not give up.

On Boxing Day, 2005, in the midst of his mental storm, Chris began the brainstorming for his memoir ***Two Sides To The Story: Living A Lie***. It started with a few ideas and slowly, from 2006 to 2010, the story came into fruition. Alongside therapy, medications, faith, and much hard work, the writing of his story became one of the driving forces in his healing, in his quest to gain a new life, a stable life. Today, while progressing towards healing, Chris continues to substitute teach full-time, while writing stories geared towards children, teenagers and adults, in a variety of genres. He plans to continue this writing journey, reaching out to those in need and giving them hope and purpose in their lives. At the same time, he aims to further educate society on mental illness and the dangerous effects that stigma has on both sufferers and their families.

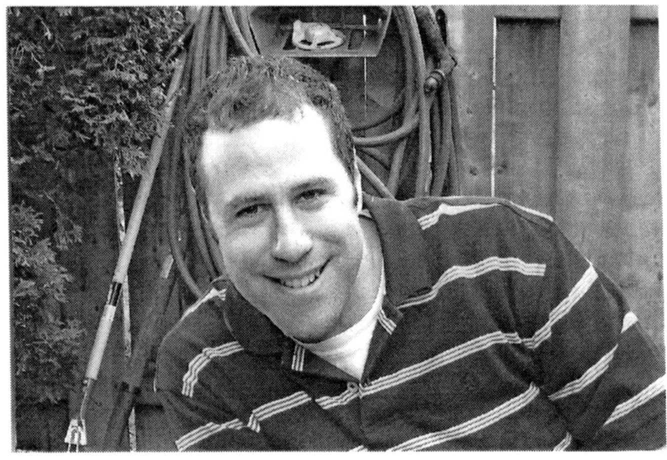

Chris Nihmey

CPSIA information can be obtained at www.ICGtesting.com
Printed in the USA
LVOW12s1822030214

372077LV00001B/1/P